... continued from back cover

"The interviews tell us of the challenges of real life, and some of the wonderful problem solving that people with learning disabilities have used to meet those challenges. Much can be learned from studying their unique stories."

Professor Sally L.Smith, Founder/Director
The Lab School of Washington DC
Head, Graduate Program, Special Education, American University

"*The Human Side of Dyslexia* helps parents see that they are not alone in their struggles, and gives teachers insights into what might be going on in their students' lives outside of school."

John Osner, Director of Slingerland Teacher Training
Charles Armstrong School, Belmont, CA

"A thoroughly positive easy-to-read book which will be most helpful to all those living and working with dyslexic learners. It is good to see an emphasis on the creative abilities of dyslexia as they are so often overshadowed by the problems. A valuable resource."

Lindsay Peer, Education Director, British Dyslexia Association, UK

"The whole area of special education will benefit from this new book. Readers can relate to the frank and detailed interviews that provide a wide range of information at a human level."

Patience Thomson, former Principal
Fairley House School, Lond **UK**

"At Shelton School, we are blessed to work with many different students. You'll find the challenges and suc their siblings, and their parents reflected in the r and inspirational book. It shows what we exp *great minds think alike.*"

Joyce S. Pickering, Executive Director, **Dallas, TX**
Executive Director, Internatio **lexia Association**

THE HUMAN SIDE OF
DYSLEXIA

142 Interviews with REAL people telling REAL stories

SHIRLEY KURNOFF

To Cherri !!
Many Thanks !
Shirley Kurnoff

ISBN 0-9703557-2-6

Library of Congress Cataloging-in-Publication data available

http://www.edyslexia.com

First publication July 2000 (e-book)

ACKNOWLEDGMENTS

My sincere thanks to those parents, siblings and college students who volunteered to share their experiences with me. With every story, I learned something new. With some stories there were tears—memories of frustration and anxiety. Other times, there was a feeling of achievement. Overall, the research project was about families, about how people cope (or not cope) with life's challenges, with dyslexia.

Thank you to my technical support team. Jennifer Berger who helped with the schematics, Karolyn Sewell for fine-tuning my commentaries, and Mary Barker for editing the interviews.

To my family, especially my husband, Mike, a special thanks for your patience and continued support.

Enjoy reading the stories!

CONTENTS

Chapter 4

THE-COLLEGE-EXPERIENCE

Chapter 5

A FINAL NOTE

INDEX

INTRODUCTION

Maybe it is your child, or your neighbor's 4th grader, or a college student you know. Someone with a different learning style, someone with imagination, someone bright and curious who isn't making the honor roll, or who isn't getting that "B+" at all. Maybe it's a co-worker, an adult, who is frustrated because of his or her "invisible" learning difference. We all know someone who has dyslexia. For me, that person was my daughter.

I don't profess to be an expert in dyslexia but I do know what it is like, as a parent, to face the obstacles of educating a child with dyslexia. Most teachers were understanding, often willing to incorporate new learning modes, and accepting of my suggestions. But there were, of course, a few who felt that my daughter's different learning style might topple their school's academic standings. Back then, I didn't have a book like this one and I really needed it.

I needed to find out how dyslexia was going to impact our family. I wanted to know more about the journey our family inevitably was going to take. What I found, though, was a plethora of information on how the student learns, suggested medication, multi-sensory programs, the legal system, scientific studies and academic analyses. But there wasn't a book written on what really matters most: the human side of dyslexia.

So, I embarked on a mission to fill that gap. *The Human Side of Dyslexia* is a book about real people with real stories, 142 of the 210 people I interviewed; a book with emotions and courage, common sense and tenacity; a book about people with different attitudes from different economic, racial and religious backgrounds. It's also a book about coping strategies that work.

As a parent, how do you cope with the emotional challenges of raising a child with dyslexia and the ensuing financial add-ons? What are siblings saying about growing up with a dyslexic brother or sister? What coping strategies are parents using to get their child through yet another school year? Is the college-search becoming a daunting task? And, what survival tactics are college students employing to get through school successfully? That, and much more, are here in this book. It's your road map to the future whatever grade your child is in now.

My goal with this book is to make your journey as a parent a lot less painful and a lot more light-hearted; as a student to show you a way to cope; as a sibling to show you a caring way to understand your brother or sister. This book will give you encouragement and de-emphasize the negativity that comes with a learning difference. It will become your invisible support system, stories for you to emulate, stories to make you laugh or cry, stories that help you open up conversations with family members.

On the surface this book taps into a highly visible audience of people associated directly with dyslexia. But these human stories also reach out to a broader audience—educators, the corporate world, even newlyweds with hereditary dyslexia. In essence, anyone who wants to know more about the social side of living with a learning difference and the social implications that come with dyslexia. *The Human Side of Dyslexia* is about life, about people.

WHAT IS DYSLEXIA?

The Oxford English Dictionary reads: "dyslexia n. a developmental disorder marked by severe difficulty in reading and spelling." There are various other definitions in encyclopedias, reference books, academic papers, or medical journals. But, in *The Human Side of Dyslexia*, I prefer to address this LD (learning disability) informally. This book is about moms, dads, siblings, and college students and their personal experiences with dyslexia. It's the informal side of dyslexia, the human side.

Let me share with you some examples from *The Human Side of Dyslexia* that best illustrate what dyslexia means in practical terms. Beginning with the younger students:

> Robert Murphy's history project on Mt. Vesuvius—showing that the ground is shaking—is more like the work of a 10-year-old. He's 7 1/2. His written words are unreadable. Troy Herbert's fourth-grade biography on Martin Luther King is right to the point and says it all in three sentences. But it takes him 30 minutes to write those few words! Nicole Vuich, 10, feels stupid in class, can't read simple Dr. Seuss *Cat in the Hat* books, and ends up being the class clown. Then, she scores 122 IQ (above average) on the WISC-111 test.[1]

Robert, Troy and Nicole are bright students with average to above-average IQ's. They are smart, analytical, creative and contributing members in class, yet they perform below grade level in reading, spelling and writing. This dyslexia is confusing to them and to their parents. Now turning to the older students:

> Jerrie Rambo says teachers don't know where to place her—she goes from being in the seventh grade English honors class to the skills class. But she hangs out with the honor students. Jerry O'Brien is gifted and is dyslexic. He's caught trying to balance what he's capable of doing and what he wants to do. Jack Peters feels like he's walking in the dark in high school—he gets a "D" in English, then an "A" in math and science. And Alex Black's TA at Stanford says her spelling errors are so distracting, she suggests using a "better" spell checker.

Students like Jack and Alex, Jerrie and Jerry, gravitate toward the smart kids in class because that's where their intellectual level lies. But discrepancies in performance—in the language arts, math and foreign language—cause them a lot of frustration. It is also unsettling for parents. Josephine Accordino feels like she has either the next Albert Einstein or an eighth-grade dropout.

These examples should give you an initial idea of how dyslexia impacts bright young people. And, for a more detailed description of dyslexia and LD issues, read the article: *Why Andy Couldn't Read*, Newsweek Oct. 27, 1997, by Pat Wingert and Barbara Kantrowitz. The authors offer a thumbnail guide to common symptoms, identifiable as early as preschool.

For information on entrepreneurs who succeeded despite their dyslexia, read the following Internet articles on Paul J. Orfalea, Founder and Chairperson Emeritus, Kinko's Inc. *Do the Right Thing: Reflections of an Entrepreneurial Sage,* by The Marshall Business School, University of Southern California. (www.marshall.usc.edu/Web/News.cfm?doc_id=2434). And, Sir Richard Branson, Founder and CEO of Virgin Atlantic Airways *Richard Branson's Virgin Success*, by John Shepler (www.execpc.com/~shepler/branson.html).

For now, though, I hope this informal definition of dyslexia has set the tone for the following interviews. The interviews are about people, about their feelings. It's not medical. It's social.

Just before you start reading, please note the following:

❑ The stories are real but the names of those I interviewed are pseudonyms. At the beginning of each interview there is a brief family description (in italic). The interviews are not verbatim, rather they are a paraphrase of what the respondents shared with me.

❑ The term "a school for dyslexia" is used throughout the book as a standard phrase for "a school for learning disabilities, a school for learning-different children, a special school for kids" or any other term to describe such a school.

❑ The college student interviews represent the personal opinion of an individual student at a specific college at that time, and are not the opinion of that particular college or myself, as author.

---

[1] WISC-111 (Wechsler Intelligence Scale for Children 111) is given to children ages 6 through 16, and measures general intelligence. This scale provides three IQ scores: verbal, performance, and full-scale, yielding information about strengths and weaknesses in language and performance areas.

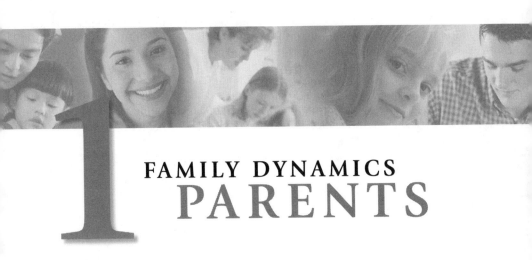

1

FAMILY DYNAMICS
PARENTS

FAMILY DYNAMICS

The emotional energy that comes from parenting a child with dyslexia is captured, right here, in this section. It is the demonstrative side of the book. It is about issues that affect the immediate family. Parents speak out about their spouses, their non-dyslexic children, and school run-ins. Siblings talk openly about their parents, their dyslexic brother or sister. They are the family dynamics and fall into two sections:

1 Parent Interviews
2 Sibling Interviews

Parent Interviews

How do parents work through this LD maze? How does it impact the immediate family? And where does school fit in all of this? I couldn't include all of what parents said. That would have taken up three volumes. What I've come up with is a smorgasbord and I've grouped the interviews as follows:

Crisis Strikes

When parents first find out their child has dyslexia, some are in shock, anger, or in denial; others are confused or relieved. Only a few anticipate it!

Working Through It

Here, stories touch on family feelings and, in particular, who is on-board and who is paddling a second boat. This is followed by turbulence in school, with stories that outline what is being said by educators, and how either a common meeting ground or deadlock develops. Finally, there are a couple of stories on cultural roadblocks.

We Finally Made It

This is definitely the warm-and-fuzzy section, but the stories aren't without trauma. Parents talk about the long journey—kindergarten through high school—and then college.

The following parent interviews give you an idea of how parents handle the breaking news, how they cope or don't cope with this "additional" baggage, and if there's light at the end of the tunnel. Parents have powerful thoughts on their spousal reaction to dyslexia. Some partners are united, others polarized, and still others bury their heads in the sand, hoping the "D" word will go away, that the bad dream will soon end. Parents also have strong opinions about their teacher-parent relationships.

Sibling Interviews

"Are you younger or older than your dyslexic sibling?" Siblings' responses reveal that attitudes are absolutely dependent on birth order. Some say: "My sibling has dyslexia and it worries me" while others say "and that's OK." Age and gender also contribute to their responses. Here, children and young adults have strong opinions about the way parents handle the LD situation, and how the family structure adapts to the learning-difference child. I hope you can relate to these stories and learn from families. For now, though, let's turn to the parent interviews in "Crisis Strikes."

CRISIS STRIKES

"Your Child Has Dyslexia." Four simple words. Four words loaded with emotion. Four words that can affect family dynamics. Some parents are relieved—now they can put a label on this "invisible" disability. Some are in shock. Others are confused. Some anticipate it, a few panic, and others are in denial and remain that way for some time.

Carol Murphy was relieved when she got empirical proof that her child was not stupid, far from it. After testing, the licensed clinical psychologist told Carol's son, Robert, 7, that he was extremely bright. His project on Mt. Vesuvius was more like the work of a 10-year-old. Robert changed 180 degrees. Once more, he was excited about life. For Elizabeth Craig her struggle was a little more complex. The principal thought her son, James, had a severe behavioral problem and suggested the family seek counseling. Instead, she worked with a private clinical psychologist who told her James didn't have a personality problem. This child wasn't crazy. This child had dyslexia. The psychologist suggested remedial help immediately, with the possibility of moving him out of his local school in due course. He gave Elizabeth several options.

For Ora Tyler, Ann Herbert and Ellen Ward the breaking news came as a shock. Ora felt as if she'd been dropped in a large ocean and didn't know how to swim, to survive. She took a crash course in reading everything and anything about dyslexia, talked with education specialists, consultants, and attended workshops. Ann and her husband, William, also were in shock. They knew nothing about dyslexia. They looked at new schools for their son, Troy, based on social rather than academic concerns. Unbeknownst to them, they "opened up a can of worms" when their oldest boy couldn't pass the entrance exam to two private schools. Troy was diagnosed with dyslexia. He was a 4th grader. Ellen wanted her daughter, Kathy, to pick up a foreign language easily in a bilingual elementary-school setting. But it didn't work out the way she planned. When Kathy took the middle school placement test, she couldn't read all the text. She was reading at a third-grade level and tested at a beginner level in Spanish. That's when Ellen was confused. She was also angry.

For some parents, though, there were no surprises. Dyslexia ran in the family. Mariellen Chan suspected something was different with Oblina at an early age. She didn't know more than five words at 22 months. But Mariellen wasn't alarmed. She'd been down the LD road before with her own dyslexia. But it took Mariellen and her husband, Len, a good 12 months before they told his father, an immigrant from China and a MIT alumnus, who believed academic achievement was a family priority.

For other families, acceptance was not the norm, denial was. Kari Brown's husband, Jason, was an avid reader but never picked up a book on dyslexia. He was curious, intellectual but when it came to his own daughter's dyslexia, he abrogated to his wife. That part still baffles Kari. This also happened in Kelly Spencer's home. Her husband, Matthew, thought this dyslexia stuff was a bunch of hooey, and that Andrew, their son, was immature and would eventually outgrow it. Katie, her daughter, also wouldn't accept that her younger brother was having school issues. Emotionally, it was a big strain on the family.

Family dynamics are not simple. They're actually fairly complex. Of the 82 interviewed parents, 39 percent were in shock, confused or in denial. They appear to be traveling along an education-track where no educator was alerting them to their underachieving child.

On the other hand, 24 percent of the respondents were relieved, that someone was actually listening to them, that there was a reason why their bright, intelligent offspring was often at the bottom of the pile in reading, spelling and, sometimes, math. They were motivated to see change and, in most cases, were eager to implement what the clinical psychologist suggested. Another 20 percent anticipated dyslexia because of past family school experiences or Special-Ed awareness.

The biggest concern, though, are the 17 percent of respondents who are angry at the school system for not alerting them sooner. So many misunderstandings, misconceptions and altercations between parent and child could have been prevented. There could have been accountability for laziness, reluctance to complete homework, resistance to writing more than three sentences and a tendency to read only thin library books. There could have been an understanding about why a young child didn't want to read out aloud in class, or at home, or was constantly erasing words on a page. Kids with dyslexia are perceptive; they know what's happening.

I hope that by reading these interviews, you will get a better understanding of why parents respond in different ways, for different reasons and with different concerns when they first hear those four simple words *"Your Child Has Dyslexia."*

CRISIS STRIKES

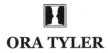

ORA TYLER

Early on, Ora realized Leigh didn't write and she wasn't moving through the normal 1st-grade transition in reading. Teachers kept telling Ora to be patient, to stop being an over-anxious parent. Ora decided to do her own research on dyslexia.

It was as if I'd been dropped in the ocean and didn't know how to swim. So, I took a crash course—reading everything and anything I could about dyslexia. I talked with education specialists, consultants and attended workshops. I'm a devoted mother. I needed to understand the problems of visual memory coordination. I jumped into the evaluation process, but the research was daunting. I was a basket case.

Gathering information about dyslexia had become my issue, not Leigh's. I invested in her success and took on the responsibility. I thought I had control. I didn't. Indeed, this was a big ocean. For the first three years—1st through 3rd grade—our problems with dyslexia were more about me than they were about Leigh having trouble in school. It consumed me. I wasn't sleeping. I felt everyone was traveling on a parallel journey without me. I felt alone.

I sought professional counseling for two reasons. First, I needed to discuss these issues with an unbiased person. It was difficult for me to accept the term "disability" with its label and permanency. Second, I've come from a dysfunctional family where my dyslexic brother was self-destructive. He caused heartache for our whole family. When I saw Leigh wasn't conforming in school, my past family history—with all its emotional trauma—surfaced. I started to think catastrophic thoughts. I remembered what had happened to my brother. It seemed like the trauma was recurring.

Counseling was my savior. I needed to go through my own therapy. I'd become so enmeshed with Leigh's schooling, my anxiety transferred to her at homework time. I also felt threatened by the fact that Leigh couldn't be a teacher pleaser. And, it was hard for me to follow through after Leigh had been tested. I sought new opinions instead of making follow-up calls. I even went to a homeopath because I thought he might have a different approach to dyslexia.

I found difficulty trusting a teacher's competency with, understanding of, and adaptation to Leigh's needs. Eventually, I went to an education consultant who advocated for me. It was difficult having a third party intercede, but it worked. In the past, I was biased about private vs. public school testing. But with help from my education consultant, I found better results in the public-school sector.

In 1st grade, Leigh wasn't reading or writing. Then, as she went through 2nd grade, I noticed a steady internal withdrawal. She started to bite her nails and didn't want to participate in group discussions. She didn't talk to me about how she felt. She was very much in her own world. Her 2nd-grade teacher basically left her to do work at her own level. Leigh didn't want to or like to do creative writing. As a result, she was the only student in her class who didn't contribute to the school newsletter. Sadly, no one thought to let her dictate her ideas. By 3rd grade, though, all this changed. Leigh was in a group of girls who all were very supportive of each other (they'd been together since kindergarten). Her schoolmates wrote her ideas for her. Leigh was happy with this. She's very creative, but putting it down on paper correctly is a stumbling block.

Although K-3 were tough years, 4th and 5th grades are much calmer. With maturity, Leigh has developed a sense of when people aren't being fair to her. She advocates for herself and seems to be accepting of her difficulties and the challenges.

I've grown through this ordeal. I'm more accepting. I'm beginning to trust teachers and even admire them. I'm definitely letting go, allowing Leigh to have her own life, make her own decisions and be her own advocate at times. In reality, I became my daughter's "protector" and it turned out to be an overwhelming ordeal. Leigh seems to have weathered the storm. Thankfully, she's a talkative, energetic 5th-grader.

MARIELLEN CHAN

The Chans have three children – Weaver, 9; Oblina, 7; and Digger, 4. Weaver and Digger show no signs of having a learning difference. The focus then is on Oblina who has dyslexia. Mariellen picked up signs of her daughter's problem at an early age because she, too, has dyslexia.

It probably was a year before we told Len's parents their only granddaughter was dyslexic. We were scared we'd disappoint them. Our kids are their only grandchildren. Academic achievement is such a priority in my husband's family. His parents are immigrants from China and, in their eyes, education is the only way to succeed. My father-in-law is an MIT graduate. Len graduated from Amherst and then from Columbia Medical School. So, we didn't know how they'd react to the news. We spent a lot of time preparing. Initially, they were stunned. But since then, I've gotten articles from my father-in-law about dyslexia, coping strategies and new theories. He's taken this on as his research project. We're delighted.

I knew something wasn't right with Oblina. Her responses at a young age were inappropriate. I didn't see the normal development you would expect from a 2-year-old. She wasn't verbal. I don't think she knew more than five words. Yet, she walked at nine months. As a comparison, Weaver was playing chess at 4. I could tell Oblina was very bright, but something was impeding her progress.

In preschool, she was saying more words but not saying them very well (she definitely has an auditory processing problem). The teachers couldn't understand her. She was missing the sounds in some words and combining two words in other instances. She'd say: "Mom, you're annoring me"—a combination of ignoring and annoying. I was able to understand but no one else did. Now, when the boys bother her, she calls them rude and totally unoxious. The words are there, she just drops some of the sounds.

I understand. And I'm not going to let Oblina grow up with a stigma. I grew up with a mother who was in denial about my learning disability. She told me I was lazy and didn't pay attention in class. She told me I saw words backwards. I know how far I've come. I got my credentials—RN and a bachelor's in nursing—but I had to work my tail off. I also know the right kind of teaching will unlock my daughter's different learning style.

I didn't want to put Oblina in a program where she felt stupid. When we moved to Maui last year, we got on the waiting list for a special school for dyslexia. She was at the church school for one year and then she made the move. We've never looked back.

Oblina started preschool at $2^1/2$ in Gainesville, Fla. But we kept her back for another year in the same class. At $4^1/2$ years, I didn't want to put her in kindergarten because she wasn't ready. We decided to enroll her in a pre-K class in a private parochial school. She wasn't even ready for pre-K. She spent a year in that program and became very frustrated. She couldn't memorize letters. She couldn't write letters. The teachers didn't really have any comments about her different learning style. We had to make some changes.

That year, I got her into a Diagnostic and Resource Center affiliated with the University of Florida. It was the best thing we did for her. The center took about eight weeks to complete its evaluation on her. They were very specific about their findings. Oblina is very dyslexic, has an inability to track properly, has auditory-processing limitations, but has a high IQ of 130. She'd never chosen to write with her left or right hand. She actually chose not to write at all.

Fortunately, they offered the Lindamood-Bell Learning Processes (LiPS) at the Center and we decided to run with it. They had never started a child that young ($5^1/2$ years). But because we were open to it and Oblina was more than happy to do it, we completed a modified program. We went every day for two hours, for four months. There was an immediate improvement. Even today, Oblina uses that method to decode words. You can see her tapping out her words, using lip smackers and tongue tappers, or touching where the air comes out. Eighteen months ago, she couldn't write her name, she couldn't sound out a letter, she couldn't draw. We now have a different child.

A lot of parents panic when they first learn their child is dyslexic. They forget to untap the wonderful strengths in their child. They focus on the negativity of the situation. Oblina is a strong athlete. At $2^1/2$, she rode her bicycle 3 miles while I jogged with baby Digger in the stroller. Then in gymnastics, everything came so naturally to her—tumbling, using the rings, jumping on the trampoline, doing flips on the mat. She also swims like a fish. Just this year, we found out she loves math and is good at it! She can do what she sets her mind to do.

So, how do I cope with three young kids, a goat, two dogs and . . . ? Our family motto is "teamwork and understanding." With Weaver, it's never been an issue that I spend more time with his sister doing homework or listening to her read. I explained to him early on that she was having problems with school. Digger, I let him play with Weaver or watch TV while I work with Oblina. I really try to remind them that they all have something special to offer. My three kids all know, you may not always get what you want, but you'll always get what you need.

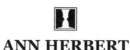

ANN HERBERT

Ann and William Herbert have four sons. They had never heard the word dyslexia before discovering three of their four sons – Troy, 17; Bryan, 9; and Austin, 7 – have this LD. Only Peter, 14, does not.

It was on a social basis rather than an academic one that we looked at new schools for Troy. Unbeknownst to us, we opened up a can of worms. We discovered our first born was dyslexic.

Troy was doing fine in his Montessori school in Dallas. Well, that's what we thought anyway. He didn't like to read, but, then, I don't like to read. Kindergarten through 4th grade was a happy time for him. He knew everyone at school, a very small, family-run place. The teachers allowed untimed classwork. Children could spend one day on math, then one day on English. It was their choice.

At parent conferences, I always was told he was doing fine. The only time I got a slight indication his written work wasn't at grade level was when he'd done a book report in 3rd grade. The teacher said it was shorter than it should be, but it was right to the point. It was a biography on Martin Luther King. Troy summarized the whole book in three sentences. She was very impressed with his analysis. What the teacher failed to tell me was how long it took him to write those few lines—30 minutes. Still, I decided not to sound any alarm bells at that time.

So, Troy moved into 4th grade. The school was so small, three grades were combined. Only three children of Troy's age were in this class. William and I started looking into new schools for 5th grade. Troy tested at two private schools.

One school called and said his test scores didn't work out. That was that. My husband and I were a little surprised with their brief explanation, especially because we thought it would be a good placement. The second school was a little more helpful. The principal called me in to look over Troy's test results. It was the first time someone had shared with me, in depth, my son's work.

There sat a page of words that made no sense, just words here and there with no sentence structure. The principal said Troy was given 20 minutes to complete the task, but he couldn't do it. Needless to say, Troy wasn't offered a place at that school. Instead, the principal suggested we get Troy tested immediately.

We found a licensed clinical psychologist who gave Troy a battery of tests. In her final days of testing, she concluded his written expression, his handwriting and spelling were well below grade level. She suggested several places to explore, including a school for dyslexia.

We had four months—January through April. William and I knew nothing about dyslexia. It was scary.

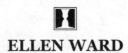

ELLEN WARD

Ellen is a single, working parent. Her daughter, Kathy, was a 5th-grader when they found out she had dyslexia. Kathy was in a multicultural school where lessons were taught in both English and Spanish. Learning a foreign language in school had been an ugly experience for Ellen. She didn't think her daughter would have the same troubles. But that was only wishful thinking.

I thought Kathy would pick up the language easily in a multicultural school setting. I specifically moved her to a rural school district in Southern California so she could learn Spanish in a bilingual school. The student population was one-third Caucasian, one-third Hispanic and one-third African American. English was the official language, but I later learned the school district had special funding for bilingual students.

It was an experimental system that started by teaching both languages, 50-50. But it ended up with two-thirds of the day allocated to Spanish. There was definitely a one-way flow—from Spanish to English. So, throughout 2nd grade, Kathy was listening to a lot of Spanish and not learning much English. Still, from 3rd to 5th grade, she was a happy student. She had friends from different ethnic groups and our house always was full of kids.

But even though report cards read "satisfactory," I wondered if the teachers were camouflaging her academic ability. I was a single mother, overworked and supporting two kids. I didn't look too deeply into my children's schoolwork because I thought the teachers knew their job. At one point, though, I did question Kathy's reading ability and Spanish vocabulary. The teachers assured me, in time, she would be speaking Spanish fluently and her reading would improve.

I found out Kathy was having problems, though, when she took the middle-school placement test. She couldn't read all the text. Her 5th-grade teacher immediately said: "Kathy needs to be tested." Kathy was reading at a 3rd-grade level and comprehending Spanish at a beginner level. That's when I got angry.

"How can this be?" I asked the principal. "Here I have report cards saying she's doing satisfactory work, but she's struggling all the time. I could have looked for a tutor on the side. We're not a wealthy family, but I would have found a young student to tutor her. If only I had known."

I was extremely hurt. My daughter was scarred. Later on, I found out that, the more kids our school district passed on to the next grade, the more money they received from the state. I realize now they weren't going to hold Kathy back a year. It was in their best interest to move her on. I decided to move Kathy to a new school district and get remedial tutoring in place immediately. The "camouflage" was over!

Ellen suggests:

❑   A bilingual school setting is a great idea for gifted kids. But if your family has any inkling that dyslexia is hereditary, don't put your child through it. Also, check out how the state funding works for that school!

CAROL MURPHY

Robert, 13, and James, 23, have dyslexia. Their older sister, Beth, is a mainstream student. Robert was diagnosed at an early age, 7. When the clinical psychologist told him he was an extremely bright child and gave him an explanation on dyslexia, Robert's school attitude changed 180 degrees.

Robert has an extensive vocabulary. We never dreamed he had a learning disability. When I couldn't teach him to read and write, I knew something was wrong. It all came to a head when he was 7. He was doing a history project, putting himself in the place of a shopkeeper on Mt. Vesuvius in Italy. He had to envision the type of pottery, clothing and architecture used at that time. Most importantly, he had to illustrate that the ground was sinking and to show extreme fear. His project was very descriptive for someone that young, by far, the best in the class. Yet, his words were totally illegible.

Robert was at a private London parochial school, a traditional UK school, where faculty didn't like to "deal with," or even discuss, kids with LD. When I mentioned Robert may have dyslexia, the headmaster responded: "No, no. It's not possible." Paul and I couldn't accept that. We asked for a copy of Robert's work and took him and his history project to the British Dyslexia Association (we found the number in the Yellow Pages). The psychologist there told us Robert was a classic case. He was a young boy with dyslexia. "He's very, very bright, very creative," the man said. "But he has a problem processing words."

The psychologist concluded Robert was three years behind in reading. I don't think he could calculate Robert's writing level because the words were indecipherable. And he didn't write very much. Robert always was erasing his work in class because he lacked confidence. After the testing, the clinical psychologist told Robert he was an extremely bright 7-year-old and his project on Mt. Vesuvius was more like the work of a 10-year-old. Robert changed 180 degrees. He was excited about life. You know, we'd have paid that man £1,000 pounds for those words of encouragement. He made a young boy and his parents very happy.

Fortunately, the headmaster accepted the test results (that was a relief) and it was agreed that the school would send me to a course titled "Talk and Word." It was a one-day class using an educational CD program and, as I'm computer literate, it was no problem. The plan was for Robert and I to work on the program 20 minutes before school started. The program pulled out random words for him to remember. For example, "The brown dog jumped over the cat." Robert would read the pre-printed cards from the CD, memorize the words and then try to type them on the computer. If he got it right, the computer made a funny, happy sound. If he got it wrong, there was a low, groaning moan. Ostensibly, the program was designed to strengthen his short-time memory. A child who couldn't touch type, though, would have found it frustrating.

Within six months, I saw recognizable improvement in both spelling and reading. Consistency played an important role in Robert's progress. We worked on these skills three times a week and, at the same time, he had a private special-needs tutor who had training in dyslexia. All in all, this combination worked well for him.

ELIZABETH CRAIG

James, 13, has been at a school for dyslexia for four years and now is mainstreaming to a boarding school outside of London, UK. His sister, Rosie, 18, and his brother, Freddie, 7, have not been diagnosed with dyslexia. James' parents, Dan and Elizabeth, both are in advertising – Dan, a company director; and Elizabeth, a creative director with a leading firm.

We were summoned to school. James was displaying anti-social behavior. What could he possibly have done? Well, he'd ripped off a boy's shirt on the playground. Fortunately, we got to the bottom of it. It all started when James wrote three short sentences with misspelled words and jumbled phrases. He couldn't even spell his own name correctly. A boy sitting next to him glanced at his work and began teasing him. The teacher managed to stop the badgering, but it continued on the playground. That was the last straw for James.

We realized then we had a confidence crisis on our hands. But the principal thought otherwise. She felt our son had a severe behavioral problem and suggested that, as a family, we go to a family counselor. My husband hit the roof.

Actually, Dan was in denial with the whole thing. We both knew James was floundering in school, but we weren't expecting behavioral problems. The principal was insistent that our son's behavior was due to our family situation. About this time, Freddie, our youngest child, was born. Naturally, we used having a new baby as an explanation for everything. James told his teacher his new brother had died. He also told the teacher we were getting divorced and he was going to live in the U.S. The school thought we were off the wall. James already was so insecure in school and now he had a new brother. The principal immediately picked up on what was going on at home and made us the guilty party. Dan refused to believe this.

Immediately, we took James to a licensed clinical psychologist who told us: "He doesn't have a personality problem. This child isn't crazy. This child has dyslexia." The psychologist suggested we get remedial help immediately and, preferably, move James out of his local school. He gave us several options.

Dan's mother stepped in at this point, offering to help finance James' education at a private school for dyslexia. She also became James' confidant, his mentor and our family peacemaker. She spoke to my husband, told it like it was. "James isn't going to follow in your path," she said. "He's not going to be a scholar, but he has so much talent in other areas. Just accept it." I couldn't have said it better.

Once my husband accepted this, he coped with it and planned for it. He gave James more of his time. They share a love of films and, certainly, sports has bonded them. He enjoys James' company. They talk a lot. They laugh a lot. Actually, James entertains Dan. Way back when James was only $7^1/2$, I didn't know how it all would work out with Dan. Thanks to Dan's mother's wisdom, we managed to survive.

Another thing that helped immensely was drama, especially Channel 4's TV Drama Workshop. As early as 8, James showed exceptional talent in drama. The program has an amazing list of patrons, including David Putnam and Richard Attenborough, and is geared to children and young adults ages 8-24. To get into it, a child has to have exceptional talent. James auditioned and, yes, he made it.

Normally, children stay in the program two years. If they're very lucky, they get an extra year. James was there four years. He wrote scripts, made films, edited them and Channel 4 sponsored them. They had regular tutors and, several times a year, well-known actors came in to give special sessions. Plus, James came into contact with children from all walks of life. That helped his social development and filled his weekends with worthwhile activities. Actually, the program became the highlight of his week.

Five years later, James won a choral scholarship to a private boys boarding school outside of London. The scholarship meant so much to him. You see, the choir sings all over the world. The group also has made CD recordings of their tours. What appeals to James most, though, is his celebrity status.

From the Kremlin to the White House to Buckingham Palace, the choir has touched many hearts. James currently is on tour in France singing in Notre Dame, Paris. The group travels with chaperones and performances usually are in cathedrals. He's singing in Latin, memorizing the words and, somehow, he seems comfortable with it. Yet, he doesn't even take Latin in school! That's James, so bright he can grasp anything if he's motivated.

WORKING THROUGH IT

Denial, confusion, shock and relief are understandable when we first find out our child has dyslexia. But, rest assured, these feelings are short-lived. The way we work through the process and get our child through school is more enduring. There is no quick fix. Sometimes, it takes 15 years. Years of planning, years of restructuring, years of negotiating, and years of re-negotiating.

Josephine Accordino and Sarah Rosen, for example, felt alone in this dyslexia maze. Josephine felt like she had either the next Albert Einstein or an eighth-grade dropout. Her mission was to see that Sal, her oldest son, didn't fail in school. Her husband, Tony, asked if she was going to hold Sal's hand all through college. The whole family heard that dad thought mom was giving too much attention to Sal. Sarah Rosen never involved her husband in LD issues. As a European, he was unfamiliar with U.S. schooling, and saw himself as a provider, not a caregiver or educator. Sarah "broke down" when her daughter was first diagnosed and went alone to a licensed clinical psychologist.

Run-ins with family members are difficult to bear, but run-ins with the school district are perplexing. Jill McQueen and Alison Vuich know how this feels. Jill's son daydreamed, didn't always grasp simple commands, took longer than most kids to master basic tasks, and had major difficulty with spelling. His teacher said there was no such thing as dyslexia, and that once "the boy" stopped daydreaming, there would be immeasurable improvement. Jill and her husband left the teacher-parent conference speechless (and this was after a private licensed clinical psychologist had diagnosed him with dyslexia). Alison, on the other hand, requested testing at her daughter's public school but the vice principal kept putting it off, hoping the request would go away. Alison learned that the school didn't want to do it because of the cost. After some hassle, the school capitulated. The WISC-111 (Wechsler Intelligence Scale for Children) test indicated an IQ of 122, way above average. Alison's daughter was no low achiever.

Dyslexia also affects after-school activities. In sports, for example, when a coach gives a left-right direction it may become confusing to the dyslexic child. The pace of learning a new language also may be too much. Ann and Bruce Berg, and Lindsay Stamos knew all about this.

Lindsay knew her son, Bryan, was struggling in Greek school, but the family came from a long line of cousins who had been that route. The Stamos have a rich culture and wanted Bryan to be part of their heritage. It wasn't an easy decision to give up what meant so much to their family. Ann and Bruce also faced a dilemma. David wanted a Bar mitzvah just like his older brother, Ben. The question was, could he do it? Most Jewish boys start preparing 6-9 months before the event. David started 18 months before. He selected the shortest portion to read, worked with a tutor who recorded every thing on tape, and encouraged David to practice every day, sometimes twice a day. David did a stellar job, but the whole family had to go that extra mile.

The process—how we fine-tune each strategy, how we approach each new hill, how we stay calm when hurtful comments come our way, how we search within ourselves to come up with new ideas, new strength and new enthusiasm—is all important. Unlike the college-search process where definitive criteria are targeted, here we have to improvise on a daily, weekly, monthly or yearly basis.

There is no one correct way to approach this. No two dyslexic students are alike. "Working Through It" is rigorous, emotionally draining and may disrupt the family dynamics. But I believe parents' perception of the journey—with ALL its challenges—and parents' education aspirations that may either flounder or stay solid along the way can affect the journey. In essence, our success depends on how we weather the storm. Do we try to stay calm and become better informed? Are we uptight? Or are we middle-of-the-road, wavering between being uptight and calm, depending on the situation?

From my discussions with parents, many are uptight initially but move to a middle-of-the-road situation as their child progresses through elementary school. Then, as they become "seasoned" parents of a dyslexic child they try to stay calm but periodically return to middle-of-the-road status dependent on ripples in the school. As you know, life is sporadically unpredictable and this is no different, here.

I hope that these parent interviews give you time to reflect on your own family's journey and to establish in your own minds, what type of traveler you are, or may want to be.

WORKING THROUGH IT

▌▐

CLAIRE HINGSTON

Claire knows that parenting a child with dyslexia can be emotionally taxing. Add to the mix a move to a special school, and family interplay becomes even more animated. Claire's daughter, Helena 13, is a 7th-grader at a school for dyslexia in Connecticut.

It's a huge goal shift. I used to think, "maybe my child can grow up to be president." Now, shifting gears, I say, "maybe my child can just graduate from high school." It's a huge adjustment. It's also sad that I'm adjusting my goals for a child at such a young age.

Helena told us in first grade that she was having trouble. Like many things, though, with children, we didn't really listen. It's unfortunate. But it's the truth. It was usually bedtime when she'd say, "I couldn't do some of my schoolwork today; it was difficult." I'd respond, "well of course you can, you're very smart, you know that." I let it ride. She was only 7½ then. It didn't seem serious. After comments like that, night after night, however, I decided to approach her teacher.

"Absolutely no. Helena's very bright." assured her first-grade teacher. "There are kids in this classroom that don't get it, and she's definitely not one of them." She said all kids progress at different stages, and Helena was no different. By year's end, though, she confessed. "Helena has fooled me, there is something not right." We alerted her second-grade teacher, who set up remedial reading sessions three times a week with the resource teacher. Again, by year's end, her teacher commented: "There's something going on. I can't tell you what it is. But there's something just not right."

Going into third grade, we requested testing by the licensed school psychologist. The battery of tests indicated that Helena was 2½ years behind grade level in reading and writing, but scored in the mid 120s in the IQ section. At that point, we really went with the flow. Pulling her out of her neighborhood school in suburbia New York, in our eyes, was a sense of failure. Helena soldiered on in third and fourth grades, with some improvement.

Everything came to a halt, though, the first week of fifth grade. Helena is a savvy girl. She sensed something was out of sync. She understood the demands of fifth grade, but she couldn't do it. She understood what was expected, and wasn't going to try. Helena has a bristly personality. I refer to her as my alpha female. But her behavior, the amount of work and the demands in the classroom were altering this spunky kid. She was sinking. My husband, Paul, and I didn't like what was happening.

I was unsettled about the whole thing. I asked the teacher for a conference but she was reluctant. Her response was that they'd only been in school a week and it was too early to tell. Paul and I had planned to move Helena into a new school at the end of fifth grade because it provided a natural break from elementary to middle school. Now, we were 12 months ahead of schedule and options were closing in; fifth grade already was in session.

I looked at several schools for dyslexia in our area. I knew I had to fix the problem. There was some admission on my part that my daughter was damaged—no longer the perfect child. I felt lost and emotionally tangled. I was working full-time in New York City. Deep down in my stomach, I wasn't sure I would see the same kids as in our local school, in suburbia New York. But when I visited, faculty and administration were caring and accepting. I still had mixed emotions, though. In truth, I felt vulnerable.

Paul's main concern was to not limit her future options. He was concerned about her being labeled and about her not following a rigorous academic track. He was not formally diagnosed with dyslexia but had all the telltale signs. Way back in elementary school, his parents and school wrote it off to poor eyesight. Paul worked extra long hours and became a successful architect. He was fortunate to excel in math—geometry and spatial design—and graduated from Cornell and Princeton.

Our extended family was largely supportive. No one was trying to tell us don't do it. My mom knew of kids at the special school. Maybe with my in-laws, there was a bit of disappointment. They are very academically oriented. Paul's parents are immigrants from Poland, and firmly believe education is critical. To take their granddaughter off the normal track was troubling for them, even though they understood she was not living up to her potential. They probably didn't say everything to me, and I'm sure my husband didn't pass it all along. Realistically, there was more said than I ever heard. On the other hand, I just had to galvanize myself and do the best thing for Helena. It didn't matter what the rest of the world thought.

I still think inside the family, there is a twinge about Helena's dyslexia. I recall once being asked "you're sending your kid to a special summer-school program . . . at Harvard, for gifted kids?" "No" I responded, "She's going to the one at the special school for dyslexia." It took, honestly, about a year until I could speak about it like anything else, with no reservation inside. If people didn't know of the special school, I didn't volunteer the information.

The move, in reality, was the hardest on Helena. She did not want to leave her friends, good friends. I don't think these were necessarily the best relationships, but she was getting their attention by acting out, not in the classroom, but outside school. She told her friends, interestingly, that "my parents are making me go, but I'm going to get kicked out and I'll be back in three weeks." She was convinced that she could do this. Her friends were very accepting of this. One of the girls in the group had an older sister who has developmental and physical disabilities, so it was no big deal that Helena was going to a special school. While everyone understood "your parents are making you do this, no problem," we ended up being the bad people.

Helena never got over her conviction that she hadn't done what she set out to do—to get kicked out and go back. She really cut off those friends, even though they tried to maintain a relationship with her. She was too embarrassed. I thought over time she might heal, but that didn't happen. We sat with her many hours, reassuring her that her friends didn't expect her to come back, and telling her that sometimes this happens. I told her "nobody is holding you to it." But, it was difficult for her to agree. That for me was the true negative of the move. By her own choice, she didn't continue friendships in town.

At the moment, I feel like it is a "work in progress." Her school advisor says she has two of the three survival skills—innate intelligence and social wherewithal. Academic excellence needs working on. A big component, too, is Helena buying into the program, and it's an emotional one. In public school, they give you the tools to succeed; here it's different. Her progress is erratic. That's been the biggest struggle. If she applies herself academically, options will open up for high school. I'm hoping this is a temporary shift.

The way I would best describe our daughter—someone with a strong personality and dyslexia—is that she sucks all the oxygen out in the room. She wants attention, she wants it to focus on her and, if it doesn't, she finds a way of getting it back. (She'll make it in this world!) As a parent, there's a lot of energy sapped from me, in the best of times. Now, there's just that little bit more.

JOSEPHINE ACCORDINO

Josephine and Tony have four children – Sal, 16; Frank, 14; Tina, 12; and Vince, 6. Sal is the only sibling with dyslexia, but this LD may run in the Accordino family. Tony, a well-known local architect, struggled in school but never was diagnosed.

I feel like either I have the next Albert Einstein or an 8th-grade dropout. My mission is to see that my son doesn't fail. My husband constantly asks if I'm going to hold Sal's hand all his life. Well, Sal is very bright, but he needs a mentor, and that's me.

For several years, Tony and I definitely were polarized in our educational goals for Sal. In 3rd and 4th grades, we got help from a private learning specialist. My husband thought that was all Sal needed. (It was just the beginning of continuous help.) Homework that normally takes one hour took Sal two to three hours. Tony felt I was giving Sal too much attention, so I distinctly remember trying to do homework with Sal when Tony wasn't around. The hardest years were 6th, 7th, and 8th grades. I can see Tony's point of view—in a way. His complaining made Sal want to become more independent. I'm kind of glad it happened.

I had to find ways, though, to cope. I became very good friends with the learning specialist, Sheila. She was my strength and her faith in Sal always was there. She kept reiterating his strengths to me. She kept reminding me that his academic years were such a small part of his life and that he just had to get through them. That's what kept me going!

My friendship with Sheila continued long after she tutored Sal in 3rd and 4th grades. I still talk with her about once a week. She knows Sal inside and out. I have talked to several parents, but it seems, all cases of dyslexia are so different. I didn't find a commonality in other families. Looking back, I was very fortunate to have Sheila as my support system.

As for the other kids, I told myself a long time ago that I'd love whichever child needed it most at that particular moment. It works. For example, Frank felt jealous of the time I was spending with Sal. They're close in age, competitive and both are very athletic. I made a special effort to have quality time with Frank, to take him shopping alone for sports gear or clothes. That seemed to do the trick. Tina, on the other hand, was afraid she was going to be dyslexic, too. She's a worrier. Actually, in 3rd and 4th grades, I knew something was different with her. We got her tested and there were some red flags. She has a processing problem. She was relieved with the diagnosis and was pleased I'd taken the time to resolve her concerns. And, Vince, he's too young to come up with any real problems. He just goes with the flow.

SARAH ROSEN

Sarah's husband, Mike, works long hours. Sarah doesn't involve him with their daughter's education. She has carried the LD load alone and, at times, it's taken a toll. Faye, 15, has been diagnosed with dyslexia and goes to the local public middle school, where the Learning Resource facilities are superior. Deborah, 13, is at a parochial school. Both are in 8th grade.

My husband leaves for work each day at 5 a.m. and doesn't return until late. He focuses on making a living and is very committed to his work, which I understand. Besides, when it comes to education, we really are from two different worlds. He's European and never finished high school. I'm totally American and more familiar with the school system here.

Mike left it up to me to make all the decisions. I don't think he understood a lot of this, but then neither did I at first. I have to say, the Learning Resource Center works hard to accommodate the special-needs kids and finds time to explain their issues to us, the parents. The decisions I've made along the way weren't difficult because I got continued support from the Center. They outlined Faye's options and the rest was up to me. I'm most appreciative of their dedication.

When Faye first was diagnosed in the 1st grade, though, was the time I felt alone. I broke down and went to a licensed clinical psychologist. I couldn't handle the whole LD thing. Now, it doesn't bother me. Dyslexia isn't such a big problem, but, still, there are moments when I get pushed to the limit. When you're in a room with six people (the school psychologist, the principal, the resource teacher, etc.) for an IEP (Individual Education Plan) meeting, you're right there alone. Fortunately, our meetings have been pleasant. But, sometimes, you have to show you mean business, too.

The school psychologist and the resource teacher in Cleveland say Faye has the most severe case of dyslexia they've seen. Yet, she made the merit roll last semester. Her writing still isn't up to 8th-grade level. So many backward letters. She's good at expressing herself in presentations and on oral tests, but writing and reading are her downfalls. For research papers, she gets help in the Resource room. Recently, she did a report on the President. She cut out articles, pictures and cartoons and did an exceptionally creative job. But when she has to type her thoughts, the creativity disappears. So, she ended up dictating it to me and managed to get an "A" on that report.

Recently, though, I kept her back in school and now she wants to return to the parochial school. I can't do this because her sister, Deborah, skipped a year and they'd be together in the same class.

Thankfully, Deborah never makes fun of her sister. They do have the normal female sibling rivalry, but they did study for the proficiency test together. Deborah, of course, passed the first time in every subject. Faye struggled and will have to retake it. But the school won't prevent her from graduating and they don't feel it will restrict her chances of college acceptance.

On the other hand, Faye is fantastic with the computer and shows Deborah how to dial into the Internet or send e-mails. She uses an Alpha Smart laptop recommended by the Resource Center. Mostly, though, Deborah and Faye's relationship is on a social basis. And, you know, I think it's healthier that way. After all, they are sisters.

KELLY SPENCER

Katie, 17, is off to New York University. She's an accelerated student. Andrew, 16, on the other hand, has struggled throughout his schooling because of his dyslexia. Dyslexia also had an impact on Kelly and Matthew's marriage. In the early days of the diagnosis, Kelly and Matthew were not united. Now, though, Andrew is a junior in the local public school and the whole Spencer family has managed to weather the storm.

For a long time, Matthew thought it was a bunch of hooey, this dyslexia stuff. He didn't get involved. It wasn't his thing. He's a physician. He thought Andrew was immature and would outgrow it. I tend to be more communicative. I'd tell Matthew about the issues in school and we'd try to work them out together. But we got to the point where we were arguing. The kids were picking up on this. There was stress in our family. Matthew didn't want to talk about it. And then Katie didn't want to accept the fact that her brother was having problems in school.

Then in 7th grade, Matthew decided to home school Andrew. At the beginning of that year, we had enrolled Andrew in a private parochial school after just moving to the Monterey Peninsula. The principal of the school was wonderful, and the teachers wanted to work with Andrew. But it was a social and academic adjustment for him. Matthew saw it as too stressful on Andrew and on our family. By Thanksgiving, Matthew took him out of school and home schooled him the remainder of the academic year. He was also privately tutored by a Special-Ed tutor. It gave father and son time to do projects together. And Andrew became very involved with the Monterey Bay Aquarium. But while home schooling worked for him, he missed the social interaction. What would we do for 8th grade?

Education is very important to Matthew and me. We looked at our choices and felt boarding school would meet Andrew's needs. He's extremely bright, has a high IQ and needs to be challenged. We looked at several East Coast schools for 9th grade. After sitting in on classes at one of them, the principal told us, "Andrew is ready for our school. You're spinning your wheels with more home schooling." Andrew skipped 8th grade and started there as a freshman. It was difficult having him away. It also was very expensive. We put all our faith in this venture. We weren't wrong.

Boarding school was a positive experience for Andrew. I'm not sorry at all that we sent him back east. But I was disappointed in the academics. He wasn't improving. His grades were poor. We didn't see him remediate his writing. He chose Latin for his foreign language. He did exceptionally well on the state exam, but didn't do the homework. Andrew needs a lot of structure.

It was an environment I wasn't expecting. There were a variety of problems —emotional, alcohol abuse and learning. Andrew isn't an assertive kid. Some of the kids were. Some of Andrew's clothes were stolen and his computer was destroyed.

On the positive side, it did help him socially. By the end of freshman year, Andrew was fitting in and wanted to go back. He made good friends, most from the East Coast. He got involved in theater. The sun rose and set on him. It was great for his self-esteem. The swim coach got him involved in the team. At the end of the season, Andrew was given the Coaches Award. He also continued his drama. He was developing into a fine young adult. His academics, though, were still mediocre.

By the spring of 10th grade, Matthew and I told Andrew we wanted to bring him home. Part of him was ready. He agreed to return. He'd enjoyed the adventure and had matured socially and emotionally.

In the summer before 11th grade, the counselor and school psychologist handpicked teachers for Andrew, ones who would best understand his needs. The local public high school has been very helpful. They recommended a counselor who was more accepting of students with learning differences. At the moment, Andrew's self-esteem is good. He's a good-looking young man and has made many friends. He's performed in three school plays and was cast right away. He seems to have the potential.

And he's doing better with his academics. Andrew's math teacher has cut the math test in half for him. Instead of extended time, his teacher condenses the test within the class period. Andrew is very capable in math, but he's slow. His teacher is looking for quality in his work, not quantity. The last couple of test scores, he's done so much better. He doesn't feel defeated. For his science requirement, he's picked oceanography. Overall, I've been pleased with the school.

We've decided to track Andrew for a two-year college. There's less stress than with the four-year route. The school psychologist retested him and concluded he's bright. She told us just to hang in there and be supportive.

It's a struggle, though, getting Katie to accept Andrew for who he is. She would like a "regular" brother. Katie felt, in our house, things revolved around Andrew. In 5th and 6th grades, I had to sit with Andrew every night and help him with homework. Katie is a B+/A student. She didn't need any help, but she wanted my attention. I tried to help her in other ways. I got involved in her school activities. I thought it was a good substitute. But I later learned it wasn't cool to have mom around in junior high!

Even today, Katie still feels we have different standards for her and her brother. For example, with the last set of grades, she felt I made a greater fuss over Andrew's results. She thinks her "A's" are just taken for granted. Katie has been accepted at NYU this fall. She's a good student, but sometimes, it's difficult for her to totally comprehend Andrew's different learning style.

LISA RIVING

Lisa is a licensed school psychologist and has two children – Charles, a 5th-grader who is dyslexic, and Jessie, a 3rd-grader who is not. Charles is struggling in the public school system. Lisa constantly wrestles with moving him to a special school for dyslexia. This may be the year it happens.

I'm tired of fighting this battle. It's been going on since the fall of Charles'

2nd-grade year. I keep telling my husband and myself: "Let's quit talking about it and do it." In all honesty, Charles needs to go to a special school for dyslexia. He's sinking at our local public school in Dallas.

It's always been a concern, though, to take him out of our neighborhood school. My main concerns are social. I don't like the idea of splitting up Charles' established peer group. These kids have been together since kindergarten. If he moves, he'll either lose his friends or have to work twice as hard to keep them. It's a shame, too, because he's in the best school district in Dallas, the best school district probably in the country. Plus, Jim and I have made sacrifices to live in this neighborhood.

Even though I'm a school psychologist, I've prayed about this move for a long time. I know I'm fighting this battle not only for Charles, but also for any other kid in our neighborhood. He doesn't know we have a three-day visit set up at the new school. It needs to be a gradual process for him so he can slowly become more accepting. He doesn't want to go to the new school because he says the kids are nerds. And, they wear school uniforms!

I don't know how the special school will work out for him. My worst fear is that he'll lose self-esteem. What person will he become? And how will be transition back into our neighborhood high school? I could make myself crazy thinking about the ramifications of everything. I don't know when he'll make the move, but I know we need to do it soon.

My heart goes out to our son. He makes decent grades, always "B's." But I'm not sure he'll ever reach his education potential. Charles just isn't getting it. He struggles to keep up with his peers. In reality, he's getting a marginal education experience.

Charles always has struggled with being different. I don't believe he's ever felt like his peers. Yet, he wants so much to be like every other child. To me, he's a hero. To get out of that car each morning facing humiliation and failure once again, must be terrifying. This year, he moved to a huge middle school —four elementary schools came together. He went from a class of 18 in 4th grade to 28 in 5th grade. Charles is mainstreamed and can go to the Resource teacher on a need basis. But I don't know how long he can last in this setting. He needs a lot of extra help and more individualized teaching.

Looking back at kindergarten, I definitely was in denial (he's my first child). Charles didn't seem to learn in preschool or in kindergarten. He just didn't seem to be achieving on the same level as other children. Still, the teachers didn't have a clue anything different was going on. But there were so many at-risk indicators. Charles didn't have any interest in language arts. He didn't have any interest in words.

He was fortunate to have a 1st-grade teacher who let him work at his own pace. In the meantime, I was trying to diagnose him. But I was probably too subjective. Eventually, I took him to an independent clinical psychologist, but I felt his evaluation wasn't very comprehensive or helpful. Finally, I got a pediatrician who put me on the right path. Charles definitely has language deficits. Spelling isn't basic to him and understanding concepts and directions is a problem.

As a result of testing, Charles was put into the Jump-Start program, which uses the Slingerland reading method. But that was frustrating because he couldn't learn to read with regular mainstream kids. And then, twice a day, he was taken out of the classroom to learn more Slingerland. Once more, our pediatrician came to our rescue. He suggested I take Charles to a speech & language pathologist for private tutoring. She worked miracles with him. She unlocked the door to his learning difficulty and after several sessions, taught him to read. But he still continues to have trouble with new concepts and spelling.

I've tried to be realistic about my kids' needs. Jessie comes home from school and, in 20 minutes, her homework is done. By contrast, Charles constantly needs my help. They're both at the same level in math and English. That must be difficult for his self-image. They've also started competing for my attention. Jessie wants me for emotional support and Charles wants me at homework time. The bottom line is, Charles needs a different way of teaching. He probably can get that at the new school. He must make the move. I just hope he'll agree.

LILY BRIGHTON

The family moved from New Jersey to Connecticut for Will's schooling. Will, is a 3rd-grader at a special school for dyslexia. His sister, Laura, 10, is a mainstream gifted student. It's still too early to tell if Will's younger brother, Peter, 5, has dyslexia.

Basically, the uneasiness of the last two years relates to school insensitivity.

The school has an excellent reputation. I'm not an alarmist, but I didn't like what was going on with Will in kindergarten. He had no interest in language arts. But his teacher advised me not to hold him back. She said he was developmentally young. We went along with it. At the end of 1st grade, he wasn't reading. Everyone still was telling me it was a developmental problem, not a reading one. It was a bad time for me.

Will was using 90 percent whole-language learning. I did a lot of research into this reading method, but I felt I needed a professional on board for additional moral support. I hired an advocate, to which the principal responded: "You're creating an adversary condition bringing in an advocate." Hey! They brought in to the IEP meetings the Special-Ed director, all his followers (five of them), the school psychologist and the school secretary. There were up to 10 people at that meeting. Barbara, our advocate, was wonderful. She fought to alter the lesson plan and to get a Special-Ed tutor. She kept faxing me the correspondence. I paid her about $600 and it was worth it.

At this time, some people were telling me to stop over-reacting. I told them: "If Will was such a bright boy, I'd let him stay at the local school. But school is affecting his self-image." I'm not here to dwell on it, but I went through a grieving process. For about a week, we had a lot of tears. Then I got to work.

My nephew, Paul, was a 6th-grader in the same school district and had a learning disability. I contacted his tutor and she gave me the name of a neuropsychologist. After a battery of tests, he concluded we had a severely dyslexic, completely illiterate child. He suggested we send Will to a special school for dyslexia. Which brings us to lack of sensitivity in the classroom from Will's 3rd-grade teacher, in particular. She demoralized him.

Information on the blackboard was erased before Will could copy it all down. Sometimes, he couldn't read what was written on the board. Will became concerned his classmates were getting it and he wasn't. The teacher thought the information was on the board long enough. She'd had no complaints from other parents. I felt simple modifications were needed. She didn't agree. We were deadlocked.

Will also felt stupid because he could hardly finish one daily edit within the time limit before there were more edits to complete. He felt everyone else could do it. This did very little for his self-esteem.

In addition, it took three notes to his teacher and one to those at the IEP meeting to ensure he wouldn't have to be in the "Reading Buddies" program. It's demoralizing for an LD child to read to a younger child. No one was listening until I banged my fist down hard.

Speaking of reading, this teacher told Will baby books were kept in the 1st-grade wing when he asked for a book to read in class. "All the baby books we left behind," she added. That's great for one's self-image. Will didn't even get to enjoy recess. The teacher kept him in when he hadn't finished an in-class assignment. One time, it was for a Mathland assignment she'd given out in the morning, with time restraints. He already missed two recesses each week because of the additional tutoring he needed. I had to make sure he wasn't held in at recess for work he couldn't complete in class. The kid was on overload. He couldn't win in class or on the playground.

Then, every night, Will had additional homework, above and beyond regular class assignments. It was to make up for lost ground. He was working way past his bedtime.

Finally, we decided to pull Will out of the local elementary school. The IEP team agreed the school never would be able to educate him to his potential because he requires a highly structured, multi-sensory, sequential, language-based approach to learning. Oral information must be presented to him at a rate he can process and with peers of similar cognitive ability. He did well within the Resource teacher's framework, but the classroom environment was a negative experience for him. His self-esteem suffered dramatically.

We moved to Connecticut from New Jersey. We wondered how Will would react. "Can you just drive me through the campus?" he asked. We did one Sunday afternoon, and he loved it. He also spent one day observing at the school. I was a wreck. So much was riding on that day. When I picked him up, he had a smile on his face. I hadn't seen that in two years. I knew, then, we were onto a winner.

Lily suggests:

❑ When it comes to your child's IEP, make sure the next year's teacher has a current copy of it and has read it.

❑ Early days in a new grade are critical.

❑ Recognize battles need to be fought. Don't take anything for granted.

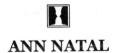

ANN NATAL

Ann is a single parent. Leonardo, 16, is a mainstream sophomore student. Lewis, 12, is in the 7th grade at a special school for dyslexia. Both children are adopted. It was a tough decision to take Lewis out of his neighborhood school.

It all seemed to start in the 4th grade. Lewis would go to the library with a friend to do a book report. After 1½ hours, his friend had written 3 pages. Lewis had written his name. He was reading at a 2nd grade level, yet the school kept checking him off as borderline. Plus Lewis started to eat a lot. He was overweight. His self-esteem was very low. I was a single parent, working long hours, but my son needed me.

We spent three hours each night doing homework, always starting it before dinner because it took so long. Lewis spent 30 to 40 minutes of that time crying. But, it wasn't just crying; it was hysteria. The quantity of homework wasn't the problem. His inability to read was. I vividly remember one time when Lewis was asked to write a one-page essay on a 108-page New England novel about the Revolutionary War. It took him 45 minutes to read the first page. He was so wiped out, I ended up reading the rest of the book. He started to become like my Siamese twin. If I moved, he moved. I couldn't even get up to get a carrot. His low self-image was wearing me down and I didn't know how to help him.

I contacted the Learning Disabilities Center in Boston. There, we got him tested privately and, through the LD network, interviewed several tutors. Lewis worked with a wonderful woman who understood this bright, unhappy young boy. After two sessions, she handed me three pages of photocopied information on dyslexia. Lewis had a classic case and was a perfect candidate for a special school for dyslexia.

I had a conflict, though. I saw how miserable it was for him in the 4th grade, but he'd been with our neighborhood kids since kindergarten. How could I move him? It was a tough decision. Lewis went to summer camp at a school for dyslexia in suburban Boston. The school offered academics in the morning and a camp atmosphere in the afternoon. At the end of summer, Lewis thanked me for sending him there. He was all set to return there for 5th grade. After evaluating my options, I cemented the decision. Lewis would start 5th grade at the new school.

But, as a single mother, how was I going to pay for this? Thankfully, my mother came up with the money. If she hadn't, the school district would have paid if we had a strong enough case. But, it would have been a costly battle. I would have had to hire a lawyer specializing in LD cases. And, it would have taken several months. Honestly, I don't know how Lewis's case would have panned out. But I do know I made the right decision.

"I have something very important to tell you mom," Lewis said, nearly bursting. "I got on the honor roll for math, social science and science." Lewis was in his second semester of 7th grade. I'm still amazed he can read perfectly. He's had so much encouragement from faculty. His English teacher inspired him to read biographies. He's just completed Jimmy Hendrick's 400-page biography and now he's moved on to B.B. King. They also have an excellent music department. Lewis is very talented on the guitar and drums and now wants to compose music on the computer. Lewis doesn't want to leave the school. Teachers are kind to him and he's made good friends.

I'm so happy he's found contentment. I've been through a lot these past few years. He's thin (on campus, they have to walk up and down the hill), he does his homework independently, he does his chores and he has a girlfriend. And, he still has some friends in the local neighborhood. I can't complain.

JANE ROSS

Jane is dyslexic, as is her oldest son, William. Fortunately, his paternal grandparents paid for his tuition at a school for dyslexia in London. Now, Jane's second son, Rex, from a different marriage, also may need special education. She's concerned where she'll get the funding.

It took a long time for William to begin talking. His nursery-school teacher said he was mirroring his words and his recall was poor. I asked, "You don't think he's dyslexic, do you?" The teachers assured me he was very bright. They were sure it had nothing to do with dyslexia. But his poor word recall triggered something in me. Maybe he was dyslexic. I knew what I'd been through.

At just that time, we were hit with a family tragedy when my husband, Ralph, passed away suddenly. William missed a lot of school, but remained in his familiar private nursery school. Then I started looking for kindergarten place-ments for the following academic year. But several schools didn't accept him. Academically, he just wasn't there. I took him to a private licensed clinical psychologist. "No," he said, "it's definitely not dyslexia. Rather, he's suffering from the loss of his father."

I relaxed for awhile, until the issue of dyslexia resurfaced. At $6^{1}/_{2}$, William was reading easy readers. His spelling was poor and his writing was limited. This time, I got a second opinion from a clinical psychologist. He confirmed William had dyslexia and suggested he get remedial teaching immediately. He didn't want to see his self-image destroyed. After networking with several friends, I located a school for dyslexia in London. But it was expensive, very expensive. I didn't know what to do. I was a single mother and a recent widow. Deep down, I knew it would be a good placement, but school fees were out of my reach.

Someone must have been looking out for me because as soon as Ralph's parents saw the psychologist's assessment, they immediately offered to pay for private schooling at the school for dyslexia. They knew how important it was at that stage of William's development to get remedial help. I felt like a 50-pound weight had been lifted from my shoulders.

In truth, though, William's father, Ralph, would have had a terrible time understanding his son had dyslexia. Academics came easy to him. He was writing a book on opera and came from a very musical family. Actually, he could learn languages by listening to opera. To see William struggling would have perplexed him.

William has incredible talent, though, as long as he believes in himself. My job is to keep him doing that. When he's having problems with his homework, banging his head on the table, I tell him I could never remember my multiplication tables. Somehow, that relaxes him. I wish school wasn't so hard for him, but he's improving all the time. I used to read to him every night, but now he loves lying in bed reading to himself.

William wants to be an inventor or car designer when he grows up. He thinks about the future all the time. He's interested in the physical world around him, in technical and science projects. He also loves computers. Ralph's father is buying him a PC next week because William wants to do graphic design and access the multi-media encyclopedia. Thanks to his paternal grandparents, William has received the best gift in life—an investment in his education, in human capital. I know he won't let them down.

Now my younger son, Rex, isn't verbalizing too well. I'm a bit worried about him being dyslexic, too, because I don't know how I'll pay for a special school. Rex's paternal grandparents won't pay for his education. They can't afford it. My parents aren't in that league either. Maybe I'm worrying unnecessarily, but it could turn out to be a problem. Time will only tell if dyslexia runs in the family yet again.

ALISON VUICH

Alison is a single parent who has two older mainstream daughters – Chelsea and Elise. Her youngest daughter, Nicole, has an IQ of 122 but it took her until 6th grade to read at grade level. She began attending a private school for dyslexia on the Hawaiian Islands and her reading increased 3.2 grade levels in just nine months.

Nicole was reading the words "neurological," "epilepsy," "residency," "neurology." This was a first. My eyes filled up as I listened to her. "Mom, what's wrong?" she asked, "Why are you crying? Did I say epilepsy wrong?" "Oh my goodness, no," I said. "You can read properly. I'm so happy you can read." I squeezed her tight. We'd come a long way.

When she arrived at the special school for dyslexia in 6th grade, Nicole couldn't tackle simple Dr. Seuss *Cat in the Hat* books. After nine months, she was able to read chapter books with complex words like "expansion," "experience," "diplomacy," etc. Essentially, the school gave her the tools to read. They recognized her specific deficit areas—auditory discrimination, phonetic segmentation and visual sequential memory deficit—and developed an individualized program to address her particular disabilities. She was taught by teachers who had in-depth training in the field. It was amazing to see her rapid progress. Honestly, before this, she was like a blind kid when it came to reading. The learning approach in the public school just wasn't working. At the school for dyslexia, they found her Braille—and just in time!

In kindergarten through the 4th grade, in public school, Nicole could learn everything, but she was impeded by her reading ability. She felt stupid and ended up being the class clown. I didn't like what was happening, but I couldn't figure out what was wrong. I knew she was intellectually very bright and could verbalize her thoughts, but she still couldn't read. I did extensive research. I needed to know how to help her.

I requested testing at her public school. The vice principal kept putting it off. I soon learned the school didn't want to do it because it cost bucks. After some hassle, they capitulated. The WISC-111 (Wechsler Intelligence Scale for Children) test indicated an IQ of 122, way above average. They put Nicole in Special-Ed classes with those kids who had varied LD problems.

Meanwhile, Nicole is so bright, she became the teacher's aid and did most of the work for the other kids. After a year, Nicole barely increased half a grade level in reading. I knew I had to make changes. We got a lucky break! Nicole was accepted at the school for dyslexia.

A child with dyslexia can make remarkable progress if diagnosed early and instructed properly. But they have to go hand-in-hand. I was determined to find a solution for Nicole and I was fortunate to find teachers who knew how to teach her. Nicole eventually plans to go into politics. To hold her back because she can't read would be an injustice. In all honesty, our Einstein kids need individualize learning programs to let them soar. Fortunately, I found a place for Nicole, just in time!

JEANNIE SMART-CHISTE

TD, 14, is both gifted and dyslexic. It has been a difficult journey for TD in the local rural school system. It's been difficult for his mother, too.

The struggle in this rural community is to introduce teachers and parents to the many shapes of dyslexia. Most people here think it's mirror-writing or reading backwards. The idea that a child could be bright, could be gifted, could read, and yet be dyslexic was unheard of. The local school district looks at these children as lazy and unmotivated. They're accused of having a bad attitude and not trying. In their minds, LD means Lazy and Dumb. The regular teachers don't have Special-Ed training and even many of the Special-Ed teachers don't have training in learning disabilities. There's a major problem brewing.

Parents who realize something is wrong, that their child is falling behind, are told, as we were, "Don't worry, the child will outgrow this." Or, the parents are blamed for having "poor parenting skills." My husband and I had always received compliments for being positive parents until we pressed for accommodations for TD's special problems. Then, suddenly, we had poor parenting skills and were labeled "troublemakers."

But our family can't move away from here because of business reasons and family responsibilities. Another problem is there is no school for dyslexia in the area closer than a 100-plus-mile commute to San Diego. So, each year, we've had new struggles with teachers and administrators. They feel special accommodations are unfair or require too much work or simply are unnecessary. I became an advocate to help my son and children like him.

I've noticed differences about TD since he was born. He was ambidextrous, double-jointed, very clumsy—he never could pedal a tricycle—had problems tying his shoelaces, and was late beginning to talk. In kindergarten, he had motor and coordination problems, poor writing skills, and difficulty finishing assignments and remembering verbal directions. I asked his teacher if he might be dyslexic. "Oh, no, TD is so bright," she said. "Boys often have these problems. Give him time to outgrow it."

By 1st grade, TD was telling me he was stupid. Spelling, writing and arithmetic were so difficult. He read aloud easily with his peers, although at home he hated to read. He frequently lost his place and made strange transpositions while reading aloud. TD judged himself far more harshly than anyone else. He was sure he was stupid and nothing we said altered his perception. His coordination was noticeably poorer than most of his classmates. He couldn't skip or jump rope, and tripped whenever he hurried. Again, I asked his 1st-grade teacher if these were signs of dyslexia. "Of course not, TD is so bright. He's a good reader. In discussing concepts, he's the class leader. He'll outgrow his problems."

School got worse for him in 2nd grade. All his spelling tests were "F's." He was showing behavioral problems and becoming self-destructive. What was going on? Right before Christmas vacation, we took TD to a private licensed clinical psychologist, where he was diagnosed with learning disabilities, but not dyslexia specifically. He suggested our school psychologist further evaluate him.

The school district's psychologist tested TD over a period of three days. After he scored everything, he called me and said, "Do you know how bright TD is?" "Yes, I know he's bright, so why is he doing so poorly in school?" The psychologist said TD had mild tracking and focusing problems, and difficulty with short-term memory. However, his IQ made him eligible for the Gifted and Talented Enrichment (G.A.T.E.) class. Finally, TD had empirical proof he wasn't stupid.

But, in 3rd grade, TD ran afoul of a teacher who didn't understand learning disabilities. She was certain if he just set his mind to it, studied harder and worked longer hours, he could do the assignments. There was no special treatment for him, no extra tutoring or extra time, no oral spelling tests, no accommodations. The teacher pooh-poohed the results of the private clinical psychologist's testing. She had her own diagnosis: I was overprotective and pushy, and TD was spoiled and lazy.

The neurologist at Children's Hospital in San Diego was the first to acknowledge TD was a highly intelligent child with severe dyslexia. None of that changed his 3rd-grade teacher's mind. She insisted TD could do it if he tried. She argued with the clinical psychologist, who had driven 100 miles from San Diego to attend TD's new IEP meeting. Seeing the teacher's mind was made up, halfway through 3rd grade, we moved TD to another school.

But when he was in 4th grade, I was warned by an administrator not to advise other school-parents on dyslexia. If I stopped, he promised TD would receive the services he needed. Unspoken but understood was the threat that, if I continued, TD would indirectly suffer.

In 5th grade, at an IEP meeting in January, the district filed to get TD out of Special Education. The 11 staff persons at the meeting said he'd outgrown his problems. Their position was that, if TD could function at grade level, it was proof he didn't need any special accommodations. The fact that he comprehends college-level material, is gifted and interested in advanced subjects, but writes less ably than a 2nd-grader, was irrelevant.

In the end, TD was placed in a Special-Ed program for one period a day, a part-time pullout class that's taught by the Resource Specialist. But she didn't know how to remediate a gifted child who also had dyslexia. Even the school psychologist told me TD didn't need to learn to read or write at grade level because technology would do this for him. He'd just dictate his thoughts into the computer using a voice-recognition program. That was her answer to TD's problems! Fortunately, with placement in this program, TD gained certain rights under state and federal law. His assignments could be shortened. He could be tested orally and given oral reports. He could have extra time on exams. Written work would be judged on content rather than on spelling. He couldn't be kept in at recess simply because he worked so slowly.

We've come a long way since 5th grade. At his last IEP meeting—8th grade —school staff members recommended TD begin taking a few college classes because his scores were so high and he shared few interests with children his own age. So, he's concurrently enrolled in high school and at the local junior college. At college, he'll take anthropology and drama (Beginning Acting). He's the first 14-year-old to be allowed on campus as a high-school student.

Jeannie suggests:

❑ Ask questions every step of the way during your child's school years.

❑ You may try to believe the educators know what they're talking about. After all, they are the experts. You know your child best.

❑ You also may want to believe your child will outgrow the problems. (A lot of parents don't want to get a reputation as a trouble-maker.) But go with your instincts. It's not an easy journey. But stick with it. Look where TD is now.

JILL MCQUEEN

John and Jill's 12-year-old boy, Simon, is dyslexic. He struggles in school with spelling, French and fundamental concepts. They also have a 9-year-old daughter, Eloise who recently has been diagnosed as a special-needs student. Jill's life has been filled with frustration and hilarity.

In primary school in Edinburgh, Scotland, the headmaster told us Simon was an intelligent boy, but there seemed to be some wall in his learning process. He also daydreamed in class. Simon could name all the planets, describe the moon and stars and tell you about his favorite TV program. But ask him to read an easy reader, and he did his best to memorize it. His teacher also said he would say things like: "Paris is the capital of France," in response to "How do you spell dog?" We told the school about John's dyslexia, but they said it was too early to tell if Simon had a specific learning disability. They did say they would keep an eye on him.

The following year, the school psychologist was to observe Simon. It never happened. She spent so much time with Primary 1 children—some had severe behavioral problems— Simon was left unseen. A few months into Primary 3, the headmaster again asked that the school psychologist see Simon. She didn't appear for several months.

Meanwhile, Simon's teacher was concerned with his poor spelling and limited speech fluency. Halfway through the year, the school psychologist finally appeared, stayed for a brief time and then re-wrote the teacher's notes as her own. Months later, we received an official report from her confirming Simon had a learning disability. But, still, there was no mention of dyslexia. The psychologist informed us that she was going on maternity leave and, if we had anything to discuss, we would be unable to do so!

We decided to take a different route. Simon met with two private licensed clinical psychologists at the Royal Hospital for Sick Children in Edinburgh. After two days of testing it was obvious that Simon had specific learning difficulties. I asked if we could use the term dyslexia and there was a pause, "Well, yes," one answered, "but . . ." Obviously, they preferred us to use the more politically correct phrase—a language based learning disability. Regardless of the title, at least some acknowledgment had taken place. Now, we could start on remedial learning.

After our visit, I was told a letter would be sent to the community speech therapist at our local hospital, to our general practitioner and to the school psychologist. It took me from the end of June until mid-November to establish who was going to help Simon first. The hospital said it was the Health Center, the Health Center said it should be the school, the school said they didn't have a speech therapist on board, the Education Board said Simon wasn't their problem. They suggested trying the Health Board. The Health Board said I should try the Community Health Center. And they said . . . try Education. Wow!!! Finally, I was told a speech therapist would be available at the Health Center for one session a week after school. At last, it seemed, we were going in the right direction.

Not so . . . when we explained our son's disability to the teacher, she promptly replied that there was no such thing as dyslexia! John and I were totally taken aback. She told us he daydreamed, was easily distracted, didn't always grasp simple commands, had difficulty with spelling and took a great deal of time attempting basic tasks. But dyslexia wasn't in her vocabulary. I looked at my husband, he looked at me and, without saying a word, we let her conclude the meeting.

I didn't want to make a fuss in case Simon got the backlash. Actually, I felt somewhat powerless in this situation. I kept asking him how he was coping in class and how the teacher was treating him. His response was, "Fine." He got on with his work, did as he was told and didn't get into trouble. She let him carry on at his own pace and I kept a low profile because Simon was getting excellent support from the speech specialist on board and the Learning Support teacher.

Then, the teacher actually did a complete turnaround! At the next parents' meeting, she talked about Simon's social integration, his awareness in class and his general overall improvement. I can only credit this to his two specialist teachers who channeled progress reports to her. Perhaps she realized I wasn't some daft little housewife with a new word to use. Fortunately, at the same time, the school psychologist suggested Simon apply for a place at the Literacy Unit that offers services for specific learning difficulties. I'm so glad he got the opportunity to go there because it opened up a new world for him. He attended his regular school most of the day and then was transferred by bus to the Literacy Unit for a couple of hours each day.

On the home front, close friends are aware of Simon's dyslexia and accept him as he is. I'm wary, though, to tell non-family members of Simon's different learning style.

LINDA BARDEY

Linda's daughter, Maureen, 24, is no longer a college student. She's back in the workplace trying to make it without a college degree. It's hard for Linda to stand by and watch. Linda has a Ph.D. in education, her husband has two under-grad degrees, and her daughter, 26, has an electrical engineering degree from Georgia Tech. And the list goes on.

If only she'd been diagnosed sooner, Maureen wouldn't have felt so stupid for so long. We learned late—in 10th grade—about her disparity. Her intellectual ability was way up, but her comments on paper were grammatically poor. She struggled with this right through high-school graduation.

We weren't sure Maureen was going to college because high school was such an enormous strain. She spent every waking hour doing her schoolwork, pulling only average grades. She didn't want to talk about it. My recollection is that she wanted to be done with school, was turned off with more school, and was thinking she could do it her own way without a college degree. Sometime during her senior year, though, she went through feelings like: "they're all going off to college and I'm not."

We worked with her, whatever she wanted to do. Her college counselor in the local pubic high school suggested she go away for school, move out of Atlanta, her hometown. He seemed to think we were holding her back, and didn't feel she would grow and develop at home. Maureen didn't want to leave home. She was sure about that. We took the lead from her.

Maureen started entry-level jobs—as a day-care center aide, a waitress, a cashier—when she wasn't attending commuter college. She thought if she worked hard, a boss would notice and, with time, she'd get promoted. But these basic jobs made her feel inadequate and stupid. As a cashier, she floundered with change. Her self-esteem was slipping. Her licensed clinical psychologist told her: "the easy, no-brainer jobs play directly into your weak areas." That did it. She decided to change her focus.

She woke one morning—three years into work—and announced she was going back to college full-time. She felt she could make it. She knew it would be difficult, but she was done with minimum-wage jobs. I'd heard good things about a small branch campus of a research university here in Atlanta. I encouraged her because this school is noted for its caring and concerned faculty. It's a teaching institution, not a research one, and has a total of 600 students. It seemed to be the ideal place. And Maureen could still live at home.

Maureen began there 18 months ago—she was 22—enjoying the small campus feeling. That's what led us to think it would be an ideal place for her to grow. But, the reading was voluminous. So, too, was the paper writing. Even PE required papers. Some friends thought because she was asking for special accommodations, she was taking watered-down courses, basically trying to do less work. This crushed her. I watched her disintegrate.

The whole experience was a big eye-opener for us, a real disappointment. Maureen decided to throw in the towel. Yes, given her choices, we thought we'd made the right decision. Tuition was a big issue in all of this, though. I couldn't afford to send her to Landmark College in Vermont—a school specializing in LD—because tuition was in excess of $18,00, plus living-away-from-home costs. She could apply for a HOPE scholarship at any state school, but most campuses are fairly large and informal. Those were our choices.

Looking forward . . . Maureen needs time to find her own way. At the moment, she feels pressured. Our job is to help her ease into a new life, take small steps at a time, without falling again. She needs to rebuild her self-esteem. Our biggest concern is how to move her out of our house, in a gentle way. She needs to figure out her expenses—insurance, rent, car payments etc. She's never been happy outside of home, at work, or in school. But luck is on her side. She's landed a full-time position as a marketing associate. She seems reasonably happy and is intrigued that some of her superiors don't have a college degree. She already checked that one out.

I'm giving her time to grow and develop. Maybe in five years she'll try college again. By that time, she'll be independent and possibly look to go out-of-state, to a college that has a strong LD support program. I just hope these experiences haven't scarred her.

KATHRYN CHILDERS

Nichole is a gifted student and also is dyslexic. Being in the Gifted & Talented Enrichment program (G.A.T.E.) in high school worked to her advantage. She graduated from the University of California at Santa Cruz in Theater Arts.

Nichole always has marched to the beat of a different drum. She has so much sparkle and so much creativity. But, in 1st grade, I noticed some discrepancies in her intellectual capability. At the end of 2nd grade, it was standard procedure for those in her class to be tested for gifted tendencies. The licensed school psychologist called her back in to redo the visual section. She told me, "Nichole definitely is gifted with an IQ of 138, but she can't spell and can't organize words." That was when we found out she was both gifted and dyslexic.

In grades 3-6, she always was in G.A.T.E. classes. These were small groups of bright kids. She was verbal and got along well with her teachers. Most of the children in the G.A.T.E. program didn't know she was dyslexic. Naturally, all her teachers knew. Nichole compensated by being smart.

But, in junior high, she was very unhappy until I let her go to this alternative high school. It's a Magnet School. She was in the gifted program at a Creative Performing Arts school. That's the only reason Nichole survived high school. The program works like this: In the San Diego school system, the G.A.T.E. program calls for seminars of 15-18 high-school students. Nichole had to be above 135 (IQ) to be termed "gifted." She was part of an elite group on a large school campus. That school saved her.

The G.A.T.E. program took care of her academic problems. There were few multiple-choice tests. Most of the work was projects, presentations, papers and discussion groups. She also could do extra non-writing projects.

Nichole would self-advocate with teachers. Since I work with dyslexic students, it wasn't a stigma for her to be labeled. (I'm a Special-Ed teacher in grades 7-12.) Also, when it came to writing up her IEP, it was no big deal. We included all possible options. I don't hate IEPs. Kids and I write them up all the time. They know what they need. Nichole was no different.

Nichole did hate school enough, though, to combine her junior and senior years. She'd gone to summer school to get rid of classes she didn't like. She also had a knee injury and was exempt from P.E. She then took more required classes, which got them out of the way. Nichole took a year off after high-school graduation. She worked and played. She was still very young, 16.

Looking back, if Nichole hadn't been in the G.A.T.E. program, she would have had a very different experience. Maybe her creativity and zest for life would have been dampened. Who knows? Certainly, our family is thankful a G.A.T.E. program was in place.

JANE BROWNE

James, 11, attends the local secondary school in suburbia London, UK. He has dyslexia. His older sisters, Kate, 16, and Ann, 13, are mainstream students. Superior support from the school has been the family's survival kit.

We chose to live in an area with a good school system with plenty of support for Special-Needs kids. It's a place where administrators and teachers are willing to listen to our requests.

James was fine in the infants class (5-7 years) because there's a wide range of ability. Obviously, the older he got, the more we noticed changes, but I never suspected dyslexia. They were gradual, though. I had his vision and hearing tested. James had a private tutor in his top infant year (7), but that didn't make a difference. The school encouraged parents to help in the classroom and I went in on a regular basis. One time, his teacher said, "Just watch James, what he says and what he does. He knows all the answers. He's one of the smartest kids in class. But ask him to spell 'house' or 'school' and he can't." At that point, I knew the school needed to step in. At our request, they gave him extra work and kept an eye on him. It was no shock to us when he was diagnosed a few months later as a Special-Needs student —they didn't use the "D" word. In fact, if they hadn't come up with anything, I would have been more surprised.

We didn't actually meet with any one person to create his "Statement"—a legal contract between the school and parent. Instead, five different sources contributed. I wrote a report, the school included theirs and the Special-Needs teacher, the licensed school psychologist and James' physician made their recommendations. Then they also asked for Social Services and Special-Needs Nursing to comment. The Statement took about six months to come through. Primarily, we wanted James to be part of the off-campus Specialist Unit. We felt it would be the best placement for him. Although we were worried about the move, James was fine with it.

At the Specialist Unit, he's in a group with three children, all of the same ability. The students are from the same Borough, but not necessarily from the same school. James goes there five hours a week and is bused back and forth to his regular school. Group tutoring is given by a Special-Needs teacher and, recently, he was offered one-on-one help in spelling and reading. So far, Ken and I are confident about the remedial program. The teachers seem to be keeping a watchful eye on James. More importantly, his self-image is great.

It's going to be different, though, in Secondary School. The system changes. Two Special-Needs teachers come into the regular class and offer help to seven or eight students. James will be in a mainstream classroom and, obviously, this help will be only in select subjects, probably English.

Recent testing shows James' reading level is two years below his age group and his spelling level is at 8 years. James is 11. But he's in the top 5 percent for IQ. Despite these statistics, he's in the top group for math, loves science and is a computer whiz. His real talent is in fixing computers. We recently purchased an IBM computer. When we got it home, James suggested he assemble it with us. Ken didn't have a clue what he was doing. James was holding down the fort. Still, we were terrified. This is expensive equipment. James told us not to worry. He doesn't actually read the instructions, just does it by intuition. Now that the computer is up and running—thanks to him—he's our expert on software and the Internet. He's also put a screen saver on our neighbor's computer. And he's only 11.

Overall, James is a happy camper. He's bright, sensible and street smart. We're thankful he's into computers and that the school system is supportive of his special needs. We've heard some horror stories from friends in other school districts.

LINDSAY STAMOS

Bryan, 9, is having a tough time learning Greek. He has dyslexia. Lindsay wrestles with the idea of letting him abandon Greek school. But the Greek Church is full of their heritage. Bryan's sisters, Athena, 12, and Gianna, 6, are mainstream students.

Bryan is struggling with the Greek alphabet. I'm afraid to tell them at Greek school in San Francisco that he has a learning disability. Instinctively, I know his teacher won't understand. She's from Greece and she's a traditionalist. Dyslexia isn't in her vocabulary or in her web of experience.

In Bryan's class, there are 15 students, all of mixed abilities. He's the youngest; most are 5th and 6th-graders. These are kids who didn't start Greek school in kindergarten. Rather, they started late in the program and are trying to whip through the material at an accelerated pace. Bryan is dying in class. The material is over his head, way over his head. In reality, he needs to be with 1st-graders, but then he'd be with kids three years his junior. Plus, his sister, Gianna, is in that class.

In his eyes, Greek school is a total failure. The work is boring and the teacher doesn't call on him. Bryan begs to leave. But it's an opportunity to learn about his heritage and to learn a foreign language. LD experts say he's already having trouble in English, so why complicate matters? For us, though, it's not merely a language issue, it's a cultural one.

My husband, John, has mixed feelings about Greek school. He knows it's not working for his son, but he desperately wants Bryan to be part of the Greek community. You see, his father was born and raised in Greece and is one of the founding members of our Greek Church. And Bryan comes from a long line of cousins who have gone to Greek school. We have a rich culture. Children are taught about festivals, family traditions and Greek food. It has a strong supportive community and John wants Bryan to be part of that nurturing environment. At the moment, though, it's damaging his delicate self-esteem.

We're looking at alternatives. The school has offered tutoring. Another possibility is to find an LD specialist who knows Greek. That's fairly rare in our area (New York would be a better bet), but we could pursue it. A second option is for Bryan to go back into the 1st-level group that has mixed ages and is based on ability rather than age.

When he started at Greek school, at the age of 6, Bryan was brimming with enthusiasm. But he was the only kid who got a zero on a Greek test that year. He remembers the incident well. Everyone saw his grade and he felt humiliated. We eventually let him drop out because he was in tears every Saturday morning. Instead, John taught him for an hour at home. For awhile, that worked well.

But for purely social and cultural reasons, we suggested Bryan return the following year. After much persuasion, he agreed. Again, he didn't do very well on the tests. But he was able to stand up in front of a large audience with his group and recite a well-known Greek poem. At that point, we were delighted with his progress.

We're also pleased with his progress in regular school. He's at a private parochial school where the Slingerland multi-sensory learning method is taught. His teachers are understanding of his special needs and continue to support him. Now with the Greek school crisis, I don't want to add anything negative to his self-esteem. Life at home is troubled enough for him. He's the middle child—between two girls. He stands out anyway because he's different, and then the girls seem to bond. To complicate matters, Bryan and Gianna are on the same reading-level books. He's nearly finished the book; she's just started. Gianna is in 1st grade and he's a 4th-grader.

I desperately want Bryan to remain at the Greek school. I need to find a tutor who understands this child, a tutor who appreciates a student with a different learning style, one who can teach Greek in a fun way. I hope I'm not looking for a needle in a haystack. Our Greek culture is just so rich in history. Bryan would be missing out if he quits now.

ANN & BRUCE BERG

Brian, 13, just celebrated his Bar Mitzvah, the traditional Jewish ceremony for boys. He was a great success but, because of his dyslexia, it took months and months of planning, preparation and practice.

Early in 5th grade, we started talking about David's Bar Mitzvah. We had to plan way ahead of time. His brother, Ben, 17, had a Bar Mitzvah, so why shouldn't Brian have one, too? But would it be too much for him? Would he be able to read the Haftorah? How long would it be? Wow. All these issues. Did he really want to put himself through all this? But it was very important to Brian to be like his other friends.

At Hebrew school that year, the Bureau of Jewish Education brought someone in to teach the Bar Mitzvah and Bat Mitzvah classes. He was a great teacher, but could he teach a student with a learning difference? We had our doubts. I networked with many in the Jewish education field. Finally, we made contact with Paul Gold, who had a son with a learning disability. Paul understood our needs. He agreed to work with David. He certainly knew how to motivate kids. One of his techniques was to have David read in Hebrew, hear him make a mistake and say, "Oh, let me just hear this again." He always used positive reinforcement. He even integrated a football game into his teaching. (He knew David was a keen sportsman.) He'd tell David the ball was on the 50-yard line. If David did that portion without a mistake, he'd be at the 40 . . . the 30 . . . the 20 . . .

Although Paul helped David prepare, our son still was worried about his Bar Mitzvah. How much of the service would he do? The whole Torah? Just his Haftorah? What about any other Hebrew prayers? Paul recorded everything on tape for him. A day never passed when David didn't practice. Over and over again. He started 18 months before the special day. Most kids start 6-9 months before.

David signed up to be the first of the Bar Mitzvahs in his Hebrew class. There would be no comparisons. When he signed up, we purposely chose the shortest Haftorah. We tried to find something early in the year. We decided on the first Saturday after school started, the beginning of September.

David did an amazing job. He has something always to look back on. Two years before his Bar Mitzvah, it looked like he couldn't do it. Now, his Bar Mitzvah was one of the high points of his life. It was tremendous for his self-esteem. We got the help he needed. He invited all his school friends to the Synagogue to hear him recite his Haftorah portion. They went to the party that night. David was riding high that day.

WE FINALLY MADE IT

It must feel like crossing the finish line of a marathon. Doubt, questioning, exhaustion, elation, all the emotions that tag along during our journey. Christina Petersen and Kari Brown know the feeling well.

Christina was sapped from the frustration of knowing she had a very bright son who was performing below grade level. She saw a steady decline in his self-image. She doubted his goals. This all came to a head when Allan, 18, told her he wasn't going to college. But four years later, he graduated from USC with a business degree. For Kari, 11th grade wasn't a great year for the family. Brenda, her daughter, was getting nervous about college, and Kari was getting tired of the whole thing. It had been a long haul since first grade and it wasn't over yet. Six years passed, and Brenda graduated from the University of Arizona with a bachelor's in psychology.

Betsy Wass remembered feeling elated. Ella, her daughter, a fourth-year doctoral student, couldn't read in the second grade and struggled through math and Spanish in high school. In the past, Betsy, a professor at Stanford, waited for Ella to finish reading a page. This time, Ella turned the page with her. They were at the same reading level. Betsy smiled quietly; the journey had been worth it.

One of warmest, fuzzy stories in this section came from Mae Robinson. She told how the Boy and Girl Scouts of America dramatically influenced her son, Scott 18, and daughter Michelle, 16. She wrote: "Wherever we can, we've tried to diminish the dyslexia issue and use the Boy and Girl Scouts to build and maintain our kids' self-esteem. In return, it has expanded our horizons. When I look at Scott and Michelle, I'm so proud of them as young people, as U.S. citizens, as caring teenagers. They did it despite dyslexia."

It's a lot easier talking about feelings once the journey is over. Still doubt, questioning, exhaustion and elation linger. The journey can be nerve wracking, the process painful, holding on to your spouse difficult, holding on to your sanity strenuous. But in the long haul, it seems every doubt, every question, is worth it. In my research, 92 percent of college students with dyslexia said family support was crucial in maintaining their self-esteem.

WE FINALLY MADE IT

BETSY WASS

Betsy is a professor at Stanford University. Her son, Jeremy, is a Yale alumnus and a recent Stanford MBA graduate. Her daughter, Ella, has dyslexia and grew up on Stanford's campus with high academic achievers. Ella pursued her own dream, receiving her bachelor's degree in psychology from Pitzer, CA and her master's in social work from the University of Washington. Ella now is a fourth-year doctoral student in Sociocultural Anthropology at the University of Washington in Seattle.

As part of her annual physical, Ella's pediatrician asked her to read. She couldn't. She was a 2nd-grader. The doctor knew immediately there was a problem. I knew she couldn't read, but I thought it was developmental. I hadn't heard about dyslexia. In fact, I don't even recall the word being used. But that was in the early 80s, long before the Americans with Disabilities Act was passed in 1990.

I had to trust our pediatrician implicitly. But I did my own research, too. Ella was tested by two private licensed clinical psychologists. They both said, "She'll learn to read, just be patient. She's so smart, she'll figure out the words eventually." I also talked with her 2nd-grade teacher at our elementary school. She was insulted and outraged that I had questioned her ability to teach my daughter to read. She actually told me I was a meddlesome parent!

Ella also was tested at school, but her dyslexia wasn't severe enough to warrant federal aid. "Not bad enough" I told the principal, "Ella can't read at grade level." I was furious. So, I began looking for a reading tutor, without much luck initially. Well, as I was ranting and raving about it at my son's AYSO soccer game one day, one of the moms overheard me and said, "You see that mother by the goal post? She's a reading tutor." Yes, I'd found what we needed. Ella started working with her immediately. Within a few months, she'd learned to read. Someone was looking out for us.

Still, quite honestly, the family dynamics were awful. When Ella was young, I tried to be the mediator and it was a mess. Ella had arthritis, both kids had asthma, both kids had problems. Ella's father was unable to deal with this LD stuff. He couldn't understand her math limitations. He thought she was putting it on. Jeremy, I think, also got frustrated with her and withdrew.

Finally, Ella's father left us when she was 12. He had a major life crisis. I was there by myself. The amount of time I spent with her on homework, editing papers, preparing for tests and giving her love and support was endless. As a single parent, it took a lot out of me.

Ella wasn't disabled enough to qualify for the Special-Ed classes in high school. So, she was put in the low stream, with kids who really needed help. She usually got "D's" in math or foreign-language courses or, sometimes, she couldn't even pass the course. One time, I asked her sophomore math teacher if he could let her retake a test. "That's totally out of line," he said. He felt he'd have to do it for everyone and that wasn't going to happen. She ended up taking tests and exams just like everyone else, with no special accommodations.

Fortunately, the following year, Ella was able to satisfy the 11th-grade math requirement by taking it daily at a local private school. She got extra help from a wonderful teacher who told Ella this after the first exam: "You know, Ella, you have a lot of untapped talent." Ella passed the math test every time. She finally found someone who understood her.

Back at public school, though, there was no such thing as an exemption in a foreign language. Ella took Spanish and struggled. She got so stressed out studying for tests. I recall one time when we were sitting at the dining-room table preparing for her test the next day. Ella crawled under the table and we talked to one another from different levels. That way, she didn't have to look at me face-to-face. She was so embarrassed about her limited Spanish ability.

In October of her senior year, Ella refused to go back to the public school. It wasn't the academics that were the stumbling block; it was the social issues. I think two forces were at work—she was taking math daily at the alternate school, so she was able to compare the two schools; and she really loves diversity, but all the kids at her local high school were from the same socio-economic background. It was getting to her.

I listened carefully to her reasons for wanting to leave and the next day, I took her to the alternate high school. Ella graduated nine months later. Even as recently as two years ago, though, she still had trouble with numbers. She got a summer job through a temp agency as a receptionist, but left after three hours. Why? She was reversing telephone numbers because of the speed of incoming calls.

I would like to end with my favorite anecdote. It was last Christmas. I was with Ella at our local bookstore selecting possible gifts. In the past, I would wait for her to finish reading a page. This time, she turned the page with me. She and I were at the same reading level. I smiled quietly. The journey had been worth it!

KARI BROWN

Brenda, 22, has dyslexia and recently graduated from the University of Arizona. Her sister, Annica, 19, is a sophomore at Penn. Brenda's different learning style took an emotional toll on the Brown family.

Both Jason and I were highly academic students, so it was difficult to see Brenda struggling in school. Everything came easy to us. When Brenda was first diagnosed, we were in shock. I didn't know about dyslexia. I didn't know about learning disabilities. All I knew was we were going to have these perfect children. We'd had an easy life so far. When we got the test results, we panicked. Jason and I never meet for lunch—he's a busy physician and works 40 minutes outside of San Diego. But that day, we met for lunch. I was crying. He looked ashen. The thought of what could be in store for Brenda, and us, was horrifying.

Brenda was only 4 when my mother noticed she was daydreaming. I thought nothing of it. A year later, she was having nightmares in my parent's Florida home. I sought advice from a private licensed clinical psychologist. It turned out the nightmares were normal, but Brenda also wrote some of her letters backwards. Once we had an inkling she may be dyslexic, the psychologist performed a battery of tests. The results were affirmative. Brenda was 5.

Annica and Brenda are opposites: tall and short (the younger one is taller), gifted and dyslexic. They lived parallel lives. Character-wise, they were like day and night. The dynamics weren't easy with two extreme students. I distinctly remember one November evening when Annica was an 8th-grader and Brenda was a junior in high school. My life was in turmoil. Brenda was finding it difficult to keep up with schoolwork, prepare for the SAT and play on the varsity tennis team. She talked about being very depressed. That night, she was at her lowest. Both girls needed me at school and Jason was unavailable. He had an important medical meeting. Annica was competing in the Science Fair and Brenda needed me at "College Night." I couldn't be in two places at once. I should have been happy for Annica's keen interest in science, but, in reality, I always focused on Brenda's needs first.

I told Annica that Brenda wasn't as responsible as she was and I needed to be at "College Night" to give her additional support. I also told her there would be plenty of school events we could attend together once Brenda was in college. The sale was over. What I didn't know was that Annica would win first prize in the Science Fair and her photograph would appear in the local San Diego newspaper the following day. The news was all over town. Friends were calling. It was crazy. I was at an amazing high with Annica's success and worried sick about Brenda's state of mind. Was I torn or what?

Brenda's 11th-grade year wasn't a great time for our family. She was getting nervous about college. I was getting tired of the whole thing. It had been a long haul since 1st grade and it wasn't over yet. Brenda had many tutors in her life. But in 11th grade, reality hit us. I worried if she'd make it to college and then how she'd cope without her familiar tutors. Obviously, there was discomfort for our family. I would praise Brenda with encouraging remarks. Jason, on the other hand, doesn't like to be a phony, so he didn't make a fuss. In fact, he said very little about her grades. That caused some undercurrents.

Actually, in all the years, Jason never picked up a book on the subject and he's an avid reader. That part still baffles me. He's a curious person, an intellectual and he treats people for medical ailments. When it came to his own child, he totally deferred to me. He was working 18-hour days and had a heart condition—the guy was exhausted. Still, I'm surprised he never researched this LD. But just before Brenda went off to college, Jason and Brenda became close. "He's more in touch with the real world," she'd say. "He told me the real world wasn't going to feel sorry for me. I'll have to fight for what I want and not let my LD get in my way."

As for Jason and me, we have a strong marriage, but, at that point, he did think Brenda's LD was saturating me. I was doting on her and feeling sorry for her, and for me. Despite this, he still let me run the show. He never questioned my knowledge on school placement or tutors. Brenda didn't switch schools and I didn't approach the school for any accommodations. I always believed we weren't going to change the world. We were the ones who had to change. We did our own accommodations. We got all the tutoring. We empowered ourselves.

In retrospect, I think we missed out on enjoying "the moment" with Brenda as a child. She wasn't allowed to sit around and do nothing. We wouldn't let her watch much TV. I read a lot—so does Jason—and I read to the kids. We expected her to enjoy reading, too. We tried to steer her in the right direction so she'd reach her education potential. But in doing so, I think we muffled out other parts of her, qualities we don't have that she has. She's more playful and casual about life. But she didn't have the practical savvy we were used to. Brenda often felt she was the weak link in the family. Jason and Annica are high achievers. They work long hours and set extremely high standards for themselves. I'm also very determined and focused. Brenda was the opposite. In all the years, we never talked openly about these issues and I regret that. To me, she kept a lot of sadness inside.

There was a lot of sadness on my part, too, terrible sadness about her dyslexia. I felt like something was broken inside her. I think pain always will be there. I felt guilty she always was being challenged. But I knew she could make it in school and I was always there for her, both academically and emotionally. Brenda graduated in the top 10 percent of her senior class!

Then, last year, Brenda graduated from the University of Arizona with a bachelor's in psychology. The best years of her life were in college. She got a good education, made wonderful friends and met a serious boyfriend. She plans to get her master's in education within the next few years. Brenda is a true success story. And to think, I worried all those years!

CHRISTINA PETERSON

Christina's son, Allan, 22, recently graduated from the University of Southern California with a bachelor's in Business Administration. Allan's different learning style had an impact on the whole family, on Christina in particular.

There are definitely two sides to this child—the side he showed to the outside world, and the side he showed to me. He left his public image at the front door and took his frustrations out at home. I was his main target. For so many years, I always was there for him. But it took an emotional toll on me. I was sapped from the frustration of knowing I had a very bright child who was performing below grade level.

Allan's learning disability also was disruptive to other family members. His sister began to resent the attention I was giving him, especially at homework time. She needed me because middle school was causing its own set of problems. Thankfully, David was levelheaded about it all. But time and energy absorbed us. I just told the family: "We all have to pull together; it's a family affair, period."

Besides family, Allan's self-esteem was in question. He knew he was very bright but that he wasn't achieving academically. It became more noticeable once he returned to a mainstream setting, in 5th grade. I carpooled several boys to school and they would talk about their test results, mainly their "B's" and "A's." I could sense Allan was feeling inferior. I constantly had to remind him: "Allan, everyone is different and you're trying your best. You have so many other talents. Don't think of yourself as a failure." It wasn't easy convincing him. He only wanted to be like his friends.

By the beginning of 8th grade, there was a steady decline in his self-image. As a parent, I was upset watching him. Allan didn't want anyone to know about his dyslexia. He didn't want to feel different from his peers, yet he wasn't performing at grade level. He covered it up by having this real cool facade, by being very popular and social. He always was on the phone or looking in the mirror. He was a big cool athletic football guy and people were drawn to him because of his charisma. Anyone looking at this boy thought he was very together. But they couldn't see his inner struggles. (This attitude is much more prevalent in teenage boys and probably almost always in boys with dyslexia. With girls, it's a lot easier because they seem less concerned about the LD stigma.)

I thought maybe the attitude might change in high school. Not so. His teachers didn't know how to deal with him; they didn't understand the emotional aspects of his academic standing. To them, he was a very good-looking, verbal, popular, bright guy. But something wasn't right. Allan didn't want to self-disclose and be different. By mid-year, we started serious testing and it was clear he had a very high IQ. But he didn't test well. He had slow reading skills and had trouble concentrating. Bottom line, his current school was way over his head. Academically, the lower school—6th through 8th grade—was OK but in high school, he was sinking. His saving grace was to play JV football. But he didn't get that far. By the spring of 9th grade, the principal, faculty members, David and I all agreed it wasn't the school for Allan. We had no choice. The school asked us to leave. The writing was on the wall.

The next school didn't have a football team. We took Allan away from the thing he loved most. Entering this new school his sophomore year had a tremendous psychological effect on him. It was a big compromise—small student body and no football team. I questioned it if was the right placement, but at the time, we had very few high-school options.

Allan was halfway through his junior year when he came into the kitchen and said: "I'm not going back." Gulp! At that point, I was exhausted. I think I arrived at a stage in my life, looked at this young adult and gave up. His only choice was to go to the local public high school. I worried about him getting in with the wrong crowd. The school was economically diverse, with students from low-income families mixed with kids whose fathers were CEOs of public companies. Graffiti littered the school walls and there were no doors on the toilets. David's take on this was: "Allan has had a very good education. Let him go simply because he's got the background of good schooling. He's been formed as an individual. He has his morals and standards in place; they've been with him a long time. That won't change overnight." I listened and let him change schools.

Allan entered the public school his junior year the second semester and loved it. Fortunately, with his weight and height, he was able to hold his own. Academically, he was doing OK. He took the SAT with mainstream students on a Saturday morning. He didn't take the extra time because he was too embarrassed to let anyone know.

But Allan didn't graduate with his senior class. Instead, he had to attend summer school because he didn't turn in two English papers. He didn't even go to graduation. He told me: "I'm not going to college. I'm getting a GED certificate." "OK," I responded. "It's your life now. I've done all I can for you. There's a big world out there." I left it at that. Inside, I was absolutely dying. I felt he wanted me to cut the apron strings and get off his case. It was one of the most difficult times in my life. I hid my feelings from him. Actually, I couldn't look at him. I was very scared.

The good news is the summer after his senior year, Allan was accepted at Marymount College, a two-year private junior college in Palos Verdes, CA. Faculty and advisors were supportive of his different learning style. They maximized his potential. Allan received his AA degree and then transferred to USC as a junior. He graduated from USC with a bachelor's in Business Administration (Entrepreneurs Program.) What a relief!

MAE ROBINSON

Mae and Anthony have two children – Scott, 18, and Michelle, 16. Both are dyslexic. They attend a private school for dyslexia in San Diego. The Boy and Girl Scouts of America have dramatically influenced their lives. They have kept their self-esteem high when schoolwork has seemed unbearable.

"He needs to find his self-esteem away from school and the Boy Scouts is a great way to do that." That's what a private licensed clinical psychologist suggested we do 11 years ago. We never looked back.

Scott started in Cub Scouts in 2nd grade. At 11, he went into the Boy Scouts group. Anthony went through the Boy Scout ranks as a kid and then, as an adult, becoming a scout leader for Scott's group. I decided to get Michelle involved in Girl Scouts and then I became her scout leader. That was eight years ago.

From then on, it's only escalated. Last August, six girls (Michelle was one of them) and two adults (my co-leader and I) went to Europe for 21 days. We met with international Girl Scouts from Australia, Canada, the UK and the U.S. As you can see, the Boy and Girl Scouts of America have impacted every member of our family. We owe a lot to that psychologist.

Scott is now an Eagle Scout. He's earned 21 merit badges, 12 of them required. That is, there are set projects he had to do, such as community service, family living, citizen responsibility, disability awareness. Because of this, he's a well-rounded, informed person. For one merit badge, he did a project on family living. He had to keep a budget on everything he spent in three months. He looked into banking and credit-card payments. Thankfully, he came out thinking credit cards aren't a good thing.

Another project was for the Citizen and Community merit badge. Scott went to three City Council meetings. He then had to pick an issue that was discussed and take a stand. He chose the increased traffic problem at his high school. He wrote a letter to the City Council indicating what he felt and what improvements could be made. He had to play the role of a responsible citizen. It did him a lot of good.

Scott wrote to Baden-Powell House, the Boy Scout hostel in London, asking to work there for six months. They agreed. He's going after high-school graduation. The hostel is right around the corner from the Victoria and Albert Museum, in the heart of London. He gets a free bus and underground pass and it won't cost us an arm and a leg because food and board are included. He'll work 35 hours a week doing housekeeping—making beds, cleaning toilets and washing dishes. A large part of the job will be setting up for conferences and meetings and then cleaning up after the events. This will give him some time to grow up and experience a new culture. Knowing Scott, he'll also travel to other parts of Europe.

Meanwhile, the Girl Scouts has given Michelle so much confidence. Last year, she applied for a leadership course at the Leadership Institute, Macy's Center in New York. Michelle was picked as one of 24 girls from all over the country to be part of this course. They discussed contemporary issues such as teen suicide, bulimia, anorexia, teen pregnancy and AIDS. It was an amazing opportunity.

The Girl Scouts also encouraged Michelle to be outgoing and confident in front of an audience. Two years ago, at a dinner dance to raise money for our troop's European visit, I suddenly saw my daughter up, on stage, about to read the winners of the door prizes. I froze. I was hysterical. She couldn't read the names. She couldn't pronounce the big words. And I couldn't fly across the room. What happened in the next few seconds was a blur. Thankfully, Jennifer and Lindsay, two girls in her group, stood behind her and whispered the names. I regained consciousness. (These are the joys of having a child with dyslexia.) Michelle wasn't fazed. Jennifer and Lindsay thought it only natural to help Michelle that night. They knew how she struggled with reading and spelling.

I forgot to mention that when one of the merit badges was about disability awareness, Michelle spoke to her group about dyslexia. She told them how she coped with this learning disability. She just came out with it, no inhibitions. I was so proud of her. Since then, she's had a lot of support and understanding from these girls.

Wherever we can, we've tried to diminish the dyslexia issue and use the Boy and Girl Scouts to build and maintain our kids' self-esteem. In return, it has expanded our horizons. When I look at Scott and Michelle, I'm so proud of them as young people, as U.S. citizens, as caring teenagers. They did it despite dyslexia.

Crisis Strikes

Parents react in different ways when they're first told: *"Your Child Has Dyslexia."* Depending on past teacher conferences, education goals for the child, personal school experiences, genetic information, Special-Ed knowledge etc., answers from 82 parents fell into these groups:

39% were confused, in shock or in denial
24% respondents were relieved that there was a specific learning problem
17% (approx.) were angry at the school system for not alerting them sooner
20% anticipated dyslexia because of genetic factors or because they were
       Special-Ed teachers

It's refreshing to see that we're not alone in our responses. I, for one, was in shock when my daughter's first-grade summer schoolteacher suggested I get Emma tested. I was probably in denial for two to three years. I tried to put a Band-Aid on the situation until, eventually, in fourth grade, with so many book reports to complete, Emma hit a roadblock. The Band-Aids were no longer adhesive. A licensed clinical psychologist tested her, and there, in black and white, was confirmation that our 9-year-old was 18–24 months behind in reading, spelling and math. The psychologist suggested we send Emma to a special school for dyslexia. I was definitely in denial once again.

But not for long. That fall Emma started at the special school. It turned out to be a wise choice. After 10 months, she was reading at grade level and writing more cohesively. Her math was still an area of concern but there was minor improvement. I have to say, though, that two factors came into play for her: (1) she had a caring 4th/5th grade teacher who encouraged her to soar, to think creatively, to be a happy 9-year-old; (2) she was determined to be at the special school for only one year. Emma put her heart and soul into each project, every day, every week for 10 months. She achieved what she set out to do. Then again, she is determined.

What I did pick up from my research, was that a substantial number of parents —39 percent, like myself—were in shock, confused or simply in denial when they first heard those four word *"Your Child Has Dyslexia."* It's a natural reaction. But I think you'll see these numbers drop over the next decade. More parents will be alerted to this "invisible" LD. More parents will be aware of telltale signs as early as infancy. Questions will be asked at the kitchen table about grandparents' schooling (if known), and parents' school experiences. And, what about aunts, uncles and cousins? How did they perform in school? If this happens, progress will have been made.

Further progress will be made if 17 percent of the interviewees, who are angry at the school system for not alerting them sooner, is lowered. If parents learn to detect early warning signs of dyslexia in K-1st grades (see Newsweek Oct 27, 1997, page 57) then the "developmental" theory put out by some 1st-3rd grade teachers will no longer hold. (This happens when a teacher believes that a child's difficulty in school is solely related to social or emotional development, and not to a different learning style.) And, in the past, especially those parents with sons, have accepted this theory.

Parents are becoming more informed, too, because more is out there on the Internet, on talk shows, and in national periodicals, newspapers etc. With hope, then, the data I've gathered—39 percent confused, in shock or in denial and 17 percent angry with the school system—will be reduced. This in itself will make a big difference in how parents handle "Working Through It."

Working Through It

Parents' perception of the journey and their educational aspirations for their child definitely affect the process. It's like running hurdles. How the runner approaches each hurdle is paramount. Let me explain.

At one end of the scale, we have parents who stop in front of the first hurdle, look at it for so long, compute negative thoughts, become paralyzed, often overwhelmed, lower their aspirations and struggle with the first and subsequent nine hurdles, similar to the kindergarten-through-12th-grade process. We could say they are somewhat uptight about the whole process.

By contrast, we have parents who leap over the first hurdle, feel confident and finish the race with few interruptions. In their minds, nothing will stop them. They're fighters, looking for ways to get over the hurdle, be it more speed, a different angle, an improved breathing system, or more height. They'll work out the stumbles, and work on maintaining high aspirations, whatever that takes. They tell themselves to stay calm with the challenges that pop up periodically and unexpectedly.

The final group, middle-of-the-roaders, are those parents who clear the first three hurdles, have high aspirations, but stumble on two or three hurdles before the end. These mini setbacks slow them down, inject insecurity and vulnerability and reduce their aspiration level. The bulk of parents land here. Parents start off in kindergarten with high educational goals, but along the way, get toppled by what is said in school. They bounce back again when they clear more hurdles, but this becomes a precarious game until their child graduates from college. Fortunately, parents who try to remain calm represent a significant number too, while only a few are uptight.

I'm not suggesting that there will only be 10 hurdles along the way. But, just knowing that this isn't a 400-yard dash, a flat distance to cover, will make us better prepared.

Other factors affecting "Working Through It," I've included below:

Family Dynamics

In some families, a young child with dyslexia sets the tone for other members. Patricia Carlson said Taylor controlled her family, though not consciously. When he was frustrated or angry, they would all hear about it. Her nerves were on edge. From nowhere, he would have a tantrum. Patricia and her husband, Doug, talked about Taylor's issues constantly. But, Doug kept a lot of his feelings inside. He didn't express himself as much as she did. "I know he'll be fine" he told himself, over and over. "If Taylor ends up driving a garbage truck and he's happy, then that's what it'll come to." She and Doug agreed on basic values for Taylor but often disagreed about the day-to-day management of it. The journey for this family was tough. Taylor has recently transferred to a special school for dyslexia where, with hope, his inner frustrations with reading and writing will be addressed. In the meantime, "Working Through It" is making Patricia understandably uptight.

Other stories show lack of spousal support. 20 percent of fathers believe their son's school problems are related to emotional or social development, not learning ones. More than 2/3 students with dyslexia are boys (these figures are within the normal range of previous research on dyslexia). Plus, 51 percent of first-born children have dyslexia. This is a hard nut to crack when dad just wants his son to follow in his footsteps—academic and athletic.

Parent-School Relationship

More than 40 percent of the interviewed parents had run-ins with the school. The "D" word was not mentioned. LD testing and special accommodations are linked with meddlesome and/or over reacting parents! Where there was a comprehensive resource center in a school district, though, I rarely heard parent complaints. What I did observe in Hawaii and parts of the UK was that teachers and school personnel were falling behind their U.S. counterparts in Special Education. This was due to lack of funding for both teachers as well as for diagnostic testing. In some instances, students with dyslexia worked alongside physically disabled, visually and hearing impaired, and mentally disabled students in a Special Needs class.

Gender

I didn't target gender as specific criteria, although in parent conversations, those with sons who have dyslexia seemed to experience more emotional highs and lows from 7th through 12th grades. Here personal image is so critical. Teenage boys with dyslexia don't want to raise any red flags and often go mainstream to look cool.

Severity of Dyslexia

Yes, severity of dyslexia plays a major role when the child is severely dyslexic. Fortunately, help is out there. But, it's important to remember that the majority of students with dyslexia are in the realm of average. Only a few are severely disabled, while another few are gifted and dyslexic.

Let me leave you with one thought. The way you respond to those four simple words "*Your Child Has Dyslexia*" and the way you handle "Working Through It" (i.e., what type of traveler you'll be), will become your family's road map.

Regrettably, there was no prototype when this mother was a school-age child. Kathy, her daughter, wrote:

I was sent to the principal's office, 8th grade, for trying to forge my mother's handwriting. The principal didn't believe that an adult woman couldn't formulate complete sentences and couldn't spell correctly. But, then, she didn't know my mother. Mom didn't help me with homework, and didn't help me with college applications. Rather I spent time reading lease agreements and newspaper articles to her. (That's maybe why I'm applying to law school.) Despite this, I consider my mom to be one of the smartest, astute and savvy women I know. She's made it in this world, only she did it blindfolded!

POINTERS FOR PARENTS

For The Crisis

❑ Realize it's the norm to feel angry or confused, shocked or in denial when you first find out your child has dyslexia. Only 20 percent anticipate "it" coming.

❑ Accept that extended family members and close friends won't understand your LD issue and may even criticize your actions.

For Working Through It

❑ We don't live in a perfect world. We can't return our kids. Don't fight reality. Accept the situation. Then you and your child will move forward.

❑ Be realistic about your child's different learning style. Remember, parents of an "A" student aren't always better off. They, too, have their own set of problems.

❑ Gather facts, dialogue with other parents of an LD student, join an LD support group, research the Internet. Just get informed. It's no longer OK to say your child's school problems are emotional or social. Once you've got the facts, discuss your findings with your spouse in an objective manner.

❑ Seek professional counseling if you're getting uptight about the whole LD thing. It helps to look at the situation from a different perspective.

On The School Scene

❑ Don't expect to hear the "D" word used in public schools—it's not politically correct.

❑ Don't accept the developmental argument put out by elementary school teachers—especially if you have a son. You know your child best. Then, educate others in a non-threatening manner.

❏ Realize that a bilingual school setting may not be the best placement for your child.

❏ Plan different schooling if your child is not fitting in, or self-esteem is slipping i.e., home-schooling or transfer to a special school for dyslexia. But put closure on the proposal.

❏ Know that first grade is the optimum time for testing. Kindergarten is too early in most instances, and second-fifth grades will require major intervention. Look for telltale signs in kindergarten and action in first grade.

For Your Child

❏ Use the Internet for you and your child to become more informed about dyslexia. Check out these sites:

LD Online WETA TV/FM (www.ldonline.org)
Learning Disabilities Association (www.ldanatl.org)
National Center for Learning Disabilities (www.ld.org)
Schwab Learning (www.schwablearning.org)
The International Dyslexia Association (www.interdys.org)
British Dyslexia Association (www.bda-dyslexia.org.uk)
Learning Disabilities Association of Canada (www.ldac-taac.ca)
The Dyslexia Institute (www.dyslexia-inst.org.uk)

❏ Find somewhere—other than just academics—to put your child's passion. If you're having a hard time finding his/her attributes, talk with other parents, network, resource the Internet. Find stuff that is not mainstream that may be appealing.

❏ Find out what makes your child happy. Surround your child with people, outside of school, who believe in his/her attributes. Work on that first.

❏ Set up criteria early on, as soon as the diagnosis is verified.
1 Happiness overrides all; that leads to healthy self-esteem.
2 School work is secondary

❏ Research has shown that students with good self-esteem and communication skills are their own advocates in college and the workplace. "A's" and "B's" aren't the only answer.

❑ Don't prevent your LD child from being part of your family traditions. Find ways to decrease the amount of information or lengthen preparation time for a special event.

With Your Partner

❑ If you can create a united front with your spouse concerning your child's educational goals, that's a major bonus. Polarized views only drive a wedge between parents, and staying together is difficult enough these days.

❑ Discuss LD matters privately with your spouse to prevent an alarmist attitude in the home. Children pick up on innuendo and sense worrisome attitudes. Have a clear plan before you include your non dyslexic child in the discussion. Their contribution may only add more fuel and controversy to the family situation.

❑ If there's denial on your spouse's part, don't try to win him/her over immediately. It will take time!

FAMILY DYNAMICS
SIBLINGS

SIBLING-INTERVIEWS

I wanted to see whether a different perspective surfaced when I asked the question "Are you younger or older than your dyslexic sibling"? My findings definitely lead me to conclude attitudes are dependent on birth order.

Children Who Have a Younger Sibling with Dyslexia tend to be more bothered by their siblings' differences. They dispute their parents' methods, question why the younger sibling is not reading and/or spelling at the same level as other kids the same age, and are concerned their sibling most likely will not follow the same accelerated academic path as they.

"Why is my brother/sister struggling so much in school?" they ask. "Why is s/he not doing as well in school as other children of the same age?" "How will s/he possibly handle college and, besides, what college would even accept him/her?" Nichole Courser, Athena Stamos and Katie Spencer, for example, have specific concerns about their younger brothers' academic development.

Athena, 13, sees her relationship with her younger brother deteriorating because he relates more closely to his 7-year-old sister, both academically and emotionally. Nichole, 14, is concerned about her 8-year-old brother's middle-school years because he's not reading or spelling at the same level as his peers and he isn't a high achiever like Nichole. She worries he'll "slack off." She worries he'll be labeled LD. Meanwhile, Katie has gone cross-country to NYU and now is becoming concerned that her brother is taking the community-college route. In her eyes, that means he won't have a prestigious college degree to help him after college.

All three girls take on the "mother" role by worrying about their brothers' "normalcy" and ability to keep up with grade-level work.

Others, however, have the utmost respect for their sibling's differences. Anne Finestien and Bobby Berg, both of whom were accepted to very selective universities, admire their younger brother's social, intellectual and athletic talents, even though the younger siblings aren't top students. Anne is amazed by her brother's grace and poise in social situations and expects a first-tier university's varsity crew team will recruit him. Bobby knows his brother will do just fine, with his strong character attributes—charisma, perseverance and sense of humor. Bobby believes Bryan can win anyone over.

From their responses, more than half the siblings, especially those over age

13, worry about their sibling's differences and take on a parental role—most noticeable among older sisters wanting to protect a younger, dyslexic brother. In some cases, they want significant input into their sibling's education, even going so far as to question their parents' actions.

On the flip side, those kids who looked for positive characteristics admire their sibling despite birth order. They accept their siblings, highlighting their brother's or sister's talents and, sometimes, even broadcasting them.

Children Who Have an Older Sibling with Dyslexia illustrate more confidence in their siblings and respect them despite their different learning style. They talk openly about their older sibling's character attributes (tenacity, determination), interpersonal skills (friendliness, charisma, networking ability), strength in the arts and sports, logic and creative-thinking skills and business savvy.

Birth order dictates that the younger sibling has an innate respect for the older child. Most of the kids with whom I talked felt optimistic about their older brother or sister's future. They were aware of their siblings' limitations, but tended to avoid focusing on their shortcomings, rather accentuating their talents, intellectual and otherwise.

Julia Stone, Theresa Jacobson and Lynn Curtis are very impressed by their siblings' adeptness in certain areas, yet remain cognizant of their obstacles as well. Julia, 21, admires her sister's people skills and creativity in marketing. But, when it comes to taking the standardized test for graduate school, Julia worries her sister's score won't indicate her true abilities. Theresa, 26, praises her brother's logical mind and strategic planning, despite his difficulty with conventional testing. Lynn Curtis, 12, believes her brother's superior athletic ability, coupled with his excellent communication skills will make him a successful sportscaster.

Even within this birth-order construct, though, there were a few respondents who had a concerned, almost parental tone to their interviews. Ross Accordino and Debora Rosen, both in their early teens, seem to doubt the future direction of their dyslexic siblings.

Ross, 14, a high-achieving student, knows his brother works hard to land average grades. Grades are of the utmost importance, though, for teenagers, which may be why Ross views them as a strong measure of future success. Debora, 13, has the same view of measurements of success. She is sympathetic about her sister's difficulties with middle-school criticism, obstacles she feels surely will follow her sister to high school next year.

Overall, I was pleased to see these young people were encouraged by the prospects for their older brother or sister. There was respect, confidence and pride. This feeling of "looking up" to their siblings gave them a more positive perspective on the whole LD situation.

The two types of interviews that follow—children with an older or younger sibling—should give you an idea how these siblings feel and how birth order impacts their perception. There are pointers for both siblings and parents at the end of the section. They touch on the children's emotions, relationships with their siblings and parents, and feelings about being part of a family that includes a dyslexic child.

Children have some strong opinions about the way parents handle this situation, how the family structure adapts to the learning-disabled child and how they feel left out. That parental focus on the dyslexic child, results in a number of reactions from siblings—jealousy, the desire to effect change within their families, frustration about how to deal with their siblings, as well as strong acceptance, tolerance and a sense of freedom. In some ways, these feelings are part of everyday life with any brother or sister. But, with dyslexia in the family, it changes the role-playing dynamics of each individual family member.

I hope you will read these interviews with the understanding that, like all human emotion, age, gender, personal experiences and views of the outside world complicate these siblings' reactions. You may see some reflections of yourself and children in their stories.

"MY YOUNGER SIBLING HAS DYSLEXIA"

NICKI CARLSON, 8th-grade

Nicki, 13, attends a local public middle school. Her brother, Taylor, 8, is a 2nd-grader who transferred out of his local elementary school this year. He now attends a special school for dyslexia.

My parents knew it had to be done. As much as he was accustomed to his teachers and friends at our local elementary school, Taylor had to go to a special school for dyslexia. It was hard for me to see him crying. It was upsetting for the whole family. But I know my parents made the right decision.

Taylor doesn't like change. Neither do I. I've become more nurturing and protective of him since he switched schools. You see, last year, a few kids made fun of him. Taylor's facial muscles aren't strong, so he drools a lot. The kids called him "drool face." I keep telling him the kids at his new school won't tease him. So far, I've been right.

Still, I wish Taylor was like a regular 8-year-old. So many things are hard for him—reading, writing, sports. My mom keeps looking for new activities that don't involve any of those things. A friend suggested Boy Scouts. I really hope that works for Taylor. He needs something to feel good about himself. I'm not so much like my brother. I have so many things going for me. I play soccer and basketball for the school team. Then, there's the theater. My favorite.

Recently, Taylor's behavior has become a problem in our family. Out of the blue, he'll have a huge fit about nothing. He argues with mom and dad about his homework. I don't think it's for attention. I think he just gets frustrated. My mom is pretty patient, but my dad tends to lose it sometimes. It seems like Taylor gets their attention because he does bad things.

In some ways, I wish Taylor didn't have a learning disability because it would be easier for me, for selfish reasons. He gets a lot of attention from my parents and from our baby-sitter. I need attention, too—I'm a teenager and I have a lot of questions. Mom tries to make special time with me, but it doesn't happen that often. Sometimes, dad takes Taylor to the movies or a basketball game. Then, I have time with mom. We go to the mall or out for lunch, but it's only for a little while.

Mom usually talks to me about Taylor's behavior. We both know that when he's good, our family is fine, but he can ruin things in a minute. Mom knows I think it's hard to have a little brother like Taylor. He constantly wants to be with her. She's his security. He doesn't talk much about school to me. He talks to mom about it in his bedroom.

He also loves to listen to mom read. Pippi Longstocking is one of his favorites. Sometimes, he doesn't seem like he's paying attention, but he's been taking it in the whole time. He knows exactly the color of Pippi's odd socks and how many pancakes she ate for breakfast. He has an incredible memory. Like the time in the summer when we were driving to a place we'd been to before. Taylor told us to look for a yellow sign and then turn right. He was right. For a kid who has so many learning problems, he remembers a lot.

But Taylor can't read very well himself. He'll pick up a book and want to read to mom. But, even though he remembers things really well, he still forgets words. He'll read: "The cat is smart." But, when he turns the page, he can't read: "The cat is black. The cat is under the table." He can't read all the words. He doesn't remember what he read on the other page. I don't get it. I try to help him, but I get frustrated. I'm a really good reader, but I don't understand how to help him. I don't understand how someone can't read. Sometimes, I think I'm too hard on him. I can't expect him to be really mature. He's only 8.

On the weekends, Taylor runs off with mom to do errands. I'm left with Dad or I go out with my friends. But, sometimes, I feel left out.

KATIE SPENCER, senior, college prep school

Katie, 17, is worried about her brother, Andrew, 16. He is a high-school junior who is planning to go to a two-year community college. Katie thinks that will limit his chances for success. She wishes he would follow the traditional, four-year college path.

Growing up with Andrew has taught me about people's differences and about how to be more compassionate. There are many prejudices in the world about dyslexia. But I'm not embarrassed at all to talk about it. Actually, I did a term paper on it for a biology class this semester. I learned a lot from the research. The problem of dyslexia lies in the emotional, not the medical side. It touches on the whole family.

We knew there was a problem with my brother in the 5th or 6th grade. I was 13. Mom would sit up with him every night and help him with his homework. I didn't understand what dyslexia was at the time. My parents tried to explain, but I didn't understand. Because my dad didn't come home from work until midnight—he's a physician—Andrew and I competed for mom's attention. My mom tried to give me attention by becoming involved in my school activities. She thought it was a good substitute. But it just wasn't cool to have mom around in junior high.

There's constant competition between us. Andrew gets away with low grades and, sometimes, with his poor behavior. I'm the older one, so my parents expect more of me. My brother's dyslexia plays on my emotional side, too. Andrew comes to me with homework questions, but I'm not very patient. I really don't help him with the assignment. It's just me being there that helps I think.

I got one bad grade this year in calculus and you should have heard them. There seem to be different standards for Andrew. There's also different punishment. One time, Andrew was late getting home on a school night. He forgot to call us. I thought my parents would make a bigger stink. I think he leans on his learning difference. He kind of gets away with more.

When I was younger, though, I was sort of on the outside. It was sort of hush-hush about Andrew's difficulty. Mom and dad were learning about dyslexia and the different testing procedures. But, when my parents decided to send Andrew to boarding school, they told me all about it. It was easy to understand because my school is half-boarding. But finding the right school for him was the worst two weeks of my life. During spring vacation, we took a family trip to the East Coast. Every day, we looked at different schools. I kept asking myself: "Why is he even going to boarding school? This is going to be a big mess." I remember that time he went to camp and it really didn't work out. He never remembered to brush his teeth and he didn't know how to do his laundry. How was this going to work 3,000 miles away? But Andrew flew out to Massachusetts at the beginning of his freshman year to start the fall semester.

My parents kept in constant contact with his teachers. They knew what was going on. I don't think they were any more relaxed while he was at boarding school. But that school worked well for my brother for the first 18 months. In the spring of his sophomore year, though, my parents and I had a big family discussion about Andrew. I agreed with them to bring him home from boarding school. I knew how expensive it was for our family and I thought

Andrew had gotten all he could get from that school. It was time to move on.

Going to an east-coast boarding school was a huge step for Andrew, but he handled it well. He made good friends. He came back after two years with definite improvements. He was social with his peers and more confident with his schoolwork. His being away brought us closer. We had a lot of catching up to do. I think a part of it, too, was that he grew up. Our age difference doesn't matter anymore. He's not so much a little brother now, just a good friend.

I'll be going to NYU in the fall, a prestigious East Coast college. My parents already know that Andrew will go to the local two-year, community college. I think Andrew's path is going to be much harder. I know how much weight the name of a college holds and he won't have the prestigious college degree to help him start off. And, if he doesn't get great grades, I wonder where he'll transfer after two years. I know, in the long run, he'll do fine. I just think it's going to be harder.

NICHOLE COURSER, freshman, high school

Nichole, 14, worries that her brother, Michael, 8, is different. He is only a 2nd-grader attending a special school for dyslexia, but Nichole worries about Michael's future.

Why isn't my brother reading like the kids I baby-sit? It's not fair. They're his age. Daniel and Michael are both 8. They've been to preschool and pre-kindergarten together. But Daniel is reading at a 2nd-grade level. Why isn't Michael doing that? Then, Eric, another boy I baby-sit, isn't having any trouble finishing his spelling homework. Why can't Michael spell the words so well? I could read and spell in 2nd grade. And, when I baby-sat Brittany, she was reading at Michael's level and she's two years younger. Why Michael? Why my brother?

It seems to have calmed down now, but last year was a hard time for our family. I was an 8th-grader in a public middle school. Mom spent a lot of time going to conferences. A lot of energy and attention was focused on Michael. She was always busy getting him tested or going to a school meeting. Sometimes, probably five or six times, she couldn't pick me up from school on time. I'd wait until she was done. I guess it bothered me more than I realized. There was also trouble with Michael's homework. He would start crying. I didn't really need Mom's help—I'm an "A" student—and I knew she would help me if I asked. But she always was busy with my brother. Sometimes, my dad would help him when mom took me for a haircut or to buy schoolbooks or to go to the library. But Michael was getting all the attention. I wasn't used to it. Even when he wasn't in the room, my parents talked about him all the time. They were concerned. My mom was frustrated, too. She's a Special-Ed teacher. She'd talk to my dad and, sometimes, she'd cry on the phone with a friend. I just listened to her. I tried to help her, to show I care about her.

In return, my parents included me in their discussions. They told me why Michael was getting tested. I read his test results, but I didn't understand all the stuff. Still, I thought, he should stay at his school. If he moved, it would be his third school in three years—preschool, kindergarten and first grade, and, now, another school? I was thinking about myself. I wouldn't want to move. I told my parents what I thought, but my mom tends to take it personally. You know, it's really only about Michael that mom and I argue. There isn't a problem with grades or curfews or friends. Mostly, my mom and I are great friends, just not when it comes to Michael.

I think he should be doing more homework and learning to read faster. I think he should be more disciplined, too. Mom says I'm trying to be his second mom. She says I'm making it worse when I tell him what to do. I guess you could say I have ideas about him, how he should act. I'd be more strict about bedtime, watching TV or homework time. I wish he'd do his assignments right when he gets home from school. Usually, he does them after dinner or whenever my mom can help him. I think it's because his brain is too tired.

Michael and I are very different, but it's OK. In a store, he'll talk to the assistant and ask questions about what he's going to buy. And, he's persistent. He's very outgoing. I'm just the opposite. He's also really smart. He knows a lot if he's interested in the subject. In history, he knows all about knights, pirates and Egyptian hieroglyphics. I'm blown apart. He knows which commanders won which fights in the Civil War. The other day, we shared my 9th-grade history book. He loved the Civil War section about weapons. That's really neat because a lot of kids his age don't even know about the Civil War.

Oh yes! He's really good at chess, too. We learned to play from a Christmas book mom gave Michael. He has good moves, ones I wouldn't think of.

Getting good grades, though, isn't so easy for Michael. My parents praise me for my grades, but they would never go on about it in front of him. Usually, at the dinner table, I share about my schoolwork. Michael talks more about recess. I'm always aware of Michael's feelings. I would never go up to him and show him a paper I'd done. He already feels I'm better than him. I remember when one night I was watching Junior Jeopardy with Michael. My mom kept saying, "Good job, Nicole, good job." You could tell he was getting upset. He thinks we should be equal. I keep telling him we're six years apart. I don't want to hurt his feelings. I'm sensitive and protective of what other people think of Michael, too. I wonder if he'll get teased when he's in junior high. I try to imagine what he's going to be like when he's 14. I see other kids at my school who slack off. I hope it doesn't happen to him. I guess I'm worrying too much. But, you see I'm more aware of different factors that can affect people. Not everyone learns the same way or at the same time.

At first, it was hard for me to accept that my brother was different from the kids I baby-sit. I'm more understanding now. I also know he's really bright and wants to learn so much. OK. He's not into chapter books yet, but he can play a great game of chess!

ANDREW BROWNE, freshman, Stanford University

Andrew's brother, Sterling, 16, is a high-school sophomore. They are close, but they're very different when it comes to schoolwork.

When it came to grades, it was like rolling the dice. I rolled the 8s and 9s. Sterling ends up with the 4s. He did all his assignments and showed great effort. But something wasn't right. Sterling tells a great story about his school friend, Craig. All three boys in Craig's family were very bright. It's a fairly strict family. One Christmas, Craig's parents announced the family was going to Hawaii for spring vacation. But, if anyone didn't get straight "A's," they were canceling the plans. Sterling said: "Thank goodness we don't have that in our family."

Sterling wasn't interested in books the same way I was. At an early age, about 2nd grade, I noticed he didn't read very well. Sterling went to the local elementary school and I was enrolled in the G.A.T.E. (Gifted and Talented Enrichment) program. I remember wondering in 5th grade and then again in 6th when Sterling was going to come to my school. I thought it would be fun to have my brother there.

As brothers, we play the classic roles. We bicker and fight, but we respect each other. We have the same values, we joke about the same things, but he's become less interested in school. There's definitely a perception that he's not academic. That's what frustrates me. I wish he would find more direction in his schoolbooks. He'll spend three hours on the phone and 30 minutes on his homework. But I get to be too pushy with him. I just want us to be similar. Now Sterling thinks he should invest more time in acting. I'd like him to invest more time in studying. He's become very involved in a local acting group. This is his new group. Overnight, he's started to identify himself as the actor. He's more interested in girls. Just the other day, he told me: "You're the brother with the brains and I'm the brother with the looks." I wish that wasn't happening.

But this has taught me a lot. I'm much more aware of different learning situations now. I cut out articles about people with dyslexia who've gone on to do great things. I understand better what my brother is going through. Just recently, in math class, I didn't understand a concept. Normally, I can follow most things. This time, I was presented with something I couldn't grasp. For my classmates, the light bulbs were going off all around. There was a frenzy. With some embarrassment, I had to ask a friend to explain. Instantly, I realized what Sterling was going through every day at school. I guess I've had it easy.

PENELOPE BANKS, recent college graduate, Georgia Tech

Penelope, 26, got her degree in electrical engineering and now lives/works in Chicago, Ill. with her husband and newborn. Her sister, Maureen, 24, is a freshman at Emory University in Georgia. Penelope remembers Maureen struggling in school. Even now, she continues to struggle. Penelope has strong opinions about her sister's attitude toward dyslexia and about parenting a child with this LD.

Sometimes, I think Maureen is trying too hard to be like everyone when, in reality, she would be better off just being herself. She is dead set on graduating from a four-year school. I wouldn't look down on her if she got a trade-school education or a two-year degree. She's very good with children and, with a two-year degree, she could get a good job as a nanny. I think this would suit her very well, but she's insistent on getting her four-year degree. I think she's trying very hard once again to follow in my footsteps. I admire her struggle to finish school, but I also see how down it gets her and I believe in doing what makes you happy. I just want her to be happy.

For awhile, I was worried Maureen would hide behind her LD. Part of me still worries. At times, it seems like she uses it as an excuse to avoid doing things or to put things off. I have asthma and I know I used to get out of P.E.

I know this is not the same, but I still see it as similar. Sometimes, I think that, since she was diagnosed, she doesn't work as hard as she did before she found out.

When we were in grade school, I used to drill Maureen on her spelling. I'd get so frustrated because she was slow and kept switching her "B's" and "D's." We drilled her by spelling out loud and writing the words down on paper. It drove me nuts. Of course, we were in grade school at the time and didn't get her diagnosis until much later. When she was diagnosed, in 10th grade, I felt real bad for the way I had treated her. And, I was mad at myself for not picking up on it earlier.

Maureen wants to be a writer. I think she can. She just needs to dictate her thoughts onto a tape or to someone else. I notice she tends to put off doing her school papers. I know part of it is procrastination in doing something she doesn't really enjoy. But I think if she would focus on just writing as ideas flow, rather than nit picking about the spelling, it would get done much faster and she'd enjoy it much more. She focuses too much on getting things perfect. Part of that is her school. The teachers don't just let her write something and turn it in and get a grade. They keep giving it back for revision until they're happy. I also think they give her too much time to complete assignments. At one point, she was only on the second paper of the semester, the semester was more than halfway over, and she still had four more papers to write. I don't believe they should decrease the number of required papers for her just because she has a LD.

I've come to resent the way my parents handle my sister and brother, who has ADD, with their respective problems. I don't believe in hand-holding or sheltering children. It's almost as if they're encouraged to hide behind their problems. Maureen needs to accept her LD and move on. I've accepted I have asthma. I resent the fact she's still allowed to live at home at 24 years old. I realize she is a big help at home, but I think there's a lot to be said for real-life experiences outside the home.

Growing up with Maureen, I was pretty self-sufficient. I didn't really pay attention to how much time was spent with her. While my parents were busy with her, I read. I read a lot of mysteries. I read the Bobsey Twins. Then I read Nancy Drew/Hardy Boy mysteries. From there, I got into the Alfred Hitchcock and the Three Investigator series. And, finally, I got into the Trixie Belden series. I also read Judy Blume and Beverly Cleary books. I had this desire to read all the books written by an author.

I never felt guilty that Maureen got dyslexia or that our brother got ADD. I got asthma, bad allergies and poor eyesight. We all have our problems. But we've learned from each other. I've become more patient tutoring my sister. But, I still get exasperated. Part of that is our different learning styles, not her LD. She always asks "Why?" I never do. I don't think it's her lack of confidence, unless it's a lack of confidence in accepting things. I think it's more that she is a visual learner—she has to be able to "see" something to understand it. On the other hand, I just tend to accept things.

What I never really understood was that it was OK for Maureen to get "B's," but not me. I guess my mom sensed I was better than "B's." And, in helping Maureen so much, she realized "B's" for Maureen were like "A's" for me. But, to an elementary-school kid, it was hard to comprehend.

I do admire Maureen's determination and writing ability. I remember she wrote a story shortly after she was diagnosed. It was about how it had been to grow up with me. She said everything seemed to come so easy to me. The story made me cry because I realized how hard it must have been to follow in my footsteps—probably harder than it was for me to live up to my mom's expectations. I also admire Maureen's ability to act. I've never been one for performing, but she's really good at it.

I've become more aware of dyslexia and, now that I know it's in my family, I'll watch for it in my own child so it gets caught early. I still find it hard to believe Maureen went so many years undiagnosed. I applaud her for struggling all those years and making it.

COLIN ADAMS, junior, high school

Colin, 17, has two brothers, Camden, 15, and Clark, 13, an 8th-grader in the local middle school. Clark, who has dyslexia, recently has mainstreamed. Colin believes his brother always will struggle.

My parents are doing the right thing. Clark would be struggling more if they hadn't sent him to the special school for dyslexia. If I thought it was a bad decision, I would have told them. But, I trusted them with their research capabilities, especially my mom. She was confident and kept me posted. Being the oldest of three boys, I cared. There's definitely a calmness in the family now. The strategy to send Clark to a special school for a few years is working. Now, getting him through high school and college is the next task.

Before he went to the special school, our family had a lot of discussions about dyslexia. We all knew about Clark's situation, how it was affecting him and how he processed work differently. He couldn't process info like Camden, 15, and I. Suggesting that Clark move out of our neighborhood school was a big issue. There was no other choice. He didn't really talk to me about it, but I knew he was worried about not being with his friends. I told him he'd keep in touch with his old friends; he just wouldn't see them at school. It ended up that the neighborhood kids still hung out at our house on weekends, to play basketball or football. And, Clark made a new set of friends at his new school.

I admire that he went to a special school. I would have a problem with that one. He decided to get help and I respect him for this. Plus, he learned so much there and didn't give up. Now that he's in a regular middle school, and getting "A's" and "B's," his struggles and concerns are under control.

Clark is low-key about school. But sports, that's a whole different ball game. Most days, he needs help from my parents with his homework. It's a lot easier for me and Camden to figure out that stuff.

I'm kind of concerned for Clark. It's definitely harder for him to get through school. Deep down, I know he'll be able to do it because he's done it so far. He struggles, but he also perseveres. Come to think of it, he probably would have been this way—very determined—even without dyslexia. It's in his character.

ATHENA STAMOS, 7th-grader

Athena, 13, has a sister, Gianna, 7, and a brother, Bryan, 10. Bryan goes to a parochial school where the Slingerland Multistory teaching approach is offered. Gianna and Bryan are reading the same books.

I wish he was more mature. Bryan and I would have more in common if he wasn't so childish. He still plays with toys and babyish stuff. Really, he's closer to Gianna when it comes to maturity and schoolwork. Bryan is a little better at reading, but they're sharing the same level books. Books that Bryan is just completing, Gianna is just starting. She's in 1st grade. He's in 4th. Mom usually helps Gianna with her homework first. Then, when Bryan needs a lot of help, she works with them together. I'm actually happy that I don't need to ask for help. It's easier for me to get my homework done without waiting for my parents.

Mom told me a little bit about dyslexia. She said it's like numbers or letters are backwards or upside-down. She gave me a few books and pamphlets and I read them myself. They're mostly for parents. I kind of skimmed through them. No big deal. Now, I have a little more understanding of kids with a learning disability. I know it's not their fault. They didn't want to be this way. It just happened. Actually, my second cousin is dyslexic, too. She's going to high school this year. She had to repeat 1st grade. But now she's fine. I see her every Sunday at Greek school. I think she's a real smart kid.

My brother is a smart kid, too. But reading isn't his thing. He does have an incredible memory, though. At home, he likes to play the game "Memory." Yeah, he beats everyone in our house. At Greek school every week, he has to memorize Greek poems. When he memorizes a poem, he has to say it in front of the whole church. He does a great job.

RACHEL MASON, freshman, high school

Rachel, 15, always has been close to her sister, Sarah, 12, who attends a school for dyslexia. Now that's changing. Sarah wants to be less dependent on her sister.

When we were much younger, I was like Sarah's mother. I protected her. I did everything for her. We had a very close bond. As an infant, Sarah took a while to speak. Her speech wasn't very clear, but I could understand her. I would tell mom what Sarah was saying. When Sarah got older, about 3, we played school together. I was 6, so I was always the teacher. We'd write stories on the plastic desks about animals. Sarah only would write two or three sentences. We'd do some flash cards. I'd read stories to her. We kept play-acting like that until Sarah was 9 and I was 12. Once Sarah had confidence in her own abilities, she told me: "I can do this by myself now. I don't need your help." That was really hard for me. I struggled with her new attitude. I felt rejected.

Still, I help her out when she needs it. She still has trouble reading and spelling. She always wants things done quickly, like in 10 minutes. Usually, she is supposed to write one report a month. She dictates her thoughts. I type it for her. After I type, she leaves. She goes downstairs to have some hot chocolate, to take a break from the work. She doesn't hate school, but she dreads doing homework. I've noticed lately that she gets a lot more frustrated. Now she just wants to be by herself in her room. When I ask her what she's thinking, she says: "Oh, I'm making a book in my head." But she's just staring at the wall. You can't attribute everything to a learning disability. Part of this is growing up and maturing, too.

I do wish Sarah was a little more mature, especially when we're with my grandparents. I want her to be perfect and I know she can't. She acts stupid in front of them. I've learned how to act in their company—good manners, calm behavior and respect for elders. I'm the favored granddaughter because of this.

I still want to protect Sarah. She gets teased a lot at school. She's chubby. But, there are great things about her. She can be really funny at times, usually when she's not even trying. She also has amazing determination. I admire that she keeps going to karate. I never stuck with anything. And, when it comes to her career choice, she's always known she's going to be a veterinarian. I remember when we used to play house, she'd save the animals. Maybe the animals couldn't see she had dyslexia.

ANNE FINESTIEN, sophomore, Stanford University

Anne, 19, believes her brother, John, 15, will soar despite his differences. A 10th-grader at a local school in San Francisco, John is on the varsity crew team and probably will be recruited by a top university.

I'm not at all concerned for my brother's future. He'll probably end up making more money than me. He loves cars and computers. He's charismatic, honest, nice and tall. His odds for success are very high. And, as for college, my brother gets good grades and will be one of the No. 1 crew rowers in the nation by the time he's a senior. He'll probably be recruited by Yale, Princeton or Stanford.

My brother's dyslexia wasn't diagnosed until his freshman year at high school. By then, I was a senior in high school. It wasn't really a problem for me because I'd already developed effective study habits. Once he was diagnosed, any "A" he got was praised for weeks, while the straight "A's" I'd been bringing home for years were taken more as the norm. This occasionally annoyed me, but I wasn't too upset about it because my parents didn't ignore my grades. I'm a gifted student and so "A's" came easily. I'm also the oldest, so any expectations were independent of those they had for my brother. If anything, John felt pressured to be an "A" student because we went to the same K-8 school and all the teachers expected him to be like me.

But he wasn't. He had dyslexia. My parents talked about John's difficulties with anyone and everyone, including me. My mom went out and got herself a plethora of info on the subject. I didn't really want or need books. I had several friends with dyslexia and I, myself, have a minor learning disability in spelling and exact order memorization. It was diagnosed in 2nd grade because my spelling wasn't as good as my performance in other subjects. I never felt bad about being gifted because I also had this minor learning disability. But, just because my brother has dyslexia, doesn't mean he isn't gifted, too. He's really smart.

I respect him for his intelligence and his athletic talent. I was so proud of him when he made the varsity crew team as a sophomore. He's the only sophomore ever to make the team. Then, his varsity crew team was the first West Coast team to win the junior national championship. He's also the strongest on the team. He's an awesome guy. I admire my brother's charisma, too. Everyone likes him because he's one of those people who is totally genuine. He doesn't try to be cool. He's nice to everyone and honest with his teammates. He's not afraid to stick up for his friend, even if everyone else thinks the friend is a dork. He ends up being cooler because he doesn't try to be cool.

I've learned tolerance from growing up with my brother. I've learned not to be impatient. And, I've learned not to jump to conclusions, because there can be a lot more under the surface.

SCOTT JACOBSON, graduate, Duke University

Scott, 28, grew up in a family of five and only Natalie, now 22, was diagnosed with dyslexia. Natalie recently graduated from Brigham Young University. Natalie's different learning style didn't affect Scott because they took different school tracks and they were four grades apart. But he's very proud of her achievements.

Natalie's report cards got posted on the refrigerator with everyone else's. My parents told us not to be judgmental and to be a little more patient with her because of her learning disability. But Natalie would comment to me about how different her report card was from mine. She'd joke about her grades. She was so excited about getting a "B." But, for me, that wasn't good enough. I realized early on we were on very different education paths.

I guess I've always felt fortunate. Natalie is less fortunate, but only when it comes to academics. She's compassionate in her work, especially with the deaf community. She's outgoing and has an abundance of confidence. That wasn't always the case.

I think dyslexia attributed to Natalie's unhappiness in middle school. She's very dramatic and she let it be known in our family that school was difficult. She and mom worked long hours on homework assignments. Natalie probably would have preferred to be on stage. I'm not sure I spent a lot of time with her because we're six years apart and we have very different interests. And, I have to admit there were times in high school when I wrote off her dyslexia as an excuse.

But my parents kept telling me not to hold Natalie to the same standards as I held myself. We knew she had more challenges with schoolwork than the rest of us. And, yes, she did get extra attention from my parents. But we accepted this. In return, Natalie was expected to be part of the family troupe in our music, theater and church activities. There, she certainly excelled.

BOBBY BERG, freshman, Yale

Bobby, 18, was a National Merit student in high school, senior class president and a talented musician. He and his brother, Bryan, 14, who has dyslexia have a good relationship.

In some ways, we're opposites. He's a sax player. I'm a trumpet player. I don't learn well from repetition. I get it the first time. Flash cards drive me insane. Actually, Bryan's study habits annoy me to no end. We definitely have a different style of memorizing. But, I don't think this has scarred our relationship. We try to meet on the level as brothers. We get along well most of the time. We let our tensions out by being able to "smack around" in our bedroom.

I've never felt guilty that I'm an "A" student because Bryan and I are equal, just in different ways. Bryan's got a lot of perseverance. I've watched him keep going even when assignments are difficult. He also has the ability to "talk to a wall." I've learned a few tricks from him about how to get the most out of people. Once, our family was on a long plane flight. Bryan went off to the bathroom and, 15 minutes later, I went to check on him. He was sitting in the back of the cabin, talking with the flight attendant. He had the whole thing under control. Bryan has the ability to talk to anyone, any age, any gender. We think he might end up a sportscaster. He loves most sports and he's very proud of his hockey achievements. This year as team captain his hockey team won the season playoffs. As he skated around the rink holding the trophy, he was beaming. That made up for those gloomy days in front of a thick textbook.

When he's studying, my mother is Bryan's designated study partner. He takes up a lot of her time. In English and social studies, she's definitely the expert. My dad steps in for science and presentations. My little brother and my mother go in cycles. They work well together and then they fuse up. I don't need a lot of help and guidance. I'm independent and self-motivated. I'm usually on autopilot. The only time we come into conflict is when I'm writing a paper. My mother is my proofreader. At those times, Bryan and I kind of vie for her attention. But we work it out.

The only complaint I have about my parents is that they should be more willing to look at different learning approaches for my brother. I understand that someone with dyslexia may use it as a block in learning. But there are so many different ways to experiment with new information. For example, Adam Robinson, in *What Smart Students Know*, has a 12-step approach to looking at a textbook assignment. He also talks about rehearsing for a test. At first, I wanted to share it with my brother. My parents didn't think this was a good idea. I don't agree with them.

Bryan still asks me for the meaning of a word or how to say a certain word. He's very comfortable using a word processor and he's very techno savvy. But there's a lot of frustration in him with schoolwork. Once, he said to me, "I wish for one day you would have to work as hard as I do to take this test, then you'd understand." In the long run, I'm not concerned for him. But I'm concerned in the short-term. It's that transition from the long umbilical cord to 9th grade and independent work. He's also worried about me leaving for college soon. But we're talking about communicating via e-mail and then eventually using video conferencing. One thing I'm taking to college, though, is the perseverance I've learned from Bryan.

LAURA BRIGHTON, 4th-grader

Laura, 10, is the oldest of three children and the only daughter. Her brother, Will, is two years younger and a 2nd-grader. He attends a special school for dyslexia. Laura soon learns that dyslexia is a family affair.

I didn't believe my mom at first. We'd lived in New Jersey forever and now we were off to Connecticut. There was a special school for Will. And dad wouldn't have to drive so far anymore. But it came so suddenly. Mom said Will would get better help in his new school. She always talks to me about my brother's disability. I knew he was having difficulty with reading, spelling and writing. She said the special school would really help. I believed her.

Last year was tough for our family. Mom was trying to figure out the best plan for Will. Dad was working a lot in Bridgeport. I could see mom was worried about Will's schoolwork. She spent a lot of time reading to him and helping him with assignments. I don't need a lot of help with homework anymore. If I can't figure out my assignments, I usually read a book to Peter, my younger brother, or play on the computer. I've learned to wait my turn to have mom help me with homework. Sometimes, I feel left out because she spends more time with Will. But it's not a lot. And then we do have time together. I love to go shopping or play Monopoly, checkers or hangman. We also play tennis together. Sometimes, we can do all that. It would be great to have more time with her and I know she wants that, too. But she is mom to all of us. Will needs her attention a lot and so does Peter.

Mom told me I was a good sport to handle the move so well. The first day of school, I was very, very nervous. It went OK. One girl was really nice to me. Then Will started his new school a week later. He seemed sort of happy and sort of nervous. We talked about it. We both were worried. Now, five months later, we've made a few good friends and we like the new house a lot. It has a big yard and woods to explore in!

Will and I get along well. He's nice to me. He makes up jokes and makes me laugh. I'm proud of him for trying so hard in reading. It's not easy for him. I feel bad for him in spelling because, a lot of times, he has no clue what the spelling words are. But this year, he's improving. He has spelling tests to see how fast he can copy them down. He's getting most of them right. This new school is really helping him. I guess the move was OK after all.

MARCUS OAKS, sophomore, college preparatory school

Marcus, 15, thinks his brother, Dylan, 12, a 6th-grader in the local public school, will have some challenges getting through high school. Long term, though, Marcus thinks Dylan has what it takes to become someone great.

Helping with homework is just an extension of our friendship. It's just like playing catch or "hanging out" together. Dylan and I share a room, we're two years apart, and that's just how it is.

I usually type Dylan's stuff for him, then edit his work. Sometimes, I'll read to him. Other times, I'll get him to read to me, but he doesn't like that. It's not a problem to read to him. It kind of makes us closer. I suppose I'm like an anchor to him.

We play football together or shoot basket. So, helping with homework is no big deal. Sometimes, I joke around too much. He tells me to stop. He just wants to get his homework done so he can go and do cool stuff like talk to school friends in the chat room, watch TV or play Star Craft or Oregon Trail on the computer. It's a nice feeling that I've helped.

But he's also helped me in a different way. He picked up some neat strategies from a tutor that he shared with me. One was for multiplication tables; the other for word association.

This works only for the 9s table:

$$9 \times 10 \quad \begin{array}{l} 10\text{-}1 = 9 \\ 9\text{-}9 = 0 \ (90) \end{array} \qquad 9 \times 8 \quad \begin{array}{l} 8\text{-}1 = 7 \\ 9\text{-}7 = 2 \ (72) \end{array}$$

For the word associations, he showed me these books—*Yo, Millard Fillmore!* '97 to memorize all the presidents, and *Yo, Sacramento!* '94 to memorize all 50 states. Both are written by Will Cleveland & Mark Alvarez and published by Milbrook Press in Brooksfield, Connecticut. They worked for me.

When it comes to my homework, I usually do it on my own. I've just learned to do that. When I've needed help, I've been told: "Just be patient. Hold on." I've tried to work through it, but I get frustrated at times. This has happened for about five years. I've spoken to my parents about it. I tell them that they do Dylan's homework for him. They need to let him do it more on his own. I don't really want them to help with homework. I just want their attention. But my dad and I still have a close relationship. We talk about football and sports all the time.

This year, I was having trouble in Algebra II. I talked to friends, but most were in Algebra I. None of them could help. Both my parents are numbers people—they're accountants—but mom was heavily tied up with Dylan all night long. In the end, I got some help. I kept asking. I didn't get as much as I probably needed. Yes, there was a little bit of resentment. It's not a big issue. It's just that all humans like that little bit of recognition.

Through all this, I've become more independent, more resourceful. I do my own research, find my own answers and don't rely on others for information.

In the end, Dylan will do OK. He's got a good sense of humor. He makes jokes on the phone to my friends and teases my parents. Dylan is a hard worker, too. He gets "A's" and "B's." He's still working on homework after I go to bed at 10 p.m. He's definitely not lazy. He gets his research projects done. And, once he sets his mind to do something, he's very determined. He wanted to be the best player on his soccer and basketball teams. He worked out in the gym with me on a regular basis to get into better shape and did a lot of practicing. He became an assistant coach in basketball and, last year, was chosen as the MVP on his soccer and basketball teams. It helps that he's a great athlete.

Short-term, I have concerns for him in high school. Long-term, I see him as a CEO of a company. I see him succeeding. He tries so hard. Whatever he wants, he'll get it. Dylan certainly has got what it takes to be great!

CURT WESLEY, recent college graduate, University of Colorado

Curt, 23, graduated with a political science degree. His brother, Russ, 18, is a freshman at the University of Oregon. Curt says his brother is such an "altogether" guy, it's irrelevant if he has a different learning style.

Our relationship was purely brotherly—no schoolwork, no math, just pure fun. I just knew Russ had some problems with learning, period. I never helped him with homework and he never shared strategies with me. I never went into too much detail about his LD thing. We didn't talk a lot about "it" in the family.

We, as brothers, are equal in many areas—scuba diving, basketball, baseball and swimming. Sometimes, it isn't even fun competing against each other. Although, being the first born, I feel there should be privileges, such as getting the better bed on vacations or having the first choice when choices are offered. Russ, of course, disagrees and wants to deal with these situations on a more democratic level.

I admire Russ for his popularity with everyone. He is a leader among his friends. He stands up for himself and his friends. He is very loyal and has a lot of courage. Let me explain one incident to you. Last summer, when we were scuba diving off the coast of Honduras, we lost track of time. I ran out of air even though my gauge showed I had plenty left. Quickly, I got Russ' attention by signaling to him by tapping my mouth with two fingers. My regulator was out of my mouth. I had only about a minute of air left and I started buddy breathing off Russ' regulator. Russ didn't panic. He just signaled to me that he'd get us back safely to the surface. We floated from 60 feet up to 30 feet. I was holding onto him and sharing air. He signaled me to make a "free ascent" to relieve him of air, then he quickly swam to the nearest person in sight. Thankfully, we both made our ascents. I could have panicked, but I stayed calm because Russ gave me no signs of panic. I just knew he could do it for us.

Looking down the road, I'm definitely not concerned about his future after college. "The Kid" is better off than the rest of us, that is, us mainstreamers. He has good friends, a girlfriend who really cares about him and he's just a likeable guy. You know, even when I josh him about his different learning style, he's too secure and smart for it to "get under his skin."

CAMDEN ADAMS, sophomore, high school

Camden, 15, has two brothers, Colin, 17, and Clark, 13, an 8th-grader who has dyslexia. Clark's dyslexia isn't an issue for Camden, though, because he thinks Clark will be a success in whatever he does.

Clark gets the most attention. It's just been accepted that he gets more help with homework. It's no big deal. I kind of don't need much help. Colin, 17, definitely doesn't need help. If I need my parent's help, I just ask. Dad is a high-school teacher and mom a substitute teacher, so they're pretty understanding of our homework needs. Actually, there's no sibling rivalry about homework issues. It's more about allowance, curfews and chores.

Our family spontaneously talks about Clark's learning disability, about how it's hard for him to spell and read. My parents said he was going to a special school for dyslexia, maybe for one or two years. I was just 12 at the time and had my own pre-teen issues, so this didn't really mean much to me. OK, I thought, that's change for Clark, but it didn't really affect me.

In our home, we're pretty casual about the whole LD issue. Under the surface, though, there's a LD issue. I know mom is concerned. She is more aware of it. Dad knows about it, but it's mom who's more informed, more organized and talks to Clark's teachers about his needs. I'm casual about the whole thing.

So, what's my brother really like? He's very determined, definitely in sports and, most especially, in basketball. Almost daily, we shoot baskets. We just go out to have fun, but he's still very determined to win. Clark isn't going to fall in any cracks and I don't think he'll have problems in college. Because of his character, he'll get through it. He could end up in business. Definitely, he'll be a success.

He's kind of shy at times and modest about his achievements. But, if it's important enough, he'll speak out. When he got a perfect test score, he wanted to be cool about it, yet share his excitement with us. To him, schoolwork has to be done. It's a task, period. Now, sports, is another issue.

As for me, I have thought about the dyslexia issue in our family. Clark got unlucky. He was the one who got it. In the end, though, he'll get something better than Colin and I will. Because of his determination, he'll try harder than us. Colin and I get what we want in school now—4.0 GPAs—and it's harder for Clark now. But, later on, he'll soar. He's learned to hustle at an early age and we haven't yet.

Clark has made me more aware of kids with a different learning style and I've learned to be supportive of my brother even though he's not "perfect." Bottom line is that I'm a guy, I have a brother, Clark, and, by the way, he has dyslexia. It's no big deal.

COURTNEY HENNEN, sophomore, high school

Courtney, 16, has twin brothers, Michael and Matt, 14. Michael is an 8th-grader who has been diagnosed with dyslexia, while Matt has a learning disability, but not dyslexia. Courtney sees no problems for Michael in the future. With his good looks, friendliness, conversation skills and doggedness to get homework done, she knows he'll be a success.

If there was no dyslexia in our family, there'd be a lot less yelling in the house. "Do your homework Michael," my mom always seems to be yelling. There's also a lot of fuss because of the twins. They're vivacious, outgoing and cause a stir. It's a double whammy. No wonder I'm in the corner. I have no say at the kitchen table. Dad is quieter, too. He and I sit and observe.

But I don't feel resentful because my days are packed full with cheerleading practice. Plus, I work for my dad in his busy produce business. There's really no time to see what's going on with the twins. I get my attention because I'm the only daughter and the first child.

About five years ago, the twins and I got tested for dyslexia. When we got the results, we discussed, as a family, the pros and cons of Michael going to a special school for dyslexia. I gave my input, but then I was still only 11. It didn't really affect me.

I told Michael I'd be scared if I had to go to a new school. I also told him I admired him for having to go through the new-friends routine. But he's more outgoing than I am. Since then, I'm more aware of dyslexia. It runs in our family. Our cousin also has this LD.

When I think of sibling rivalry in our family, it's not with me or one of the twins. It's more between the twins. In grade school, Matt would say things like: "You're more stupid than me. You can't read right." Sometimes, I tried to stop the arguments. Now the tables are turned. Michael is getting the higher GPA because the study skills he learned at the special school for dyslexia have projected him further in school. Matt is tailing him now.

It's interesting about the twins. Michael has the higher IQ, the higher GPA (2.8), yet he's the one stuck with this dyslexia. Last year, I was so proud of him. He got the award for the Most Improved Student in 8th-grade social studies. That was quite an accomplishment because it was his first year back in mainstream school. We talked about it at the dinner table for several days.

I became the substitute helper when Mom was at a meeting or doing school stuff. Most of the homework time was directed to Michael. Matt could pretty much do his own work. When Michael read, he struggled with words and then got frustrated. Sometimes, we'd take turns reading. I've always been somewhat patient, but these sessions tested me. My patience level improved.

Michael's future will be full of fun and excitement. He's got a good sense of humor, is able to laugh at himself and is very determined. He keeps going until his homework is done and he doesn't complain. He's friendly, great with people, good looking, strikes up a conversation very easily and isn't shy. (I'm the shy one in the family.) I'm not too concerned about schoolwork. He might struggle in the beginning, but, once he gets used to it, he'll be fine. It'll be fun to see where he is 10 years from now.

"MY OLDER SIBLING HAS DYSLEXIA "

DEBORA ROSEN, 8th-grader

Debora and Faye are two years apart, but they're both in the 8th grade.
Debora is 13 and attends a parochial school, while her sister, Faye, 15, goes
to the local middle school. Faye's school has an excellent resource center for
students with a learning difference.

I feel bad that Faye got stuck with the disability. I know how lucky I am to
be gifted. Faye complains that schoolwork is hard. I can't help her with math
because she uses a different technique. I can help her, though, with editing
papers and reading English-Lit books I've already done reports on. I'm a fast
reader. I try to help as much as I can, but I get frustrated. When we're
working on a paper, I get impatient and finish the sentence for her. Other
times, I help her come up with words. Sometimes, she writes words
backwards or misspells them. I'll overhear her say: "Oops." She knows she's
goofed. That's my sister.

So, it was really a surprise to our family when she made the honor roll with a
3.5 GPA her first quarter of 8th grade. You could hear us screaming in the
kitchen. Faye was really proud of herself. She hung the report card on our
fridge. There was a big stamp saying that she'd made the honor roll.
Fortunately, my parents care more about our effort than our grades, so Faye
and I aren't competing. Faye never feels like she's trailing behind me. She
has a lot of courage when it comes to schoolwork. Even if she doesn't do very
well on a test, she'll go back and try again. She never gives up. I used to
worry about her because she was really sensitive to criticism. But now that
she's nearly a freshman in high school, she's getting tougher.

She seems to have so much strength, too, when it comes to children who are
less fortunate. We both volunteer in an organization for Down-Syndrome
kids. She handles the situations much better than I do. Maybe it's because
she's older, or maybe it's because she has a better understanding of people
with disabilities. She works so well with these kids, especially on creative art
projects. One time, she made a big flower, almost 6 feet tall, out of
Styrofoam. The kids were amazed. She always gives me ideas. She seems
to have them up her sleeve.

Before my mom explained dyslexia to me, I couldn't figure out how Faye could be so creative and still have trouble in school. I didn't really understand that it was difficult to read. Back then, Faye needed mom's help with reading. I was OK with that. Actually, I'd rather not have all the attention Faye gets. Now she's having trouble with algebra. I try to be patient and understand her concerns. But one thing that did bug me recently was when I had to take the Proficiency Test and Faye was exempt from it. It just didn't seem fair. Still, I've learned so much from my sister's experiences. Living with Faye has helped me understand my close friend.

ROSS ACCORDINO, 8th-grader

Ross is 14. Sal is 16. The brothers are competitive and very athletic. Maria, 12, and Vince, 6, are the two other Accordino children. Sal is the only sibling diagnosed with dyslexia. Ross is concerned about his older brother's grades.

We're an Italian-American family. We talk a lot at the dinner table. So, everybody knew dad thought mom was giving too much attention to Sal. Everybody knew there was a problem with Sal's schoolwork. We knew because it seemed like mom was never home for weekday dinners. She was going to a lot of meetings on dyslexia to find out what it all meant. Sometimes, dad went with her. But it didn't bother me because I could do my homework alone.

Well, I thought it didn't bother me until one day when mom was just about to leave for another meeting. I said to her: "You need to be home and cook dinner. Last week, we had dinner without you and dad cooked the meal. It was awful. I'm not upset that you give Sal more attention or drive him to his tutor. It's just that I'm missing your home-cooking." Mom listened. She looked like she had tears in her eyes. I'm not the jealous type and I have a lot of friends. I just enjoy my mother's cooking. Now, before she goes to one of her meetings, she always makes a good Italian meal for us.

Mom and dad learned at the meetings that dyslexia is not a disease. It's like a kind of illness that doesn't go away. Sal gets confused in his reading and spelling. They say he needs a lot of help to get him through high school. He just doesn't get the "A's" and "B's" I'm getting, except in math. He's really smart in math and wants to get a business degree at college. He's really smart, so I'm not worried for his future. He'll be fine.

But, last semester, he talked to me about my grades. He was real proud of me and said: "At least you don't get D's or C's." He didn't actually say he was dyslexic, but I could tell that it was hurting him. I'm glad I know that because, sometimes, I think he gets away with not getting better grades. My parents seem to have a different set of rules for him. They expect me to get a perfect report. But after talking with Sal, I know what he's going through now. He works real hard like me, but only comes out with "C's" and "B's."

He's really good at mechanical stuff, though. He can fix cars and do things I have no clue about. It's just natural for him. I go to him when I need help with anything mechanical. He also helps me with my algebra homework. I'm in first-year algebra, so I don't understand everything. He explains everything. It's great having a brother who gets the X's and Y's.

Mom doesn't go to so many meetings anymore. And we don't talk about Sal's schoolwork at dinner so much anymore. He's a sophomore now and he's doing really well.

JESSIE RIVING, 3rd-grader

Jessie, 9, attends public school. Her brother, Charles, 11, is a 5th-grader at the same school. Day by day, Jessie says, school is becoming more difficult for her brother. It's affecting his self-esteem. It's changing things at home.

I hear Charles crying to mom. Lately, it's practically every single day. He needs to talk to her more now because he's having hard times with his schoolwork and he gets into trouble a lot. Some boys tease him, too, even his best friend, Drew. Drew circles his hand at him to say he's stupid. It makes my brother feel sad. Charles is not stupid; he's really smart.

When we play chess together, he thinks up really good moves. And we have a fort down the street. Charles came up with the idea of having a ramp. He planned it out and made it. And it works.

When I hear Charles talking with mom, I stay up in my room and try not to listen to what they're saying. Sometimes, when I'm standing by her and listening to her shouting at Charles, she tells me to go up to my room. That makes me mad. I don't like her shouting and crying. I say, "Mom, snap out of it." She starts laughing and, sometimes, she cries. This happens once a week, mostly after school.

Mom often asks if I'm feeling sad because she's with my brother a lot. Sometimes, I do. She promises to find time with me and she does. The other day, we stuffed a toy animal for our church. This morning, she took time to make a skirt for my white bunny. Next week, she's trying to work on some pants.

Homework takes me about 20 minutes. But, for Charles, it takes like two or three hours. Sometimes, I try to help him on his math. I know multiplication, addition, subtraction and division. But he gets a little bossy. I try to help him, but it's really not working out.

Sometimes, when we're not doing homework, I like to follow my brother around the neighborhood. I like to be his buddy. Sometimes, we're happy and then, other times, we're mean to each other. But, he's my brother.

MARIA ACCORDINO, 7th-grader

Maria is 12. Her older brother, Sal, 16, is dyslexic. She has two other brothers, Ross, 14, and Vince, 6. Maria is especially sensitive to those with learning disabilities.

I know I'm a worrier but when I was in 2nd grade, I was sure I had dyslexia like my brother, Sal. I have a hard time memorizing words and facts. Sometimes, I feel stupid. I get words mixed up and I can't work very fast. Sal is a lot like me. We both take after my dad's side. My dad, we think, is dyslexic. He's a brilliant architect.

I saw something happening to Sal in 6th grade. Mom said maybe I was sympathizing with him. Then they did some tests and found out I'm not dyslexic. I was relieved but I do have a learning problem. It's just not dyslexia.

There was a lot of tension in our family at that time. Maybe that's why I got worried about having dyslexia. Dad thought mom was giving Sal too much attention. It was pretty bad when Sal was in middle school. Now Sal is a sophomore and he works on his own. Mom and dad told me then that Sal learns a different way. It's a mind thing. When he reads a word, his mind switches it around. Or, when he spells, he doesn't remember the order of the letters. When he does his homework, he wants everyone to be very quiet. Nobody can talk. It doesn't bother me. Ever since we found out Sal has dyslexia, mom got really involved in meetings. She's trying to find out how to help Sal. She tells us at the dinner table about famous people who are dyslexic. We're a family that talks openly and that's helped me understand my brother's dyslexia.

I also understand better because, at school, we have a reading buddy system. I'm a helper. A bunch of 2nd-graders were having trouble reading. The learning specialist found 7th-graders to help four 2nd-graders. We listen to them read every Monday during our Study Hall. I noticed right away that my reading buddy wasn't reading very well. It reminded me of Sal when he was little. She told me she doesn't like reading. She pretends to read the words. Sometimes, she wants to draw a picture instead of reading to me or she wants me to read the story.

One time, I asked her what book she was reading. "Oh, it's like Homeward Bound," she said. "What's it about?" I asked. "It's about a dog and a cat," she said. "What's it called?" I asked again. "The . . . I usually don't read the title because it's not important." She's already 8 and having trouble. I told my mom my buddy doesn't like to read and guesses at words. Mom said maybe she has dyslexia. I'm supposed to tell the teacher and maybe the school will test her. My buddy needs some help, and I understand.

LYNN CURTIS, 7th-grader

Lynn, 13, and Mitch, 14, an 8th-grader, are 18 months apart. Lynn is an honor student. They are in Algebra I together. Lynn is the family's "house editor." She types and edits Mitch's research papers.

When I started to get work that was at Mitch's level, my parents talked to me about dyslexia. They said it's part of our family—my mom's dyslexic, too—and we must help Mitch any way we can. I'm a 7th-grader in 8th-grade math and 9th-grade language arts. Mitch and I have been on the same math and English level for quite awhile. It's been hard for both of us, but we have a good sibling relationship.

My family calls me the "house editor." I'm good in English, so I like helping Mitch proofread his work. Usually, he has one or two social studies assignments a month. He does all the research in the library. He's good with computers. Actually, he's better with the technical stuff than I am. The only trouble he has is doing the typing and proofreading. Since 7th grade, he's said his thoughts to me and I type away. He also has trouble sounding things out. But, we talk it through and the paper gets done. When we were younger, I would help with his spelling words and he didn't like that. Last year, we really started to get along much better. He wants my help now and I like it.

Mitch's hardest subject is reading. When I see him in the library, he'll ask me to spell a word. He doesn't like to read that much and I seem to have a large vocabulary. Actually, he thinks reading is a waste of time. He also has trouble with letters. He confuses them. Even when he talks, he'll say words backwards or say things mixed up. Like, he'll say "red crushed peppers" instead of "crushed red peppers." And, one time, I had a social studies project about Bakersfield, California. Mitch knew all the answers, but he kept calling the place Boxerfield. The most embarrassing time, though, was in our math class. Instead of saying a "condominium," Mitch said "condom." At least, our teacher had a sense of humor about it.

Even though he said that in math class, my brother is good with numbers. He helps me with math assignments. We're in the same Algebra I class. At first, he didn't like that his little sister was in the same class, but now we use it to our advantage. We help each other. The only thing that's hard for him is understanding the lesson. Sometimes, when the teacher explains it, he doesn't always get it the first time. But, at least at home, we can chat about it. He also helps me with history. Mitch has a great memory. And, he taught me a way to remember names, events and facts in chronological order.

One time, Mitch got an "A" on a poetry book he wrote. I never helped him with this project. He used spellcheck on the computer and just wrote what he felt. Another time, he got an "A" on his social studies test. He had to memorize all the states and capitals and spell them correctly. He was beaming. You know, Mitch could do so much better if he liked to read. But he thinks reading is a waste of time.

Usually, I get better grades than Mitch. But I try to be supportive because I know it's so much harder for him. He seems to need more attention now than he did in elementary school. And he'll need even more help when he goes into 9th grade next year. Sometimes, I feel left out because Mitch gets more attention from my parents. They help with his reading assignments or buy him special books. I never really need any help with my homework. But, when I feel really left out, I'll come in to ask questions about my homework. Mom will say, "Not now, I'm helping Mitch." So, I'll just sit and wait until she has a free moment. I've learned to be patient. Other times, I'll come into the room to see what they're doing, just to be part of the family.

I'm not concerned at all for Mitch's future, as long as he doesn't get a job as an editor! He'd be great as a TV sportscaster. He knows so much about sports. He's always wanted to be an architect, too, so who knows? What I do know is that he's a great athlete and he makes people laugh. When he plays soccer, he always does his best. He's a real good team player. He's also an excellent tennis player and is on the school's varsity team.

If I don't become a famous actress—drama is my thing at the moment—maybe I'll start a school for dyslexia. I now know how it effects everyone in the family. It's been a team effort for us.

JULIA STONE, recent MBA graduate, works for an Internet media company

Julia, 25, and Hope 27, are 22 months apart. Hope graduated from Boston University in Marketing and Advertising. They have a younger brother in the 7th grade. Hope was the only sibling diagnosed with dyslexia.

I predict bright prospects for Hope. She is so talented, not only in her professional career, but in her personal endeavors too. Hope is the Director of Marketing Communications for a telecommunications research company. Her colleagues respect both her work ethic and her ability to achieve results. To me, she will be successful in any business field where she is acknowledged for her skills and personality. In reality, she has the ingredients for success; she's a hard worker, a fighter and strong willed.

My sister is also a caring and loving individual and most of all, sensitive to other people's situations and differences. With maturity, she has developed superior people and communication skills. In fact, I remember when she presented her capstone research project at the end of 12th grade. This was her defining moment. Her presentation "Dyslexia: A Way of Life" was empowering. Hope crawled out of her shell and became a voice for an important cause. On that day, my sister spoke with confidence, despite her nervousness to speak publicly to an audience of 100 plus people.

Although Hope and I share similar interests—both in the social and intellectual arenas—it became quite apparent early on that academically we were very different. While I "breezed" through high-school math and English courses, Hope struggled with those subjects. In fact, she spent many afternoons with the math and English teachers, getting that "extra" help while I participated in after-school activities—drama, athletics. Not that Hope wasn't the extra-curricular or "sporty type," she just had to factor in tutor sessions in between tennis and swim practices, and peer counseling. I didn't.

Aside from school, Hope was never treated differently in our family because of her learning style. Sure, there were many Sundays when my Mom spent extra time with her, going over history test questions or editing English papers for mis-spelled words or grammar mistakes. But equally, I recall study sessions of my own with Mom—they just tended to be shorter.

I do, however, recall my parents worrying about her schooling, but any serious concerns were voiced privately, without me knowing. I would say my parents focused their efforts on both daughters. For Hope, they made sure she was placed in small, nurturing schools where the faculty got to know her as a person, for her qualities as a human being and not just for her academic ability. For me, they encouraged my interest in the arts and foreign languages. They always supported me in the high school plays and musicals, as well as encouraged me to become fluent in French and Spanish. Despite Hope's dyslexia, it was never a big deal in our home.

Now that we're both working professionals in the high-tech industry, we have a mutual respect for each others' accomplishments. We're still very close as sisters. We spend time together on the week-ends whether it be hiking or "hanging out" or ordering sushi. My sister will always be my best friend, dyslexic or not. I've always looked up to her, even to this day I do. I guess that's one of the "perks" of being a younger sister—I continuously learn and grow from my older sibling.

THERESA JACOBSON, graduate, Duke University

Theresa, 26, grew up in a family of six children – two brothers and four sisters. One brother, Jacob, 35, was diagnosed with dyslexia. Theresa recently married Scott and the issue of children has surfaced. Dyslexia runs in both families. Scott's sister also has dyslexia.

I know dyslexia is hereditary, so the overwhelming question is: "Will we have a dyslexic child?"

I know what it means to have it affect my family. My family dealt with it through education. It's always been the main focus in our family. For my mom, it was the key to getting out of a poor childhood situation. For Jacob, it was a way to manage dyslexia. But, I know he has deep-seated feelings about his education. I think Jacob feels resentful that my parents didn't give him enough opportunities to excel in other, non-academic areas. They basically took the approach that they were paying a lot of money to send him to a private school. They thought that it was the school's responsibility to help him. I think these education issues came up when my mom was pushing us to go to the UC schools. She had gone to Berkeley. Jacob got into Brigham Young University as a freshman.

I was definitely aware that Jacob was different from us. But my parents are very private about these things. They didn't want to make Jacob an issue. It was between the three of them. I don't think my parents were hiding anything from us. They just didn't tell us very much about dyslexia. Not until I was older, in middle school, did I push the issue. Being the youngest, I was probably more precocious and less inhibited than my siblings. I wanted to know. I also wondered if I had dyslexia. I didn't. I questioned how Jacob got it.

Even with extended time on tests, school wasn't easy for Jacob. So, when he got accepted at Harvard two years ago, I was so proud of him. I'm not surprised he got into the master's program in Public Administration. He's so strategic and very cunning. For instance, in Dungeons and Dragons, the computer game, he maps out everything. He's a schemer. I'm so unlike him. His ideas blow me apart. Jacob also has a very different sense of humor. He catches people off-guard. You have to be awake when he's around. When he was at Harvard, I think that sense of humor got him through the rigorous master's program.

I'm much more alert about learning differences now. My ears perk up when I hear information on the radio. There's more to life than just academics. "A" students go down one education track, while students with dyslexia take a different route. They have to make things happen. In some ways, I think their lives are richer.

TALIA LAURANCE, 4th-grader

Talia is a talkative 9-year-old parochial school student. Her sister, Erika, 12, is a brilliant artist but suffers from severe dyslexia. In the past, Erika has helped her younger sister, but now the gap is narrowing.

Our neighbors raved so much about the painting. One even wanted to buy it. Erika had done a still life on silk, from memory. My sister is an amazing artist. Just last week, we went to a place where you can paint on pottery. People in the store were stunned by her design. They asked to buy it. Then the store manager asked if she would do this for them on a regular basis. I got upset. One reason was because they asked her. The other was because I hated my pottery. At the end of the school year, Erika had several paintings displayed in the art gallery. Two families asked to buy her sunflower painting. Another time, a friend's mother came to our house and raved about a picture of a sea umbrella on silk. The compliments just kept coming in . . .

Mom asks if I'm tired of hearing that my sister is an amazing artist. I'm relieved that she understands. It's confusing to me. Erika needs a lot of attention with schoolwork. And then she gets a lot of attention because of her artwork.

Actually, I'm really happy for Erika when this happens because school is so difficult for her. She can barely write, can't tell the time and math is a jumble of numbers. For reading, she has to listen to books on tape. When I was younger, she helped me with my homework but now I'm a bit ahead of her, even though I'm in the 4th grade and she's in 6th. It's mainly in math. The only time we were both on long division was this year, but now I'm doing decimals. I don't think she's started that yet.

Now she helps me with my growing-up problems. A few girls at school tease me about my body. I'm a little chubby. She gave me good advice. She also helps me with my anxiety. The other day, I'd just gotten up from a nap and I had so much schoolwork to complete. An anxiety attack hit me. My sister sat down on the bed, rubbed my back and sang a little song to comfort me. She made me feel so relaxed. You know, she's such a caring person.

PATRICK MORGAN, 4th-grader

Patrick, 10, attends a local elementary school. His brother, Matthew, 11, is a 5th-grader at a special school for dyslexia. But, to Patrick, his older brother has a great memory and knows so much about history and geography. In Patrick's eyes, Matthew is a champion.

Matthew is smart. He's better at building models and knows more about history than me. The only trouble he has is putting stuff down on paper. His spelling is really bad. That's when mom and dad help out. I know Matthew is getting a good education at his special school for dyslexia. But, sometimes, I feel guilty that he's not a regular kid in a regular school like me. But I understand why he needs more attention and I'm OK with that. I keep myself busy while mom and dad are working with him. I play outside with my friends, watch TV or just hang out in my room. I don't feel jealous in any way. My parents treat me the same as my brother. I know they love me the same as Matthew.

The interesting thing about my brother is his great memory. He can remember things we did a year ago. He also memorizes history and geography facts. When he came in 10th in the Geography Bee at his school,

I was really proud of him. That takes a lot of concentration. I was also happy for him when he won first place in his school soccer tournament. He's not as athletic as I am, but that's OK because he has lots of friends. And, if he wasn't my brother, he'd be one of my best friends.

BRENDAN MANNING, 5th-grader

Brendan, 10, attends a local elementary school. Brendan loves magic. His brothers are Wesley and David. Wesley is a 2nd-grader, while David, 13, attends a special school for dyslexia. Brendan and David work together on editing papers and math homework.

David can't spell too well. But I'm always happy to help because then he gives me math hints. He'll write stuff like: "The wolf trailed of" instead of "off," or "Well have to stand here" instead of "we'll." "Their" and "there" are also confusing to him. But his ideas are amazing.

I learn a lot from his stories. He just wrote one called "A Fine Day to Die." He really likes those War Hammer models. When he paints them, they look like real-life people. He also changes their facial expressions. David had this idea and then he started writing. He wrote a three-page story in a few days. He did a really good job. And, he didn't get mixed up with "where," " were" and "wear." Sometimes he can get a little embarrassed because I'm smaller and younger than he is. He would probably feel better if I was his older brother helping. But he helps me with math homework. His teacher helped him in 4th grade and now he's showing me. One was on Long Division. He told me to remember that Dead Mice Smell Bad. In Long Division, that means Divide, Multiply, Subtract, Bring down the number. So you do DMS check B. And, it works!

Even though David and I really get along and he helps me with my math, last year I felt kind of left out. David needed mom's attention a lot. So, she got somebody to teach me magic. I really like doing tricks. Now, every night about 6, the whole family sits down and watches me. I do one or two tricks. There's not that much time because we have to eat dinner. And, then, when I have to wait my turn with homework, I just pretty much practice my magic. I want to become as good as my teacher. Mom and David help me out. Mom watches me do the tricks over and over again and David gives me good advice on how to set up my show.

Everyone in our family knows my brother is having trouble with spelling. So, when my teacher showed us a video on dyslexia last month, I was kind of happy. I want to know more about David's problem. Four kids said they had a brother or sister who has dyslexia. I didn't raise my hand. I didn't want my brother to feel bad. Actually, a boy in our class who is a little dyslexic keeps one of those pocket computers in his desk. I asked my teacher if a person can outgrow dyslexia. Maybe, that way, David's spelling problem would go away. She said that a kid just learns to live with it.

ANNICA BROWN, sophomore, University of Pennsylvania

Annica, 19, has a sister, Brenda, 22, who is a senior at the University of Arizona. Annica says her sister has so many attributes that are unrelated to school. Brenda has a good sense of humor and can laugh at herself, a virtue Annica respects. Annica believes her sister will be a great teacher because she has an understanding of people's needs and an abundance of determination.

I never tried to make Brenda feel inferior. Even though work came easy to me, mom never wanted me to say I got 100 on my test. I was subtle with my report cards, too. Mom is always protective of her. I think dad is more realistic. Both parents are smart in different ways. My dad is the scientist (he's a physician) and my mom is the literary buff. My sister had a great support system.

But, I felt bad for Brenda because school was difficult. Taking tests was really hard. When she was studying, if she didn't grasp the information the first time, she'd walk around the house memorizing facts, over and over again. She'd say them out loud, repeatedly. She used index cards. She studied with the music on loud. It seems kind of strange because I thought she needed perfect silence. But we're totally different sisters and that's OK.

What wasn't OK was when Brenda went off to college. There was a void. Suddenly, the attention focused on me. I wasn't used to this and I didn't like it. I like my freedom. I'm self-motivated, I work for "A's," and I do my own homework. When Brenda needed extra help with assignments, I completely understood. I knew she definitely got more attention, but I didn't want that type of nurturing. As a gifted student, I didn't need my parents' help, except for maybe reading over my papers.

I know I'm fortunate. And, yes, I felt sorry for Brenda. With only two siblings in our family, why is it Brenda with a learning difference and me as the gifted one? I think she just accepted who she was. She wished me well in my achievements. I've definitely grown more compassionate from my experience with my sister. I'm not a very patient person by nature, but, last semester, I took a biology final and a classmate was taking it with extended time. I understood. And my best friend goes to Amherst. She's ADD. LD doesn't mean a person isn't as intelligent. It just means a person processes words differently.

Aside from all the academic trappings, I really respect Brenda. She's carefree —I wish I was less inhibited—and she has a great sense of humor. When she makes inappropriate comments, she laughs at herself, a virtue I respect. She's also able to flirt with guys and get neat boyfriends. Brenda wants to teach English as a second language to Spanish-speaking children. She'll make a good teacher because she's got talent and determination. She also has an understanding of people's needs. But, like every college student, she's worried about her future.

I've learned it's possible to get close to a sister who seems totally opposite to me. We never really competed academically, only physically. I passed her up in 4th grade. Now, I'm 5ft 10" and she's 5ft. But, now that we're both in college, there's a commonality. We both have uncertainty about the future. We both have guys and that stuff. And, we're from the same family, with concerns about parents and grandparents. College has definitely brought us closer.

WHAT SIBLINGS SAY

27 siblings (young children, teenagers and young adults) contributed to this section. None of the siblings have dyslexia. I asked them about their relationship with their dyslexic sibling, with their parents, and their feelings about dyslexia in general. Their interviews reveal a number of interesting patterns, not only regarding birth order, but also age, gender and parental attitudes toward dyslexia. Let's look briefly at them all.

Birth Order

From what siblings told me, birth order absolutely alters sibling relationships. An older sibling often tends to be more protective over a younger child with dyslexia. They want to have input into the parental decision-making process surrounding homework and family issues related to dyslexia. They also appear to be concerned that their sibling doesn't conform to their preconceived standards. Instead of feeling comfortable with their sibling's differences, they can't understand why he/she doesn't fit into the "normal" box. The respondent's age and the parental attitude toward dyslexia may have contributed to this negative thinking about their sibling's futures.

Without a doubt, the younger, non-dyslexic siblings are less concerned with different learning styles. In fact, they seem to see their brothers/sisters through rose-colored glasses, almost completely eschewing any negative feelings. More importantly, they applaud their accomplishments. For them, "different" doesn't mean "better" or "worse."

Age

The age of the child affects how they perceive their sibling's different learning style. College students respect differences and see promise in their sibling's future. Often, they are close in age and have witnessed a track record of mini-successes (non-school related) from their dyslexic sibling. They also no longer are in a parenting role.

Teens, meanwhile, with a younger dyslexic sibling say that grades are most important and are the only measure of success. They have some strong concerns about differences.

At the other end of the scale, 9-12 year olds don't seem particularly concerned with differences. In essence, they see only the positive side of their dyslexic sibling. Young kids also lack the intellectual understanding or depth of experience to make supportive comments. Essentially, they take their brother or sister at face value.

Gender

The child's gender seems to have an impact on his/her thinking and to strongly reinforce birth order. Teenage girls who are older siblings, for example, take on a protective, parental role, a behavior that appears to come from love and caring.

Family Views and Influences

The home atmosphere significantly affects kids' attitudes toward dyslexia. In families where there is calm and a sense of control, optimism prevails. Where there are concerns about differences and academic limitations, where the family's issues regarding dyslexia haven't been mapped out, where there is parental confusion and uncertainty, the non-dyslexic child seem to be worried and confused.

It seems that, if parents get "their" plan under control early and keep any concerns to themselves, the family has an easier time coping with the challenges. Just like the rules surrounding dating, drinking and friends sleeping over, the parameters of dyslexia must be discussed early on. It's just one more part of the daily routine.

While birth order, age, family views and influences are important in this section, other factors surfaced along the way. These included sibling feelings, relationships between children and their parents, and relationships between siblings. Let's start with the research data.

My sampling included 27 siblings (non-dyslexic) between the ages of 9 and 28. The following is data I gathered from their responses:

67% don't resent their parents helping their dyslexic sibling with homework or projects

92% do their homework independently and don't need help on a daily basis

35% help their dyslexic sibling with homework or do a "homework exchange"

56% are confident about their sibling's future

76% are more understanding of students with a disability because of their experience with a dyslexic sibling

92% had not read a pamphlet or seen a video on dyslexia

Children and Their Parents

While less than a third of the siblings indicate they are "put out" by their parents doing homework with their dyslexic brother/sister, those who were affected—mainly 9-year-old boys and girls, and teenage girls—voiced their opinions loud and clear. For example: Jessie Riving, 9, yearns for a time when her mom will work on a project with her. It seems mom always is working with Jessie's older brother, Charles, who has dyslexia. Nicole Courser, 14, sees that a lot of time is focused on her younger brother with dyslexia, sometimes to the detriment of her emotional needs.

Only 2 out of 27 children had read a pamphlet or seen a video on dyslexia. Instead, most siblings were given fleeting accounts by their parents, often incorrect statements, about this learning difference. One child says "dyslexia is not a disease, rather it's like a kind of illness that doesn't go away." Another believes "dyslexia is when someone writes his/her numbers or letters backwards or even upside down." Now, with so much more information on LD web sites or on-line newsletters, I'm hoping that families with dyslexia will be better informed.

Sibling to Sibling

Only 1/3 of the siblings help their dyslexic brother/sister with homework, sometimes on an exchange basis. Brendan Manning, 9, trades math strategies with his dyslexic brother, for paper editing. Talia Laurance, 10, collaborated on homework with her dyslexic sister, 12, until Talia started to get ahead in math and language arts. In most cases, though, siblings prefer to work independent of each other.

Friends seem to be OK with dyslexia. Still, there is occasional teasing. For example: Jessie Riving, 9, says a neighborhood kid circles his finger to indicate her brother with dyslexia is a "thick head." Nicki Carlson talks about her brother being teased for drooling. (He has facial muscular problems.) Overall, most kids didn't feel it was an issue.

How Siblings Feel

The majority of siblings I met, consider themselves very fortunate not to have to struggle in school. Debora Rosen, 12, feels bad her sister got "stuck" with dyslexia. Patrick Morgan, 10, feels guilty his brother doesn't attend the same public school. Andrew Browne, 20, waited a long time for his younger brother to join him in the G.A.T.E. program, but that never happened. The stories go on and on. All in all, the non-dyslexic siblings realize how fortunate they are when it comes to family genes.

For the most part, non-dyslexic children understand their brother/sister with dyslexia. They start to comprehend their frustrations and they learn to become less critical and more tolerant. Talia Laurance is outwardly jealous of her sister getting compliments on her artwork. But, at the same time, she acknowledges that her sister needs that because she reads at a 2nd-grade level, can't tell time and is 12. Tyrone Begley, 19, sees his brother, Liam 20, struggling with college reading material. This is the same brother who is a computer whiz, who takes computers apart and then reassembles them, and sets up new software programs without reading the instruction manual!

For Andrew Browne, it isn't until he arrives at Stanford University that he really begins to understand his brother's challenge with dyslexia. In one math class, it's as if the light bulbs are going off around him, and Andrew can't grasp the new math concept. He realizes then what his brother faces every day, every week.

For other siblings, living with dyslexia in their family makes them more aware of this LD. Kate Spencer, 17, does a term paper on dyslexia for her 11th-grade biology class. She wants to know how it impacts the family. Kate concludes that the problem lies in the emotional, not medical, side of this learning difference. Her brother, Andrew 16, has dyslexia. And, finally, because of 12-year-old Maria Accordino's experience with her older brother, Sal 16, she knows when her reading buddy, a 2nd grader, is guessing at words and making up the story line. Maria suggests to her teacher that her reading buddy gets tested for dyslexia. And, there are more stories like these ones.

I sensed a need for sibling opinions. They are integral to the family yet so little has been written about how they feel. It's as if research focuses on the dyslexic child and sibling attitudes are set aside. I wanted to know if they felt left out, not special, and what it was really like growing up with a dyslexic brother or sister. From their straight forward, say-as-it-is interviews, I gained new insight and I hope you did, too. Thanks to all those young people who gave me their time.

POINTERS FOR SIBLINGS

About Your Dyslexic Sibling

❑ Find ways to do "fun stuff" with your sibling, stuff that isn't school-related (i.e., watch a movie, exercise or play sports, surf the Internet, play a board game).

❑ Talk confidently with your sibling about his/her future. Identify their strengths and compliment them on their achievements.

❑ When kids ask questions or say mean things to you about your sibling's schoolwork be supportive of your sibling when you answer.

❑ Try to resist making hurtful comments about schoolwork to your brother or sister.

About Your Parents

❑ Don't offer your parents advice on your sibling's study habits unless they ask for it. It's their job, not yours!

❑ Try to do your homework by yourself. This will free up your parents to work with your sibling when that sibling really needs help.

❑ When you think it's a good time to talk to your parents, let them know if you think they're not spending enough time with you.

❑ Definitely, ask your parents to spend time alone with you each week (i.e., work on a project together, go to a sporting event, theater or movie, go shopping, take a mini-trip).

About Your Feelings

❑ Every time you moan about studying for a quiz or test, or get an "A," put yourself in the place of your brother or sister. Empathy is a bonus.

❑ Try to look at differences in a positive way. Recognize your sibling's strengths and realize the talents they have that you don't. Try to balance the scale.

POINTERS FOR PARENTS

❑ Recognize "pressure points" that may crop up with your non-dyslexic child. Then be extra attentive with him or her. This may happen in elementary school when you first find out your child has dyslexia. It may occur in middle school with teenage daughters who may feel neglected with too much attention focused on the dyslexic child. And, it certainly happens when SAT preparation and the college search is in progress.

❑ Use the Internet for you and your child to become more informed about dyslexia. Check out these sites:

LD Online WETA TV/FM (www.ldonline.org)
Learning Disabilities Association (www.ldanatl.org)
National Center for Learning Disabilities (www.ld.org)
Schwab Learning (www.schwablearning.org)
The International Dyslexia Association (www.interdys.org)
British Dyslexia Association (www.bda-dyslexia.org.uk)
Learning Disabilities Association of Canada (www.ldac-taac.ca)
The Dyslexia Institute (www.dyslexia-inst.org.uk)

❑ Discourage siblings from working together on homework unless the chemistry is good and no embarrassment is attached. Stick to sports, board games and videos for sibling sharing.

❑ Encourage "homework exchange," provided both children gain from the experience. Remember, it's a sharing of ideas, not a one-way situation.

❑ Don't worry too much about what your child's friends think of dyslexia. It appears most kids are OK with it.

❑ Don't feel sorry for your dyslexic child. Two-thirds of the kids in the survey were confident of the future of their brother/sister. They saw talent, creativity and determination.

❑ View your child's learning experience with his/her LD brother/sister as a bonus in character building. Sensitivity, compassion and patience can't be learned from textbooks.

❑ Consistently compliment your non-dyslexic child for understanding the family's LD situation, working independently on homework and being a team player.

❑ Be aware of the time and attention you are giving to your dyslexic child. Then, listen to the needs of your other kids. If it means bringing in a college student to help with a project, hobby or sport, just do it!

❑ Don't over-analyze the homework situation. Kids are OK with parents giving more time to their sibling.

2

HOW TO COPE
PARENTS

HOW-TO-COPE

Consider this a hands-on, how-to-cope section. There is no quantitative data, no ratings, just practical suggestions. This section is about parents—35 of them—who share what's worked for their children from Kindergarten through 12th grade.

Kindergarten through 5th Grade: elementary school

Parents talk about staying up-to-date with their child's school progress, the criteria for selecting a private tutor, factors relating to their child's IEP, and out-of-mainstream issues i.e., should their child transfer to a special school for dyslexia or should they consider home schooling? (More than half feel that the decision-process is wrenching.) Parents also touch upon the financial implications of moving to a fee-paying school.

6th through 8th Grade: middle school

Strategies for homework, burnout, Special-Ed tutoring, technology use, and an incentive plan for report cards are some of the topics discussed in this section. In reality, parents look at different ways to keep their child "afloat" in the mainstream.

9th through 12th Grade: high school

Every "C" and "D" now shows up on an official transcript. The SAT and college-application process are also nagging points. Parents tend to be more worrisome here. Together, with their student, they utilize special accommodations and coping strategies that preferably don't cause run-ins with the school. For example, they try to schedule difficult classes during first and second periods (history, science etc.); create a study hall last period for homework assignments; and petition American Sign Language as the foreign-language requirement.

The how-to-cope section is jam-packed with pragmatic ideas. To all those parents who shared their family secrets, their family coping strategies, I thank you sincerely. Your ideas will make a difference for so many families.

KINDERGARTEN THROUGH 5TH GRADE: STRATEGIES

Parents look for innovative ways to help their child. Zoey Roy turned to technology - all her TVs at home were wired for closed caption viewing. Her daughter, Kayleen, 11, read along as the words whizzed by on the screen. She still enjoyed her weekly comedy shows, movies or documentaries while every day words were reinforced on the screen. Angela Yamasaki, a marriage and family therapist, drove an hour each way to have Michael, 10, tutored by someone who related to him. Angela knows that a person's personality wins over the learning process every time.

Jane Laurance and Kathleen Wilson got smart on state law. Jane got her daughter into the school district's Special Education program while still remaining in the private sector. Kathleen read up on IEP's (Individual Education Plan)—a federal contract between the school and parents. Knowing her legal rights, Kathleen felt more in control.

In other families, the question of moving a child to a special school for dyslexia or doing home schooling becomes a daunting decision—not every child will benefit from either program. Ann Herbert and her husband were torn. He didn't want his son labeled as a special kid, in a special school for dyslexia. Ann knew what that meant. She's a former teacher. Plus her mother-in-law said there are "low-achieving" kids in the special school. Ann was confused. Wayne Rose took four months to make his final decision. Moving his daughter Terry, a third grader, out of her local elementary school and into a special school caused their family many sleepless nights.

There was also uneasiness in Timothy and Rose Oaks' decision to home school Dylan, a first grader. He needed his self-esteem rebuilt. But, friends, family members and his teacher thought otherwise. Lee Fine took to home schooling because she was tired of the nonsense in school. Josie, 10, hit a confidence crisis, didn't want to be picked on to read aloud in class, and didn't want to be taken out of class for Special Ed. Lee, a substitute teacher, enrolled her in the state-run Community Home Program.

Once a decision is made to move to a special school, there's a temporary sense of relief. Then the question, "who pays school fees?" pops up. Madison Morgan and husband, John, handled the financial add-ons themselves—$3,800 per annum. They didn't ask their parents for help and didn't ask the local school district to chip in. Rather, they adjusted their lifestyle accordingly by working harder and longer hours. Daniel Sawyer needed to come up with the extra money and that was a tough call. He and his wife, Kerry, worked on getting financial aid from the local school district. That seemed to be the only way.

From what parents say, Kindergarten through fifth grade is a time to get acclimated, familiarize themselves with, and adapt to, this different learning style, and read up on the law. Going out of the mainstream vs. staying in the mainstream is a key issue. It's also a time for basic skills—reading, writing, arithmetic—to be in place. Strategies to get these in place—a Special-Ed tutor, modified homework plan, technology—become important.

KINDERGARTEN THROUGH 5TH GRADE

KATHLEEN WILSON

Kathleen learned quickly about the IEP (Individual Education Plan), a federal contract between the school and parents. This happened in first grade in her daughter's local public elementary school. Stevie 8, is now a second grader.

The main people who hold the school together, just don't get it, they just don't understand. I battled constantly with the school system—the RSP (resource specialist,) the school psychologist and the principal. Her first-grade teacher was more empathetic. I tried to educate her on dyslexia and she was receptive.

The school psychologist was another story. After he'd administered a battery of tests on Stevie, he told the principal, the first-grade teacher and the RSP — at our first IEP—"I don't see that there's really anything wrong with Stevie. She's slow, gets frustrated when asked to read and needs several explanations during testing. But, she draws descriptive pictures, shows maturity beyond her years. She knows where she lives, her birth date, her mom's name, her dad's name. She even knows her grandmother's telephone number, with area code, in Florida." That impressed him. "Stevie is street-smart," he told everyone at the IEP meeting. I think he was doing ADD testing because Stevie drew picture after picture, with little reading or writing tasks.

For our first IEP, the RSP pre-wrote it. The school couldn't know everything about my child. I was furious. I had it null and voided. I'd done a lot of research and knew my legal rights. The IEP is a contract between parents and school attendants, not something pre-written by the RSP. I had it redone.

The re-draft stated that Stevie attend a Slingerland program (www.slingerland.org) once a week because the RSP—the one who'd pre-written the IEP—wasn't credentialed in teaching learning disabilities. The program lasted nine months—it was excellent—then the school revoked it. Stevie was shattered "Mommy, I don't understand, they took my program away from me, they took Ms. White away from me." Stevie lost nine months in her reading progress, through no fault of her own. At the end of first grade, she was reading at a 1.9 grade level. Six months into second grade, she was back reading at a 1.00 grade level.

I've only been through two IEPs, but I learned fast—I had to. I learned it's a business agreement, a contract, and in truth, I, as a parent, have more control of this contract than the school. I don't have to agree with what they put down, and I can add my modifications. Thank goodness I had this learning curve at an early stage, when Stevie was still in elementary school.

Let me share with you what I included in her recent IEP:

1 Any reading in the classroom related to class work is to be read to her. Stevie is not to read out loud in class.

2 Tests are to be untimed, at all times.

3 The weekly spelling test is to be modified—a reduced spelling list with less complex words

4 Work-shop Way—an 80-word reading sheet—is to be excluded from her program.

5 Use of her Alpha Smart in the classroom, use of a spell checker and computer-typed assignments are acceptable.

Her last IEP was done in Feb—quite late in the school year—and I check on it periodically, to see that all points are followed up in school. Oftentimes, one slips through the net. Here's an interesting one.

Stevie needed to read a lengthy paragraph, as part of a skit, in front of another class. It was a combined project. She thought she'd be able to memorize the words but there wasn't enough time. We had two days to do it, plus other homework assignments, spelling words, reading etc. I went in personally on the day of the skit and told the teacher, "No way, Stevie can't get up in front of the class, she's just not ready." Guess what? Stevie was asked to stand up (by the associate teacher) to perform. She panicked, started to cry and left the classroom. My daughter was standing right there when I told the teacher that morning, "Stevie can't read out in class today." It gets a little old when I've tried real hard to implement what's on the IEP.

On a lighter note, the modified weekly spelling test that I originated for her and 12 other students works wonders for her ego. She gets 100 percent every time, and stands tall. There are no complicated words and there isn't a long list of intimidating spelling words. For example: Billy went out and got the dog. Jane is in the car.

For the Work-shop Way, I suggested she learn those vocabulary words through the reading specialist teacher. The project became too overwhelming. It's a reading sheet comprised of four squares, 20 words per square, a total of 80 words. For example, in each square is a set of sentences "Let's go play baseball. Let's go pick apples." She was expected to do it overnight. That put her on overload. I also asked for math tests to be color-coded—highlighting pluses in yellow and minuses in red. I also asked that the tests be untimed. When there's a time restraint, Stevie panics. She takes in too much and just sees one big dot.

OK, so I'm an experienced IEP writer but last year it nearly ended up in a legal battle with the school. I threatened that if they didn't do the education properly, they would pay for private tutoring, a special school for dyslexia, or anything else Stevie was going to need. I also handed them the testing we'd done with a private clinical psychologist—that was done after the school psychologist said there was little wrong with our daughter—who stated that Stevie is a bright first grader, with a very high IQ, with dyslexia.

In all of this, my husband Ray is very supportive, and lets me handle the IEPs and the school conversations. I've been there, I struggled in school, I wanted to become a journalist. I, too, have dyslexia.

I know parents like me who rewrite the IEP, are an inconvenience to the school. (They all know me by name now.) But they don't know what a struggle it is, to us, as a family, to go through this bargaining process.

JANE LAURANCE

Jane has dyslexia, so does her daughter, Erika, 12. At Erika's private parochial school (K-5), the resource teacher was credentialed in speech pathology, not dyslexia. Jane started out on a fact-finding mission to get her daughter into the school district's Special Education program, while still remaining in the private sector. She does a great job.

Erika has classic dyslexia. She can't tell the time. She only reads books on tape. But her comprehension, in terms of world events, in terms of under-standing life issues, is very sophisticated—more like a 17-year-old. She is also a remarkable artist. Will she make it to college? Emphatically, absolutely, every day I tell myself that. And it will be a four-year school, at that. I'm a determined person, I am my daughter's advocate, and I usually don't take "NO" for an answer (unless there's a valid reason).

In nursery school, teachers noticed Erika was incredibly verbal, with excellent social skills. But, she didn't show the same interest, as the other kids when they were studying reading readiness. Her teacher did a simple developmental screening test in writing. Erika was able to write anything, but it all came out backwards, including her name! She also had a hard time with single-sound letters, as if they didn't exist. For example, with the word "cab" she couldn't hear the "a", and couldn't sound it out. For her intelligence level, and for what the teachers expected of her, she just wasn't there with reading readiness. It didn't set off any alarm bells in kindergarten, though. I didn't get Erika formally tested. I'd read a couple of articles that said not to do that, but to instead wait until first grade.

In first grade, we were blessed with her teacher, Sue, who had a second degree in Special Education. Sue guided us through this conundrum. Sue worked with Erika on reading and writing, and during that time, administered a number of tests, including Woodcott Johnson. Then we were ready to go to the school board and school district and request an IEP (Individual Education Plan). I soon learned that an IEP is federal law for the public sector, but how it's written up is done locally.

I was learning new stuff each day. It helped, a lot, that I'm a certified teacher, from New York, nonetheless. I researched the law of California—law is not my background and I don't have a degree in Special Ed, either. But I became the spokesperson. It took a little bit of *chutzpah*, and a lot of law, to get where I wanted to go. Everybody kept telling me, "You go to a private school, you're not going to get help from the public school district. What, are you crazy?" Forget it. I forged ahead. This had not been done before at the school. I was the front-runner.

What I found out in Sacramento is that our local school district is totally responsible for educating my daughter. I was getting misinformation most of the time from local sources. So many people didn't know the legal rights, including Erika's school. They didn't even know how the IEP system would work in a private parochial school. After several phone calls and weekends of research, I found out that Erika could have the same services offered to public school kids. I quickly learned the steps and the process to get these services, and set out on "my mission."

I called the school district. I met with the superintendent. I explained that I knew the school district gets a certain amount of money for Special Education and is obligated, by law, to provide education for ALL children in the state of California. I also explained that I knew they had 60 working school days to test my child.

I had copies of Erika's school file including recent testing, bound together in a professional file. I had a second copy for the superintendent. I also included a list, from Sue, of tests to be done next. I didn't want to reinvent the wheel. The superintendent was receptive to my proposal. Then again, I had it all laid out. I told her I expected to have a date within 60 days. Then I called her office once a week, on Friday, to remind her how much time was slipping by. I got an appointment within two weeks of the deadline.

The test results from the school district were concurrent with Sue's testing. Erika was ready for Special Ed. But, from my research, I knew the school district only had a certain amount of money and I questioned how much they would actually offer.

"We can offer Erika one day a week in a class with four or five other kids, for 40 minutes," was their initial suggestion. I was not buying into it. Erika was going into second grade and reading at preschool level—she knew about 20 words. Now I really had to know my rights. Before signing the IEP, I asked for maximum services, but I left room for a compromise. In the end, I settled on twice a week and 40 minutes one-on-one with a reading specialist. That felt right.

The only thing I couldn't get was transportation. The state had recently changed the law. My husband and I rearranged our schedules, with help from co-workers. We became the "official drivers."

Erika started second grade with a warm understanding teacher, Pam. She had 25 years' experience in Special Education. Immediately, they bonded. We lucked out. Once we got Pam on-board, she became our advocate, and when battles surfaced, she went in and, because of her, we won them. That is the honest truth.

There are other stories, each year. The best thing, though, that I've learned from these experiences is becoming my kid's advocate—and reading up on the law!

SUSAN SMITH

Tom and Susan have two children, Matt and Anna. Matt is an alumnus of Pomona College, (Claremont Colleges) CA. Anna recently graduated from the University of California at Davis. She received her bachelor's in American Studies, with a minor in Film Studies. Susan used outside testing as a guide in parenting her daughter.

The term "dyslexia" or "learning disabled" was thrown around once in a while at Anna's school. To me, it is a pejorative term that infers stupidity. We don't use those terms in our family and, because of our religious beliefs, we prefer not to name it. Instead, we work on the strengths of the individual. In our case, we worked on helping Anna shine in whatever she did. We encouraged her to be the best soccer player or the best violinist or the best water polo player. We respected her talent and expertise in both academics and extracurricular activities.

But Anna was reversing numbers and letters in 1st grade. She also had a difficult time reading out aloud and understanding what she was reading. The first step was to find outside help, a tutor. But before I could do that, I needed to know the areas to work on. Her initial testing was a practical-skills test. Anna broke the psychologist's own testing rules by scoring at grade level; it was on an untimed basis. That gave me the first clue I would have to become a strong advocate for extended time on tests.

Anna didn't go through the regular psycho-education testing because, in our religion, we feel the teacher and parent maintain the highest expectations if a standard hasn't been established. That way, no ceiling is placed on the student. As a former high-school teacher, I had a problem with teachers passing labels around from year to year. Once that label was established, it was very difficult to break. For both religious and practical reasons, I didn't want anything more than was necessary in her school files. I don't like to be labeled and I didn't want my daughter to be labeled.

I did, however, use the outside testing results to negotiate with teachers. I didn't want to impose on the school unnecessary work or put Anna into a slow track. We were willing to support Anna with tutoring so that school still would be a good experience. We focused on tutoring in reading, math and coping strategies.

ANGELA YAMASAKI

Michael, 12, is a 5th-grader at the local middle school. He has dyslexia. David, 9, his younger brother, has no learning problems. Paul is a psychiatrist and Angela is a marriage & family therapist. The family drives an hour each way to have Michael tutored by someone who relates to him.

Being a marriage & family therapist, I think the process for Michael isn't as important as the personal relationship with his tutor. We travel 35 miles, twice a week, to visit Anne, in San Jose, CA. We travel on a mountainous, windy road with hazardous conditions. But, she's had an impact on Michael's life.

Anne made a very special connection with our child. She's Chinese American, very quiet and very tuned in to learning disabilities. She understands both the learning and social implications of dyslexia. Michael was embarrassed to be going to a tutor. He felt only dumb kids went there. One time, I overheard him tell his best friend he had a tutor because his mom wasn't satisfied with him. Another time, he told his friend he was going to the orthodontist but he doesn't wear braces. He still insisted he was going to the orthodontist for X-ray work. Anne was instrumental in putting him straight. "I'm your teacher," she said. "You don't have to call me a tutor, teacher sounds better. Plus, you don't need to tell your friends you're visiting me. They probably don't tell you everywhere they go." Coming from her, it made sense.

It's been $2^1/2$ years since we started with Anne. Basically, the session is three hours—one hour to get there, one hour for tutoring and one hour to return home. Some nights, we get home at 9. This year, we're trying a new session that gets us home by 7 so we can have dinner as a family. And, his session is only once a week now.

At one time, because of all the driving, I thought Michael would want a local tutor. I interviewed several people but he refused to meet them. "No, I want to stay with Anne," he said. I knew then, the long hours of travel had been worthwhile.

How did all this come about with Anne? Midway through 3rd grade, Michael still wasn't motivated to read. He has a great memory and that's how he was compensating. But, he'd recognize the word "chapter" (in caps) at the top of the page and, when the same word appeared at the bottom of the page (in lower case), he'd tell me he'd never seen the word before. This happened especially with words like "through" and "thought," "grill" and "girl." My relationship with him wasn't good, especially when it came to homework. I became a task master. We finally decided to do something about it—to get him tested.

That's when Anne came onto the scene. After his testing, I needed to locate a Special-Ed tutor who had a working knowledge of dyslexia. More importantly, I knew the chemistry had to be right.

In the meantime, though, David was feeling left out. He didn't like that his brother was getting all the attention. He said, "I want to have a tutor, too." Last year, Michael's learning problems became a family issue. When the clinical psychologist needed to see Michael for testing, David wanted to come, too. Then, when he saw Michael went with mom to tutoring, he had to come to San Jose with us. I planned special activities with him—shopping, library visits, an occasional movie—so he was getting "quality" time with me. There's never a dull moment being a mom.

ZOEY ROY

Kayleen, 11, still is not reading at a 5th-grade level. Her brother, Bryan, 8, was reading fluently at 6¹/₂. Two years ago, the family stumbled on closed-caption viewing on their newly purchased TV. Kayleen instantly took to this form of reading. Now, when she watches "Home Improvement" and the Discovery Channel, she reads the words as they pass by on the screen.

Kayleen's self-image is more important to my husband and me than academics. The nuns at the Catholic school treat her like their own child. They love and nourish her and foster good self-esteem. If Kayleen's self-esteem isn't there, all the academics in the world won't work.

Fast-forward a few years, and Kayleen's interest in reading has quadrupled. We credit closed-caption TV.

We'll sit with Kayleen and watch a comedy show, a movie or a documentary. She finds it exciting to watch the words whiz by on the screen. Two years ago, she started doing this, and it looked like a good opportunity for her to improve her reading level. Now, our home TVs are wired for closed-caption viewing, for all programs, on all TV stations. I found that well-known TV brands include this option, but it's not on all models.

Recently, we bought a TV for Kayleen's room. It was one, of course, with a closed-caption option. Kayleen likes to read along as she watches the words on the screen. It helps her become more familiar with everyday words. If that's the only way she'll read, I'm all for it. I don't mind that the television is in her room.

One of Kayleen's favorite programs is "Home Improvement," followed by "Happy Days" on Nickelodeon. She watches them all with the hearing-impaired option on the remote control panel. She doesn't read out loud, but I notice her lips are moving. With some of the longer movies (Wizard of OZ, Chitty Chitty Bang Band, Annie, etc.), she's exhausted from reading the text.

H

KATHRYN MASON

Richard, who works for a computer company, encouraged Sarah, 12, to use software programs for reading and writing enhancement. Sarah has dyslexia. The Mason's second daughter, Rachel, 15, is an "A" student at the local public high school.

Now, Sarah is reading at grade level and is learning with help from the computer. These are a few of the programs she loves:

1   Interactive Movie Book by Sound Source Interactive Company (www.soundsourceinteractive.com). This is an interactive movie book series based on current screen versions—Black Beauty, the Secret Garden, Babe, Free Willy, and others. The software included text, movie clips, pictures, puzzles and 3D sound animation. We liked this program because it combines kid's love of stories with movie clips. At first, Sarah used the "read to me" button. I was pleased she could follow the reader by pointing to the words. Later on, she read the text to herself. At the end of each chapter, she did a puzzle that tested her on reading comprehension. She also used the bookmark feature that marked where she was in the story. The best feature, though, was the movie clips. They made the story come alive. I could hear her chatting to herself or giggling.

2   Storybook Weaver Deluxe by The Learning Company / Broderbund (www.learningco.com). It allowed Sarah to make up her own stories using their illustrations. She selected the pictures and backgrounds and then typed in the words. It definitely stimulated her writing. She was excited to click on the illustrations. It made writing more fun.

The keys did the work for her. Once she was confident with the program, she made a book titled "Two Sisters." Rachel helped her pull the project together, and we had it bound. There was a sense of accomplishment. Writing words in a lined notebook is boring to a kid who has difficulty processing words. With this, the program was colorful and creative. It did the trick.

3 Oregon Trail and Treasure Mountain by The Learning Company /Broderbund (www.learningco.com). We encouraged her to use these programs because we wanted her to have some "fun time" on the computer. They helped her become more competent with reading, math, and with following directions.

EVELYN RHYS

Evelyn struggles with moving Bennett, 10, to a special school for dyslexia. Her husband is opposed to the idea. He thinks Bennett's problems are about immaturity, not learning. School fees also are a factor. Bennett is a 4th-grader in the local public elementary school. His younger sister, Claire, is a kindergartner at the same San Francisco school.

Should Bennett go to a special school for dyslexia? I think about it two or three times a day. He already went there for a six-week enrichment program, the summer of 2nd and 3rd grades. I was expecting something magical to happen with his reading. It didn't. He had a really good time, learned cursive writing, but he was still two years behind in reading. So, at the moment, moving him doesn't seem like such a great idea, for a number of reasons:

1 There's no guarantee of improvement. We can't just assume he'll be able to read. One of my friends sent her child to this special school for several years and didn't notice a marked improvement. Her family made a big investment of money and time. I'm not convinced it's going to be worth it.

2 My husband isn't convinced. It'll take a really good argument for William to change his mind. He thinks Bennett's difficulties in school are related more to immaturity than to a learning disability. Maturing late is a family trait. Plus, he feels one-on-one tutoring is a better investment.

3 Involvement in our neighborhood setting would be lost. It's more

isolating going to a private school. This school is 15 miles from our home. If Bennett wanted to see his neighborhood friends, we'd have to set up a special "play date."

4   It would be financial overload. We're talking major money here, $10,000 a year. What about the return on that money? Actually, I don't know where we'd even get the money. We're already paying a Slingerland Special-Ed tutor twice a week to work on his reading. Going "private" really isn't an option at this point.

I sensed something wasn't quite right when Bennett was already in pre-school. His teacher suggested a young five program instead of kindergarten. We went along with that. Then, as a 1st-grader Bennett was not recognizing easy words. The school tested him for hearing and speech—no problems there—and for language processing. He wasn't tested for pre-reading skills. I didn't panic at this point because his teacher assured me he was so bright. She said his test scores were rather low but that could have been because he's a poor test taker. The school psychologist added that the test-taking conditions could have been better, too. I bought into all of this. They were the experts. I put it down to immaturity. What did I know?

But 12 months later, as an 8-year-old, Bennett still hadn't picked up on reading. He was reading at a beginning 1st-grade level. Finally, with support from his 1st-grade teacher, we got the school to test him again in the fall of 2nd grade. The scores indicated his IQ was above average, but his perfor-mance level in reading and spelling was well below grade average. At the November parent/teacher conference, I asked the Learning Specialist: "Are you saying he's got the big D?" There was noted silence. She then proceeded to talk about Bennett's test scores and how the school could help him. But I kept asking. Eventually, she told me: "We just can't use that word." The school psychologist, the principal wouldn't use the "D" word either. We concluded no one in the school district uses that word. That still baffles me.

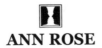

ANN ROSE

Dyslexia runs on both sides of the Rose family. Ann's husband, Wayne, is dyslexic. He is also a very successful public servant. And Ann's brother is severely dyslexic. Ann and Wayne's son, Bill, 13, is moderately dyslexic. He's in 7th grade at the local middle school. His sister, Terry, 10, is mildly dyslexic. She's a 5th-grader at a special school for dyslexia. She's been there two years.

I can talk about anything, but when I talk about my kids, the tears flow. They're so dear to my heart. The implications of moving Terry out of our local elementary school and into the special school caused our family many sleepless nights. This is Terry's story . . .

In kindergarten through 2nd grade, we got no strong indication Terry had a learning disability. We'd planned for her to go through the public school system. But at the beginning of 3rd grade, I began to see classic dyslexic symptoms. She had difficulty learning cursive, her spelling was unpredictable and her reading was slow. We decided to enroll her in the Saturday morning Scholar Program at the special school. Bill had been in this remedial program for 4th, 5th and 6th grades. Terry went for the whole 3rd-grade year. During that time, she took the admissions test for the school. The results indicated she was mildly dyslexic, with her weakest area being math.

Taking her out of her neighborhood setting was a big decision for us. Terry isn't severely dyslexic. But I saw the light early on. "Dad," on the other hand, took some convincing. It took us four months to decide. Wayne finally agreed when he saw Terry struggling with math homework. She didn't know what 6x3 was or 7x6 or 5x9. He remembered being there himself, in 3rd grade, and not knowing his multiplication tables. That following Sunday morning, in a conversation between Sunday School and church, we agreed to send her to the special school.

Let me share with you some of our concerns:

1   Kids from middle-class Texas, not kids from our local neighborhood, go to the special school. There are kids from wealthy families in the school. How would this affect sleepovers? How would Terry react to her friend's homes? One of our major concerns was that she'd be embarrassed to invite them to our modest three-bedroom house once she'd seen their homes. All these social issues never surfaced. Terry

has her own playroom attached to her bedroom and her school friends love to come here.

2 Opinions from parents and friends. When I told friends where Terry may be going for 4th grade, they asked why. Like I was crazy. Like our local elementary wasn't good enough for our family. The hardest sell was to my mom and dad. They couldn't understand our concerns, despite raising my severely dyslexic brother, Jim. They just couldn't understand. But when I looked at mom and said: "You don't want Terry to end up like Jim," the light bulb went on. Wow! It had taken weeks to get to that point. Now my parents have become great supporters of Terry and of the special school.

3 Bill's opinion – Bill would throw a fit if I suggested he go to a special school full-time. He thinks wearing a school uniform is a no-no. But he became extremely jealous when we talked about how Terry and I would carpool to school. (I work at the special school). He talked about the amount of time we would have together and how that was unfair. He also was envious of the organizational skills and time-management classes she would take. He voiced his grievances loud and clear. He treated Terry accordingly. Bill knew his sister would benefit from the math program at the special school. Still, knowing this when you're a teenager and accepting it are two different things. We resolved the problem by suggesting Bill come to summer school at the special school, specifically to take study skills and organizational classes. That hit the spot.

4 Terry's concerns – With a September birthday, Terry would be the youngest student at the special school, and by a greater margin than she'd been in the public school. A silly thing, but it bothered her a lot. But once she arrived at the special school, all her concerns disappeared. She wasn't different anymore. The truth was, most of the 4th-graders were more severely learning disabled than Terry was. Her self-esteem was high. She felt so smart. We all had worried unnecessarily.

5 Mainstreaming back into our local middle school. We knew before she started at the special school that mainstreaming back would be an issue. We didn't know exactly how it would impact our family. Now we're facing the transition. There are pros and cons. One advantage is that Terry will be in the same school as Bill. He'll be in 8th grade; she'll be in 6th. They'll get on the bus in the morning and come home together in the afternoon. I hope he'll look out for her during the day.

I have no concerns about her mixing with our neighborhood kids. She's a bright child and has a certain amount of "street smarts." She's also strong-willed. She'll handle it.

My main concern is her being labeled. It's so safe for her at the special school and not so safe out there. When I registered Terry at the middle school last week, the lady's eyes in the school office lit up. She said: "So, your daughter is a Special-Ed student." "Oh, no, she's not," I argued. "She's reading above grade level and she's already got a math tutor in place." The lady's eyes kind of dulled. She had been seeing dollar signs. Texas gives special funding for Special-Ed students. I really don't want that label on my child.

A further implication is that it's going to take a tremendous time commitment on all our parts. Instead of 30 minutes, we'll be back to three hours of homework. It's going to be hard at first to make the adjustment.

◾

LUCY DOGGETT

Oliver, 14, and Thomas, 12, have dyslexia. Their sister, Jane, 17, is an "A" student. Inefficiency—the length of time it took for "bureaucracy" to process information—prompted the Doggetts to opt for private schooling. Lucy did "charring" to help pay for school fees.

When he drew the car, he drew the windows next to it. His hand control was very poor and he didn't like being left-handed. Oliver didn't like being different. One of his nursery-school teachers who was trained in special needs suggested I carefully watch Oliver's progress in the next few years. He was only 3½ at the time, but she had an inkling his learning style was different.

Oliver disappeared into the woodwork at Infants School (5-7yrs). You're talking about 32 children in a class. Information wasn't being passed on. Oliver was on Book No. 6 before his teacher realized he couldn't really read. He was memorizing words. Oliver is a mischievous and highly intelligent child. He managed to come up with his own reading strategy in class. The teacher would ask him to spell or read a word. "I haven't got my glasses," he'd reply. "Do you wear glasses?" asked his teacher. "Sometimes," he replied. Actually, his vision was perfect.

The facade was over, though, just before his 8th birthday. I had him privately tested at the Dyslexia Institute in Staines, UK. The results indicated his reading age was 4 years, 8 months and his spelling was extremely poor. The psychologist suggested we get Oliver "Statemented,"—a legal contract between the local Education Authority and the Special-Needs student. But, the local Education Authority wouldn't accept the private testing. Instead, they got their own school psychologist to do an evaluation. They proceeded to tell me it would take a year before any help would be in place! "A year," I said. "What will become of him?"

Oliver now was in 2nd-year Primary in London. The dialogue with the local Education Authority went something like this: Once he was statemented, I could lose my choice as a parent as to which school he attended. More than likely, he would be sent to a local school with many Asian students where English was a second funded language. Just thinking about that school and the time it would take for the "Statement" to come through infuriated me. James was a sad little boy who was floundering more and more. The rest of the world was taking off and he wasn't. We had to make some radical changes. Fortunately, my husband and I were in total agreement.

We researched several schools in the London area. A special school for dyslexia in the city came out on top of this list because of its caring faculty and state-of-the-art computer equipment. But how were we going to pay for this? We knew we had the money to start him off because my husband's mother had left us some when she passed away a few years before. At that point, though, we didn't know we had a second son who had dyslexia. We thought it'd be a short-term stay for Oliver, but . . . he settled in so well. He stayed there four years and was elected Head Boy. I was getting a degree at the time, a bachelor's in linguistics at the University of Hertfordshire, but we needed the extra money for school fees for both boys. I went out charring (housecleaning) because I could push a vacuum around and it wasn't mentally taxing. Thank goodness for my clients. Their payments got us through some hefty school bills.

I was a bit worried at first about Oliver going to this private school. Relatives of Sir Winston Churchill and other upper-crust families were in class with kids from the local Council Housing. But even with such diverse socioeconomic backgrounds, there was a commonality among these kids. They all needed and wanted to learn to read and write. Oliver took to the school like a duck to water. Within six months, we saw drastic change in him. He grew about one-and-a-half inches. My doctor said it was because Oliver didn't have any stress. We were stunned. He was now a relaxed boy with renewed self-confidence. It was probably a blessing in disguise that our local school's bureaucracy took so long to implement its recommendations.

ANN HERBERT

Ann and William Herbert have four sons—Troy, 17; Peter, 14; Bryan, 9; and Austin, 7. Everyone but Peter has been diagnosed with dyslexia. Sending their first born to a special school for dyslexia caused concern. Then there were worries about the re-entry into a mainstream school.

William and I knew nothing about dyslexia. It was scary. William was in shock. His first born wasn't perfect. He also had some reservations about sending Troy to a school for dyslexia. He preferred to have him go to a place where they wouldn't label him as a special kid. As a former teacher, I knew LD students were labeled.

Everybody, it seemed gave us their opinion—invited and uninvited. My mother-in-law told us because it was a special school, there would be a lot of retarded kids there. Or, maybe, Troy would be mixing with kids unlike his neighborhood friends. She didn't know what she was talking about. If she and others had been more knowledgeable about the school and about dyslexia, we would have received more positive feedback. Instead, we got negativity all the way.

The fact that none of our friends knew about this special Dallas school also was disturbing. Our friends' kids were mainstream students in either the public or private sector. Everyone Troy grew up with was mainstreamed. William and I always had agreed the best gift to our kids was a good education. We looked to the private-school sector to service these needs. William was apprehensive about a move to a school for dyslexia, but, once he'd seen the campus and the students, he was fine. We both knew it was the right placement.

First, Troy started in the summer program. He stayed there through 8th grade. His headaches disappeared. Looking back, they definitely were stress-related. He couldn't complete a written assignment without getting a migraine. Thankfully, he hasn't had one since mid-6th grade. Plus, he blossomed in this new setting. That year, he announced he had to have a laptop computer. Our mouths fell to the floor. Now he can't live without it. He's come a long way since 4th grade.

The issue of mainstreaming to a high school surfaced in 8th grade. Fortunately, the school for dyslexia directed us where they thought Troy would best succeed. The principal offered three choices:

1 A parochial school (9th through 12th), with a program for incoming freshman with a learning disability.
2 A private, small college-preparatory school (9th through 12th)
3 Return to the school for dyslexia for 9th grade

Troy explored ideas 1 and 2 and decided on a parochial school. He told me he wanted to get lost in a crowd. He was getting ready for his college experience. I had some concerns about the move. I didn't want him to fail there when he could succeed in a remedial setting. He assured me he always could go back to the special school. That summer, he started at the parochial school. He got "A's" in most of his classes.

Thanks to that experience, I felt very calm in making the right school choices for Bryan and Austin. They are both at the school for dyslexia and will remain there as long as they need. When they're ready to move on, the school counselor will help us find a suitable place. I dread that day. I'm not addressing the situation this year. Bryan has another year to go. I feel confident, though, the school will give us good advice.

KERRY & DANIEL SAWYER

Daniel, Trent, 17, and Kyle, 14, all have been diagnosed with dyslexia. Both sons attend a special school for dyslexia. Kerry and Daniel had several nightmares about paying expensive school fees. But they made it.

{Daniel} The thought of having to come up with another $15,000 horrified us. And it wasn't even guaranteed Trent would get into the school for dyslexia. Trent was in 2nd grade when his tutor, an Orton-Gillingham specialist, told us about this exceptional school. We respected her opinion, but, in the meantime, school fees for Trent at a private developmental school with a flexible curriculum already were expensive at $8,000.

The developmental school was proving too difficult for him, so we asked friends and co-workers what they knew about parents' rights with a learning-different kid. A colleague of Kerry's recommended talking to a female attorney who specializes in Learning Disability issues. Her suggestion was, first, to get Trent accepted at the school for dyslexia. Then we could ask for funding from our local school district. Just our luck, Trent got accepted. We ended up using our retirement money to pay the school fees with the hope—and a lot of praying—the Boston School District would reimburse us. That was a major gamble on our part!

{Kerry} Meanwhile, I went on a major research campaign to find out what was offered in our local school system. It turns out Law 766 states that a child is entitled to the best education possible. I checked out all the different classes in our local elementary school. What I learned was the Special-Ed classes included students from a wide IQ range, varying from below average to above average. That was a surprise to us. Our attorney suggested we have Trent tested privately. The results indicated his IQ definitely was above average.

Our attorney was especially interested in the information about the wide IQ range within the Special-Ed classes. (The range was between 60 and 140 and Boston did its own testing.) Our attorney claimed the wide IQ range didn't provide a stimulating environment for Trent. She presented the evidence to the State Mediator. They had locked themselves in. No more was said about our son being part of a Special-Ed class. Instead, they wanted a full description of the special school. At the hearing, they suggested, "You pick where you want Trent to go. We'll pay his tuition fees." Daniel and I nearly fainted. It was difficult to control our emotions. Our risk-taking days were over—for a short time, anyway.

{Daniel} Right after we got the school fees reimbursed—we'd used up all our pension savings—the recession came. I was laid off work for 18 months. Kerry had to pay off her school loan. Kyle, meanwhile, was coming up with issues in 1st grade. He was skilled at hiding his learning disability and learned to compensate. But he started to tease children in class. He was letting out his pain on other children. We took him to a private licensed clinical psychologist who diagnosed him with dyslexia. Kyle's IQ was way above average (135) and the psychologist told us he was having a hard time with his self-image and his inability to perform at an above-average level. When I talked to Kyle about this, he actually felt relieved. He was so concerned Kerry and I wouldn't understand. I just said, "Kyle, you're having trouble in school. You're not happy there. Let's talk about it. No matter what, we'll make it together as a family. We're with you 100 percent. We'll find the right place for you, we will."

I knew then Kyle needed to go to the special school for dyslexia, but I didn't know how we were going to do it. With me being out of work, we were already stretched financially. That last year had been tough on the whole family. Then Kyle got accepted at the school. We were lucky again. But this time, we decided to refinance our mortgage because Kerry had just started a teaching job. Somehow, we scraped through again.

With more expenses on the way, once again we pulled in our savvy attorney.

This time, the school district assured us they now were fine-tuning their Special-Ed classes. There was no longer such diversity in academic ability. Our attorney wasn't totally convinced. They also knew we were seasoned parents. In the end, they asked what we would like for Kyle. Their suggestion was for us to settle out of court in a pre-trial hearing. "If you'll pay attorney fees ($1,500)," they said, "we'll pay his tuition and transportation, a total of $23,000." Wow! Life was looking good. Our gamble paid off yet a second time. I remember saying to Kerry, "No more kids, please. We won't make it a third time around with this school district."

A humorous side to this settlement was that the Boston School District wouldn't pay for Kyle's transportation until he officially started there in 3rd grade. Kyle already was in the special school for 2nd grade. So, for seven months, two vehicles followed one another to school and then came home the same way. Our boys went separately to the same school.

MADISON MORGAN

The Morgan boys are 16 months apart. Matthew, 11, is a 5th-grader and Patrick, 10, is a 4th-grader. Matthew has dyslexia and attends a special school. The costly fees are having an impact on the family.

The financial responsibilities are horrendous. The past two years, we haven't taken any extended vacations. Matthew's tuition comes first. Everything is secondary. Certainly, we didn't expect to pay $3,800 a year for a grade-school education. We also don't get any help from our families because that's the way we want it.

My husband is in the police force. The Residency Law only allows us to live in the city of Cleveland, so it narrows our options for schooling. Plus, the Special-Ed services in our school district are very poor. When it first came up that Matthew was a special-needs kid in kindergarten, the Board of Education suggested two schools, neither of which were city of Cleveland schools. In both cases, he would have been in the developmentally disabled handicapped classes. I wasn't prepared to have him bused across town or to be in a class with emotionally and physically disabled students. I didn't want to take the risk.

We took a bold step and moved him to a private school for dyslexia in suburban Cleveland. We get no financial aid from our school district because it's a private school. Matthew has been there since 1st grade. Now he's a 5th-grader and we've seen excellent improvement. My husband works part time as a carpenter and I work full time as an office manager/sales representative for a small company. Between us, we're able to make the school payments.

Fortunately, there is a united front in our marriage when it comes to Matthew's education. We usually talk about the issues together and then come to a decision. We both have the attitude that Matthew always will need more help with his work than Patrick. The best thing we can do for him is to place him in an environment conducive to his different learning style and to give him continuous support. He'll do the rest.

RUTH SMITH-BROWN

Ruth and Michael have four children—Emma, 25; twins Jane and Jason, 23; and James, 18. Jane and James are dyslexic and attended a boarding school for learning-different students. Fortunately, for the Smith-Brown family, Ruth's mother helped out with all the education bills.

Jason was the more difficult twin. He had academic ability but wasn't using it to his potential. He was lazy and an under-achiever.

Jane was just the opposite. She tried hard and persevered, but made no academic progress in the Special-Needs unit at the local state school. Actually, the teachers were too nice to her, almost patronizing. Academically, it was useless. Jane still couldn't read or write properly at the age of 10 and she couldn't tell time. Emotionally, they kept her self-image high, but that was all. The unit was made up of a small class of eight children with varying disabilities. One child was spastic, another diabetic and two hearing impaired. They all had labels. One mother actually phoned to ask if Jane was emotionally disturbed. I guess she needed a label. I hit the roof!

I nearly exploded a second time when Jane was approaching 11. I went to see the secondary school Special-Needs teacher to discuss how Jane would cope. "Don't worry," the teacher said, "someone will go into the classroom daily to read for her." I shot back, "I don't want anyone to help her anymore. I need her to read." What was this professional thinking? I was at the end of my rope.

That's when Lynn, my older sister, stepped in. She began doing her own research. She found a boarding school in Lichfield north of Birmingham, UK where students with dyslexia used the multi-sensory approach. The school had successful results with this method. Lynn immediately told my mom about her findings. There was no point in phoning me because she knew I couldn't afford it. The rest is history.

Jane learned to read and write fluently within two years. She was a boarder until she was 13 and then she and a school friend stayed mid-week with a family in Lichfield to attend classes. Jane came home on weekends to socialize with local friends and to be with our family. She did that for one more year while "Granny" agreed to continue paying for school fees and accommodations. Jane knew how lucky she was. In return, my mother saw that her granddaughter was developing into a confident and intelligent teenager. Her investment was paying off.

Turning to James, our youngest child, I had my suspicions about his dyslexia at an early age. He was fairly late in talking, riding a tricycle was a traumatic ordeal and doing puzzles only angered him. By the age of 9, he still was not reading fluently. I didn't want to wait any longer for remedial instruction. My mother, again, came to our rescue. She suggested he enroll in the Lichfield boarding school. We never looked back.

The school fees were hefty with both children at boarding school. Plus, Mom put Jason through university. I don't know how we would have managed without her help. Our kids owe a lot to their generous grandmother.

ANNE FRENCH

Anne is a nurse practitioner and her husband, Edward, a computer engineer. Edward, Andrew, 10, and James, 8, have been diagnosed with dyslexia. Anne got involved in a legal battle with the school district because she knew Law 766 in Massachusetts entitles every child to the best education possible. That was not happening for her boys. The school ended up paying private school fees for both children.

We rejected the IEP because we felt Andrew needed more help. Our suggestion was $1^{1}/2$ hours a day of multi-sensory language training in a small-group setting. The school's recommendation was $^{1}/2$ hour of speech therapy. The school came up with another solution. In September of Andrew's 1st-grade year, they proposed he be tutored for 1 hour and 15 minutes a day in the back of the classroom with another student who had muscular facial problems. They grouped both as LD students! This wasn't acceptable to us. Again, we rejected the IEP.

Nothing changed for Andrew that year. He continued to struggle. But we knew the next year had to be different. We found an inner-city Catholic school that had a special language-based 2nd grade class. There were 10 LD students and mainstream students working with one Special-Education teacher and one Wilson reading tutor. We were comfortable with our choice.

In the meantime, we took legal action against our school district because we were being forced to go private. Edward and I are strong proponents of public education and this was going against our beliefs. In a hearing with the State Education Officer, he proposed the region start a small language-based classroom. But that was rejected by a majority vote. They believed LD students must have total integration in a classroom (25 students), with some additional tutoring. What followed was very interesting. The State Mediator and the state-appointed lawyer said if the region wasn't willing to start up a more feasible program, they would need to provide an outside placement for Andrew. In retaliation, a spokesman for the school district said they'd already done so much for Andrew, they didn't think it necessary to offer anything more. I lost it. I threw my 6-inch pile of papers in the middle of the room and told them all where they could go. I left the room and they immediately called a recess.

When we returned, it was like night and day. They offered to fund a private placement for Andrew, to pay $18,000 for his tuition at a school for dyslexia (plus transportation costs; private elementary schools in our state usually range from $6,000-$12,000 a year). I was stunned at the speed of their decision. I can only credit this to the well-informed attorney we'd hired. He specializes in education/learning disability cases and was recommended by the Massachusetts Association for Learning Disabilities. Because he was firm yet confident, the State Mediator knew we would go to trial if they didn't come up with an appropriate proposal. They conceded. Our attorney fees were reimbursed, but they couldn't refund tuition fees ($2,000) at the parochial school. That was fine. It was more costly for them to set up a special language-based program for 6-8 kids than it was to buy private education for one kid, our kid. I've since learned this is happening in other parts of the country, too.

On Parents Day, the third week of school, I noticed samples of James' writing seemed immature compared to other 1st-graders. This is now our second son entering the learn-to-read-and-write zone. His teacher assured me all the children were being tested for reading ability in the coming weeks. I was impressed the school was setting up a special program to catch low-achieving readers. He told me we'd be informed if James fit the profile. Great, I thought. But we never heard any more.

James became increasingly unhappy, complaining of stomachaches and not wanting to go to school. In early December, I met with his 1st-grade teacher for a routine parent conference. A young woman started talking about James' progress. I stopped her and asked who she was. She said she was the Chapter 1 Reading & Special Math tutor who had been seeing James since late September. My blood pressure hit 200. I asked why we hadn't been informed. Everyone looked slightly embarrassed.

I asked if James needed a core evaluation—a battery of tests—for his IEP. They said their team would be discussing it. Upon leaving, I stopped at the principal's office to get a form to activate the testing. I learned the school district has 40 school days to conduct an evaluation, convene a team to make recommendations and implement a plan. I wanted action. James was evaluated in January. The school knew I meant business.

We were officially informed in March that James came within the profile of needing Reading Recovery. But they didn't place him in the program because preference was given to two other children who'd been in last year's kindergarten class. (James was at a parochial school for kindergarten). They said they took only two children from each 1st-grade class. I didn't buy it.

In the meantime, James' teacher continued to complain about James fooling around in class. He seemed to pick on James if homework wasn't done or if James' belongings weren't in their proper place. James became increasingly depressed and despondent. And we hadn't heard from the "team" about the core evaluation or what they planned for him in 2nd grade. Time was running out. James was distraught. We decided to put him back in the parochial school. He'd been in the K/1 combination class previously, so returning to the same teacher and about 1/2 the same kids provided a comfort zone for him.

The team eventually did present its report. And, somehow, the Reading Resource teacher suddenly had an opening for him. But we didn't take the school up on its offer. It was too late, James already had returned to the parochial school.

About the same time, we had an IEP meeting to plan James' remedial program for 2nd grade. The region had just hired a new Special-Education Director. During the first five minutes, he talked about his own difficulties as a non-reader in 4th grade. I had someone on our side. He then indicated he'd read all the reports on James and felt a placement in the private school for dyslexia was appropriate. And it would be funded by the region. Yes!!! The battle was over. I didn't have to recall all the incidents to him because his notes told it all. He knew it had taken three months before we learned the Chapter 1

Reading & Special Math tutor had been seeing James and that the principal said James wouldn't receive Reading Recovery because he didn't meet the profile. Yet, upon meeting with the Reading Recovery teacher, she said James had met the profile, but two other children already had been chosen. By the time the Reading Resource teacher had an opening for him, James' self-esteem was on the floor. In light of these mistakes, the wise and worldly Special-Education Director decided to avoid a lawsuit and provide an appropriate and rational solution to the problem.

Andrew started at the school for dyslexia in a 3rd-grade class of six children. He participated in a variety of activities—the Outward Bound program, arts, music, woodwork and computer design. It helped boost his self-esteem. Now he's through 4th grade and reading at grade level. His confidence is high. Andrew is a talented young boy and can build anything electronic. Yesterday, he had a lawnmower strung up in the basement. He'd picked it up at the recycle center and was dismantling the motor to use it on a future projects. He's taken apart a computer, calculator, toaster, anything with parts, including my HP business calculator worth $100. He also loves computer graphic design. Our house is always in a state of chaos with his collectibles. He's a very creative kid. And now that he can read, we're on the way to success.

James has been at the special school for one year and is in a class of five. It's early yet, but he still continues to struggle with his self-image. Academically, he seems to be doing well. He catches on quickly and is moving along well in language-based skills. He loves sports and gets lot of positive acknowledgment for his great throwing arm (he may even be a future quarterback). Recently, though, he turned rebellious. He spray-painted a third eye on his face.

I'm blessed my boys have been given an opportunity to maximize their education potential. It took a lot of perseverance on our part. But it's been worth every drop of sweat and every sleepless night. Remember, Law 766 (www.masspac.org) states that a child is entitled to the best education possible. If your public school can't offer this, be prepared to battle. It's worth it.

ROSE & TIMOTHY OAKS

Rose and Timothy have three boys. The youngest, Dylan, 10, has dyslexia. Dylan's brother, Jordan, 14, is a freshman in high school. Marcus is 12. Both parents are San Francisco accountants. Two coping strategies that worked well for their son were home schooling (to rebuild his self-confidence) and the Lindamood-Bell Learning Program (to get him to read fluently).

{Rose} Thank goodness, at last, someone is listening to me. Dylan was diagnosed with dyslexia at the Lindamood-Bell Learning Processes in Berkeley, CA when he was in 3rd grade. For two years at the Montessori School (K-1), teachers and teachers' aids kept brushing it off with me. "He's in the realm of normal for reading," they insisted. An education specialist tested Dylan at the end of 1st grade. "Cool it a bit with Dylan," she said. "He's ready to do it. He's got all the talent. Just be patient."

But Timothy and I knew Dylan had a reading problem. Dylan did heavy-duty phonics in kindergarten. In 1st grade, he knew all the sounds and was able to put them together. But by the end of the year, we didn't see much progress in his fluency. He memorized words. Often times, he recognized the word "the" or "they," but he couldn't remember it on the next page. It was puzzling. I wanted him to read out loud. Dylan didn't want to do that. He felt threatened. Definitely, there was a problem.

{Timothy} Conceptually, Dylan can read. He's a bright kid. I assumed this nonfluency was brought on by stress in the classroom because he would stutter and stammer. Dylan had so little self-esteem. He was taken out of class to work with the poorest readers. He often missed story time, science projects and other presentations. He was very uncomfortable in the classroom and, yet, very, very comfortable outside the classroom. We knew there was a problem, but we didn't know what it was. That's when we took him out of school and home schooled him for 2nd and 3rd grades.

{Rose} Dylan needed those two years out to rebuild his self-esteem. It was the best thing we did for him. He blossomed. We just followed what he wanted to learn. He's very bright, very mechanical and loves putting things together and doing science projects. We did fractions with him. He loved it. I also did a lot of reading with him. But he kept telling me, "Mom, I hate to read." I didn't understand because I'd patterned my reading methods after the programs used by my two older sons, Jordan and Marcus. Within a few months of home schooling, though, I decided to bring in an education specialist to assist with reading. Nothing came of it. No real improvement. I just knew there was something wrong. As parents, we still were very perplexed.

After two years of home schooling, I felt it was time for Dylan to mainstream. His self-esteem was high, but he also needed social interaction with his peers. I went into our local elementary school and told the principal Dylan was technically a 4th-grader, but he should put him in 3rd grade. They mumbled something about him having 2nd-grade skill levels. "No way," I said. "Socially, he's a 3rd or 4th-grader." It was agreed. Dylan repeated 3rd grade. It was the right decision at the time.

{Timothy} Undoubtedly, the turning point came when Dylan attended the Lindamood-Bell Learning Processes in Berkeley at the beginning of 3rd grade. I drove the 50-mile commute with him. We went every day for six weeks, three to four hours a day, after school. He was learning how to read fluently. In the car, I would remind him: "By your birthday, they tell me, in six weeks, you'll be reading. That's the goal. It's a lot of hard work. Then we're done with it." That worked for Dylan. I also added an incentive for the hard work. There was a prize for him, a remote-control car. He celebrated his 9th birthday. He loved his new toy. He was reading!

Not every child can achieve amazing results in just six weeks. For Dylan, though, it worked. The timing was right and the place was right. The Lindamood-Bell program (http://www.lblp.com) develops phonemic awareness. Dylan learned to visually recognize the different sounds produced from the formation of his lips, and then to connect them with an auditory sound. It helped with decoding.

{Rose} Dylan now is a 4th-grader. Socially, he's very popular and he loves school. With his added confidence in reading, he's the class advisor on reading problems. He tutors a small group. He feels important and tells his classmates how he managed to do it. Somehow, he's turned his disability into a positive. It must be his charisma and style.

Rose & Timothy suggest:
❏ You need to be your child's advocate. It's your mission as a parent to do this. It comes with the territory. Don't rely on anyone else.

LEE FINE

Three members of the Fine family have dyslexia – Michael (father), Elsie, 22, and Josie, 10. Elsie was home schooled for four years. Now Josie is in her second year of the program. Lee talked about this alternative schooling as a permanent schedule rather than a "quick fix."

I'm tired of the nonsense, so we decided on home schooling. Josie was scared to go to school some days for fear she would be picked on to read out loud in class. And she didn't want to be taken out of class for Special Ed. We had a confidence crisis on our hands. She was in 4th grade.

Now, Josie is in the Community Home Program run by the state of California. The curriculum is the same as she would get in school. As a substitute teacher, I know what her peers are learning. I also try to stay abreast of what is being offered in Special Education. I know Josie finishes her textbook. That doesn't always happen in school. Her program requires a lot of discipline. Every month, she turns in her work samples for the previous month. Every three months, she brings in all her completed work. We recently found out her teacher had trouble reading in 4th grade because she has dyslexia! Josie now has found a good listener.

I already have experience with home schooling. My oldest daughter, Elsie, was home schooled in 7th and 8th grades. I just made up my own curriculum (it's legal to do that). Initially, I tried to go through the school system, but they really weren't helpful. In the end, I had to go through the state. When I finally took her out of school because her self-esteem was suffering, the school hassled me. They pleaded with me to let her stay.

Admittedly, it takes a tremendous amount of communication and patience to home school my children. But I'm very close to my girls—I'm their mother, their teacher and a role model. They thought it was good to do this. I didn't force them at all. But I did tell them if they couldn't hack it (be disciplined with their assignments), they'd go right back to the local public school. Periodically, I ask Josie what she thinks of home schooling because I need to keep track of her progress. Her program doesn't have a set schedule, but by the end of each week, she must have finished a set amount of work. Planning and time management come into play a lot.

Of course, the downside to home schooling is the absence of social integration with kids of similar age. But being part of a religious group, we already had an established social group. Interestingly, our religion doesn't advocate home schooling at all. Fortunately, though, our church activities take up a lot of our time. We have five meetings a week where Josie interacts with other young people. She's also encouraged to help within the community, especially with the elderly members. So, at this point, her social life is pretty full.

Home schooling simply became a way of life for Elsie, too. In 9th and 10th grades, she was enrolled in a Chicago correspondence school. Her goal was to get her high-school diploma, but she quit at the end of 10th grade. She isn't self-motivated when it comes to schoolwork. The interesting part is, when she heard Bill Cosby's son had dyslexia, she was inspired to return to the program. I suggested she write to the American School and ask if she could continue. She's now in the program after an absence of five years. She needs a high-school diploma if she wants to get into computer school. Meanwhile, for the past five years, she's been running her own successful housecleaning business, earning $25,000 working part-time. She's no fool. Her desire now, though, is to become a graphic designer.

Home schooling can only work where the idea isn't just coming from the parents. The child has to want it, too. There also needs to be a strong social scene in place. Both are critical for the program to be a success.

6TH THROUGH 8TH GRADE: STRATEGIES

Homework is a huge issue. Ann Rose said "same time, same place" was the only method that worked for her family. Bill, 13, and Terry, 10, walked through the front door, ate a healthy snack and then headed to their desks around 4:30 p.m. When homework was done, there was still time for outside interests - Boy Scouts, basketball practice, choir etc. For Mara Manning's son, David 13, using headphones made homework more enjoyable, more relaxing and helped with his concentration. David selected his favorite CD, got situated on the computer, and sang along as he did his assignments.

Jeannie Smart-Chiste targeted the amount of homework for her son, TD. In his IEPS, she stipulated that his teachers graded only what he completed of his homework. For instance, of the 10 math questions (normally 15) what percentage was correct? His teachers agreed it was a sensible way to test TD's knowledge. They were looking for content. And, Rod and Louise Ferrari joined an organization that offered a pool of Special-Ed tutors for help with homework.

Gayle Curtis and Sadie Sheehan worked on other strategies. Gayle introduced a report-card incentive plan for, Mitch, 14, and Lynn, 13. The bonus system for effort/achievement was $10 (superior), $2 (satisfactory) and $0 (needs improvement). The sales promotion program was $50 bonus (straight "As" on a single report card) and $50 (superior effort/achievement in all classes). In this way, Mitch, who has dyslexia, came out a winner, too.

On a different note, Sadie worked on the "burnout" phenomenon with her son, Kevin, 14. It always happened in November and April. Kevin got sick, missed a week of school and used that time to recharge his brain. After a week, he was so fresh that catch-up work wasn't a problem. Sadie understood her son's dilemma, understood his different learning style, and worked with him.

Here, in middle school, families become more creative. A lot has to do with survival. A lot has to do with multiple teachers instructing in multiple subjects. Parents push the envelope, coming up with original strategies. If they don't, no one else will.

6TH THROUGH 8TH GRADE

H

SADIE SHEEHAN

Sadie and James have two sons. Their oldest, Sean, is gifted. Their youngest, Kevin, has dyslexia. Sadie has developed some family coping strategies through the schooling years.

I knew Kevin was different. "Kevin, you finish the story about Joe, the tractor, in the vacant lot," I suggested. And Kevin proceeded to tell the story about the "bacent" lot. He'd heard that story a hundred times from his dad. He couldn't say "banana" either. There were definitely problems with his hearing. When he was in kindergarten, Kevin told me, "Mummy, there's something wrong with my brain. I can't learn. I can't say the sounds like other kids in my class." Finally, in 2nd grade, he was lying on the top bunk of his bed, banging his head on the wall. "Mummy, there's definitely something wrong with my brain." I had to do something.

We got Kevin tested. The private licensed clinical psychologist suggested he go to a special school for dyslexia, new territory for us. Sean, our first born, is gifted! This is how we coped:

1 We listened to our child. When we suggested he go to the school for dyslexia, Kevin absolutely panicked. He refused to leave his school. He was only a 2nd-grader, but he knew he had made up his mind. He was frantic about the thought of moving. We were desperate to make the right decision. We decided on somewhere in between.

   Judy, a teacher at the school for dyslexia, became Kevin's tutor. We all agreed it'd be for one hour before school started. No one at Kevin's regular school would know. It would be his secret; even his close friends wouldn't know. For four years, four days a week, James and Kevin got up at 6 a.m. It was a special time for father and son. They made breakfast together or ate out at the local coffee shop. They chatted on the way to school. This worked so well for Kevin in 3rd through 6th grades. Judy was Slingerland trained and used the multi-sensory approach. To this day, she still follows Kevin's life, always asking how he's doing at Boston College. Judy wasn't only his tutor, she became his mentor.

2 We paid attention to Kevin's highs and lows. In November and April, he'd get sick. He'd miss a week of school. "Are you aware you do this, twice a year, always in November and April?" I asked Kevin. He thought for a moment. "I guess you're right." He said. "My brain is so tired, so tired." I knew he was burned out. As a student with dyslexia, he was concentrating extra-long hours, listening attentively, writing papers and navigating tricky hormones. He told me, "I get so tired. I can't learn any more. I need to take a week off for my brain to get refreshed." I asked him about making up the lost work. "My brain is so fresh afterwards," he said, "nothing is a problem." This child, he understands himself so well.

3 We encouraged Kevin to sail. He doesn't do so well in team sports. He can't always remember instructions. Making a left or right turn sometimes is confusing. Sailing is an independent sport. It works for Kevin, it helps him make good decisions. I noticed he developed good spatial understanding as a result of this sport. In middle and high school, he sailed almost every day with his partner. It cleared his mind. Then he was ready for homework. Fortunately, the principal at Kevin's college preparatory school allowed sailing as his designated sport.

GAYLE CURTIS

Gayle's son, Mitch, 14, is an 8th-grader in the local middle school in Cleveland, OH. His younger sister, Lynn, 13, is in 7th grade at the same school and is an honors student. Gayle says being in a good school district with an effective Resource Center makes her feel she's getting the best education for her son. Her personal school experiences as a dyslexic student also help her understand Mitch's frustrations. She and her husband, Dan, came up with an incentive plan for report cards that helps Mitch break down goals into small increments.

There are three fundamental strategies that have worked well for our family:

1 Being in a good school district with adequate funding for a Resource Center and a Resource Specialist, worked for us. Our local middle school has an excellent resource program. Mitch takes advantage of it. He takes extended time on tests and has a note taker and an editor. He has two team teachers and had a 1-on-1 tutor in elementary school. Our school district allocates $12,000 per year, per child. It's

amazing. Teachers are paid well and there's still enough money left for resource teachers. That's why we chose to live in this area of Cleveland.

In addition to adequate funding, the teachers in our district seem to understand not only children with dyslexia, but all kinds of children. There are gifted kids in the school, deaf children with their own sign-language interpreter, students with a learning disability and children from Asia and South America using an interpreter. The school's policy is to mainstream all students and add resource help where needed.

I've a lot of faith in our local school system and leave it up to the teachers to do their job. They're on target with our kids. They're on the phone if there's a problem. They keep me posted. Mitch is a B/B+ student and Lynn is an honors student. I'm an alumna of the school and it's amazing to see how many alumni also send their kids to this public school. It's a credit to our district.

2 Using my own school experiences as a dyslexic student helped to guide Mitch through K-12 and to understand his frustrations. As a child, I was the "dummy" in my family. Pretty, but thick. My two older brothers were very bright. I had a hard time in school. I understand Mitch's frustrations. I tell him about my school experiences and tell him not to be like I was. I got a good basic education, but that was all. I had to learn on my own a lot of the time. Way back in the late 60s, school for a dyslexic student was very different. Teachers thought I was lazy or "thick," or just not interested. A lot has changed.

Mitch is getting so much more out of his education. He's being taught good study habits and research skills, and he gets special accommodations where necessary. He takes school seriously and knows a college degree is important.

Mitch has an incredible memory and a very high IQ. But if I ask him to write or spell, he's lost. I've taught him to be independent in other areas. He has a laptop computer with a built-in spell checker. He uses that all the time, even in the library, to look up words for research projects. And when he decided he needed more allowance money, I told him he had to find his own job. He did just that. He got hired at McDonald's as a cash register attendant. I always tell him: "You can do it for yourself and, if you need a net, we'll always be there."

I also tell him good organizational skills will help tremendously in school, especially next year when he's in high school. I hired a tutor to teach him time-management skills. There's been an amazing difference in his ability to organize his schoolwork. And he still makes time for varsity tennis and soccer, his job and his social life.

3 Implementing an incentive plan for report cards worked well. Before we even suggested such a plan to our kids, we told them: "you must try to be the best human being you can be, that includes being kind to others; you have one job in your life right now. School work and report cards are your job."

Both kids get a minimal weekly allowance, mainly for lunch money. Lynn baby-sits and Mitch works at McDonald's. The incentive program is to add a few bucks to their bank accounts. It goes like this: A= $10.00; B= $5.00; C= No money; and D= Lose all the money earned from that report card.

You're probably wondering how this works for Mitch, as an LD student. (He usually gets "B's" with an occasional "A.") There's no reason he'll get a "D" unless he does no work in that class. That's a no-no in our family. If he does all his homework, he should get a "C." If he works harder, he can get a "B." And, in reality, Mitch strives for "A's."

We've also included a bonus system for effort/achievement/conduct. This works well for Mitch. He usually picks up extra dollars in this category. It goes like this: superior =$10; satisfactory =$2; needs improvement =$0.

Finally, we have a sales promotion program. If you get straight "A's," there's a $50 bonus. If Mitch gets all "superior" he gets $50.

Although Lynn is an honors student, she also needs incentives. She needs a little motivation. We think our incentive program is working well for both kids, in different ways. They average $50-$60 a report card.

ROD & LOUISE FERRARI

Paul, 23, and Melissa, 16, have dyslexia. They did not officialize their learning disability in their London, UK school. Rather, Rod and Louise hired outside Special-Needs tutors to supplement their learning. This was a key factor in their children's success.

{Rod} We took a round-about approach to our kids' different learning style. We decided not to go head-first into the bureaucracy. The "Statement"—a contract between school and parents—isn't quite worth the paper it's written on. There's usually a hassle. Besides, dyslexia doesn't get much recognition in the state schools now. It's still actually a taboo word. The new term is Special-Needs.

Still, we had open communication with teachers every year. On the whole, they were understanding and compassionate. Occasionally, though, a "dud" surfaced. We also were actively involved in PTA activities. Paul and Melissa have good personal skills, too, that helped them later on in secondary school. Looking back, this system worked well for our family.

{Louise} The essential link was we were able to hire private tutors through SPELD (Specific Learning Difficulties). This volunteer organization offered a pool of Special-Ed tutors. Actually, by pure luck, I saw an announcement in our local paper about a general meeting at Harrow Town Hall to start a branch of SPELD. This was way back in the early '80s. It was just what I needed. Paul was having trouble reading. I was searching for a support system out of school. I found one.

I became a founding member of SPELD. The aim of the association is to educate the public on dyslexia and to offer a pool of trained Special-Needs tutors. We meet once a month. We've developed into a "large" family over the years and have become an excellent support group for new families.

Fortunately, one of the original founding members, Mary, became Paul's tutor. Every week for an hour, she worked with him. The chemistry was right, thankfully, and Paul progressed in reading. Melissa also had success with her tutors. She would go into a session in an OK mood and come out in a great mood. Intuitively, I looked for tutors with a sense of humor and an ability to relate to the kids. Personality and age were important issues, too. In the end, though, I let the kids make the final decision.

I don't think we would have gone the tutor route if we hadn't found SPELD. I'm dyslexic, and I know how important it is to relate to a person who understands different learning styles. When it came to my children, I didn't find it helpful to give them advice on schoolwork. I'm only their mother. But, coming from a Special-Needs tutor, Ah! that was different.

CLAIRE NIELSON

Natalie is the second youngest in a family of five children and the only one with dyslexia. Claire attributes her daughter's balanced self-esteem to a strong support system: family, church and the theater.

I'd be standing at the kitchen sink doing dishes and, at the same time, quizzing Natalie on her spelling. I had the current spelling list with me at all times. I'd test her in the car, at the breakfast table, wherever. The computer was good for analytical thinking but the spell checker only went so far. To use it properly, Natalie needed to know how to spell, period. That was the problem. For me, it was a matter of pride when she misspelled words. Quietly, I hoped as long as she watched me do the correct spelling, somehow some memorization would kick in. No such luck. Drilling her on spelling was the only way to go.

I definitely spent more homework time with her than with Julie, Shauna, Allen and Thomas—my other four children. I read a lot to Natalie because it saved valuable studying time. I would read the history chapter and then make up a verbal test. I also read the assigned English literature books and we'd review them together. I showed her how to study a chapter in the biology textbook to prepare for a test the next day. I invested a lot of time and energy into this child.

Natalie definitely has an abundance of energy and comes across as a confident person. Much of this can be attributed to her strong support system:

1 Family – Fortunately, we have a solid family. Glenn and I are happily married. At holidays, we always have friends and family to celebrate with us. With seven in the family, there was always someone to chat with. We supported each other in times of triumph and letdown. Middle school was a tough time for Natalie. The whole family heard about it. And we pulled together as a team.

2 Church – We attended church regularly. Julie, Shauna and Natalie all

sang in the church choir. I lead the church choir. Natalie also performed in our church singing group and locally for various volunteer groups. There always was something happening in the youth club. Natalie definitely got positive reinforcement from our church. It was a world away from her school. They didn't give spelling tests. There was no academic measuring stick at church. Natalie blossomed in this environment. I have to say prayer also helped.

3 Theater – I encouraged Natalie to develop theatrical talents. It was a wonderful expression of her creativity in music and drama. She was part of the local children's theater group and usually played the star roles. Again, Natalie shone out of her school setting.

Will she outgrow dyslexia? I don't think so. But Natalie will learn to cope with it. She no longer thinks she's dyslexic. Yet, when she's driving, she still puts up her fingers if someone tells her to make a left or right turn (she's just making sure). Natalie graduated from Brigham Young University with a bachelor's in Early Childhood Education. She works for the California School for the Deaf using her American Sign Language skills on a daily basis. She still has an abundance of energy and is brimming with confidence.

ANN ROSE

Ann lives with three dyslexic family members–her husband, Wayne, her son Bill, 13, and her daughter, Terry, 10. Bill is a 7th-grader at the local middle school and Terry is a 5th-grader at a special school for dyslexia in Dallas. Homework is an important part of the family's daily routine.

Living in a family with three dyslexic members, everything is in a constant state of upheaval. I have to have a time and a place for everything.

As soon as Terry and Bill walk in the front door from school, they have a healthy snack and then go to a specified place to do their homework. It's usually their desk in their room. But it's the same time and same place every day. It's up to me to enforce this.

It has to be the same routine every day or else Bill will forget to do his homework. Knowing what he has to do when he walks through the door, he seems to get a second wind. Homework has to be done first because he has a music lesson and Boy Scouts on three school nights. If he doesn't have homework, he still has to do some studying.

For Terry, it's always the same time and the same place, too, but with a slight modification. I don't make an issue about the untidiness of her desk. She actually performs better if it isn't a perfectly clear desktop. I've witnessed her do homework with "stuff" piled two inches high. Right now, there are more important issues to worry about.

The strategy that works best for Terry is me just being there when she does her homework. Only for math, though. It gives her self-assurance. Terry does all her other homework at day-care or in a study hall. Math is the single most frustrating subject for her (and for me). I ask her what 7x2 equals. She won't know. I've tried getting sticks and letting her hold them in her hand. I've tried total voice moderation. She works it out in her own way. I've learned to just be there for her.

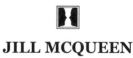

JILL MCQUEEN

Jill knows when Simon, 12, is about to "hit the wall" with homework. She is prepared to do a 180-degree turn and offer a new learning approach. Simon is dyslexic and in his first year at the local secondary school.

They are the most fundamental principles that trip Simon up. I call it the 2-plus-2-equals-22 syndrome. No amount of explaining can help Simon once he's got the wrong idea in his head. This usually happens once or twice a month with homework. He'll persist and only get himself deeper into the problem. Then he'll get more and more frustrated, yet more and more determined to solve the dilemma. Most adults would take a break or consult a knowledgeable source. Most children would give up or follow the adult route. Not Simon. He has to persevere for hours. In the end, he's exasperated and emotionally drained. Any parent of a child with dyslexia will tell you if he/she hits "the wall" at homework time, it's really useless continuing until a different method of learning is adopted.

One particular school night, Simon had to learn the names of 12 different shapes and how to spell them. Memorizing the more complex shapes (hexagon, rectangle, cuboid, spheroid) was confusing to him. "How many sides does each one have?" he kept asking. Tears came and he couldn't go any further. I quickly had to come up with an alternate approach. We ended up making the shapes out of paper and tracing the words. It turned out to be a fun project and, eventually, he identified the shapes and spelled them correctly. But he stayed up way beyond his bedtime and wasn't able to complete the mounds of other homework.

Another time, he got uptight with his French homework. He was spending every waking moment counting in French. Counting to a hundred was no problem. It was getting the numbers to come out automatically that was the stumbling block. I read the numbers to him and he responded in French. But he was exhausted from the whole process and became obsessed with learning them. I asked him to slow down. "No, I must do it," he responded. But the final crunch came when he spent from 4:30-9:30 p.m. doing his French homework. He still hadn't done all his other homework. Then at the breakfast table, he wanted to go over more French phrases. I decided at that point it was time to contact the school.

Simon's French teacher came to our rescue. He recorded an audiotape for him that included numbers, classroom commands and classroom work. I no longer had to read to him in French. He now walks around the house with his Walkman on and seems to like this independent work. He's even making progress. I've learned over the years with Simon that a "change of guard" is the only strategy that works when he hits "the wall."

JEANNIE SMART-CHISTE

Jeannie and Tony Smart-Chiste have one child, TD, who is dyslexic. When he was tested for a learning disability, TD's IQ made him eligible for the Gifted and Talented Enrichment class. TD, 14, is an 8th-grader in the local public high school.

We've stipulated in his IEP that his teachers grade only what he completes of his homework. For example, if he does seven out of 15 math problems, what percentage of the seven are correct? In this way, he isn't required to finish everything. Some of his teachers have a hard time accepting this. He got a "D" in his GATE class the second grading period in 6th grade because the teacher wouldn't modify homework assignments. By the end of the year, thanks to the encouragement from school administration, the teacher finally conceded. He got a "B" in the class, with a comment that he'd "made a lot of progress." He really hadn't. She had, grudgingly, allowed the accommodations.

None of his teachers gave him a reduced homework load without our request. Several of them, though, agreed this was a sensible way to test his knowledge —they were looking for quality in his work, not quantity. But he did receive a "D" this year in 8th grade algebra because his teacher had "forgotten" about his homework modifications.

We haven't implemented any reward system for getting homework done on time. Our problem is that he won't stop working on his homework. Eventually, he starts working in circles and has to be forced to stop. Even in 1st grade, before he was diagnosed with dyslexia and before we learned any coping strategies, TD took forever to complete his homework. I'd sit with him, but he'd ignore whatever suggestion I'd make. Eventually, it led to an argument. Finally, I told him, "Just don't do it. Tell the teacher I wouldn't let you." He would cry.

Homework time has changed radically since those early elementary years. Now we work together as a team. His reading comprehension has never been a problem, but his editing is questionable. His typing still is slow. So, on long essays, I ask him to dictate and I type it on the computer. He shuffles the paragraphs or sentences around. His thoughts aren't organized when he touch types. And if he just dictates long reports without seeing the printout, the essay winds up pretty jumbled. This system works for him now, but as he matures, I'm sure he'll want to type up his own work in preparation for college papers.

For TD, the best way to do homework is pretty much same time, same place. He likes to spread everything out on the floor in his bedroom. If he isn't using a computer, you won't find him at a desk or a table. Somehow, he inherited my preference for the carpeted floor!

MARA MANNING

David, 13, Brendan, 10, and Wesley, 8, are brothers. David has been at a school for dyslexia for 5th, 6th and 7th grades. He listens to music while he does homework. He used the CD on his computer to play Pavarotti or music from Titanic. It helps him relax and concentrate.

In summer school of 4th grade, David signed his name and forgot a letter. He just exploded. The young camp counselor calmly suggested, "Let's do the card again. No big deal." David made the exact same mistake again. Thankfully, the counselor put his arm around him and asked if he wanted to go dunk baskets or shoot goals. I got in the car and burst into tears. I had wrestled for so long with the idea David was different. It was just denial on my part. He was my first born. David finally was tested in 5th grade. No one used the word "dyslexia" in his public elementary school. At that stage, he was ready to enter an effective remedial reading program. He told me, "if the tests show I have so many problems, I'll go to the special school for dyslexia." He was wonderfully open about it.

I thought of headphones while I was working out on the treadmill. Why couldn't David use them when he was doing homework? It would block out a lot of the noise and probably allow him to concentrate better. David has an auditory processing problem and is slow when it comes to writing. He started out by putting in tapes of Liza Minelli, Elton John or Pavarotti. I didn't care what he listened to as long as it helped him relax.

Using headphones makes homework more enjoyable for David. His concentration is still strong, even with music in the background. It's interesting he doesn't use the headphones at any other time, only when he does chores—emptying the dishwasher, tidying his bedroom, talking out the garbage and homework.

Virtually all his homework is done on the computer. He learned to touch type at the special school and seems to like the speed of the computer. He uses a pencil very slowly and his handwriting isn't that legible. When he's on the computer, he uses the CD for music. Recently, he's started singing as he touch types. Just before homework time, he takes a few minutes to select his favorite CD.

Interestingly, though, David's talent lies in art, not music. That's why the headphones have intrigued us. David works on the Warhammer 40,000 futuristic 30mm models made of lead. He primes them, paints them and then applies very detailed brush work to achieve skin tones, beards, mustaches and pigmentation. So much energy and concentration go into his art work.

9TH THROUGH 12TH GRADE: STRATEGIES

High school is a new ball game. Transcripts are official, every grade counts toward an accumulative GPA. The pressure is on. It's OK to ask for special accommodations. We're talking about extended time on tests or exams, extended time on reading assignments or papers, exemption from a foreign language, or substituting American Sign Language as a foreign language. Parents soon learn that the more coping strategies the student has, the more workable high school becomes. This is what parents say:

Both Ginger Litlover and Susan Smith thought up new strategies on a regular basis. Ginger suggested: scheduling a study hall last period to start homework assignments; using a wipe-off calendar to break up long-range assignments into smaller pieces; tapping into the local community college for courses on organizational skills, time-management and writing a research paper. Susan suggested: selecting difficult classes first and second periods— math, biology, chemistry, European History; choosing a teacher who doesn't feel threatened when a student asks for minor modifications; physical exercise first, then start on an assignment or research paper.

Faye and Howard Diamond also honed in on multiple strategies. They suggested: using an Alpha Smart computer for notetaking in class (this was on loan from the Resource Center); organizing a reader from the resource center; setting up study groups for heavy-reading classes—European History, biology, U.S. Government; preparing 9-11 months before the SAT test date (non-dyslexic students take six months); taking a semi-private SAT preparation class with another LD student; and taking the SAT with extended time in a familiar setting—the Learning Resource Center—and spreading it over two days. These mechanisms prevent Beth, their daughter, and a junior, from falling into a deep hole.

Peggy Avery tapped into technology. She knew that her daughter, Lacey, was more productive in school because of her computer skills. With Lacey's Mac computer there were no reading commands, just icons; copying and pasting previous work saved time on writing new papers; graphic work was made easy; Internet and CD databases were instant resources for research papers; and handwritten assignments were history.

A stumble in all this, is when a student attaches stigma to special accommodations. (This usually happens with teenage boys.) They feel they can navigate high school alone—with no formal help.

In the final analysis, parents say: "if it takes four years to get into the groove for college where special accommodations and personal coping strategies are the norm, then it's a good time to do just that in high school."

9TH THROUGH 12TH GRADE

■I■

GINGER LITLOVER

David, Michael and Audrey all have been diagnosed with dyslexia. David is a freshman at the University of Arkansas at Fayetteville, AR; Michael is a 10th-grader and Audrey, an 8th-grader. Ginger is a high school teacher at a school for dyslexia. With years of experience in parenting and teaching LD students, she shared some of her "strategies that work":

1 Homework:

   Consistently use any tutorial times before, during or after school to complete homework.

   Do as much work as possible during study hall.

   Use an aide at school as a help source.

   Find a tutor. In my experience, there is too much of a power struggle between parent(s) and child. I have helped very little with homework.

   Tutoring 1 to 2 times a week, depending on the subject matter.

2 Research Papers:

   Divide research into small components. Here, a calendar is critical for planing. Use a large desktop or wipe-off type.

   Take a class on writing research papers at your school or community college. If a course isn't available, I recommend the following handbook: Writing The Research Report ISBN 0-03-047073-0; Holt, Rinehart and Winston, Inc.

3 Management:

   Schedule study hall for last period. My oldest son who participated in varsity football and track all four years of high school, always requested his study hall at the end of the day. He would get as much homework as possible done at this time.

   Take an organizational skills course at school or at your local college. This will help with filing and organization at home and scheduling at school.

Use a tub file to file back assignments and tests. In this way, they can be pulled out at a later date for exam studies.

Take a time-management course at school or at your local college. This will help you prioritize your time. Time management is the key to a successful college experience. Why not start in high school?

Use a calendar to break up long-range assignments into smaller pieces. Most students with dyslexia get very overwhelmed with large assignments.

4 General:

Buy your own textbooks. Writing in the margin, highlighting and defining words in a textbook are critical for comprehension. I try to buy all history and science books from the publisher. Textbooks on tape haven't been effective for my children, but reading aloud and paraphrasing often are very helpful study techniques.

Use computers on a daily basis for word-processing and spell checking. They have been the "saving grace" for our children. I have seen computers literally change the lives of children with dysgraphia, severe dyslexia, and oral and written expression problems.

Be involved in sports or an extracurricular activity. Sports have served as a great outlet for frustration in the academic area and as an area of success in our family. I trained under Dr. Lucious Waites at the Texas Scottish Rite Hospital, and he always told parents, as well as therapists, NEVER to take their LD children out of an extracurricular activity where they were experiencing success, even at the detriment of academic performance.

5 Psychology:

Be your own self-advocate. Most teachers appreciate students who speak up about their special needs. There are some who don't—tread carefully with them! Ideally, students must be proactive to be successful!

Seek professional counseling if needed. This has served a big purpose in my family. As you know, learning problems can and often do turn into emotional problems if left alone. I didn't want any problems to fester.

I hope some of these coping strategies work for your child. They certainly did for ours.

SUSAN SMITH

Anna struggled academically in grades 9-12. She was in a private, college-preparatory school with high-achieving students. But Susan, a former high-school teacher, came up with strategies to help her daughter. Anna went on to the University of California at Davis following high-school graduation.

1 Advocate for yourself and don't be embarrassed to ask for accommodations. Anna and I worked closely with the Academic Dean who had a personal interest in LD students. Her own child had a learning disability, not dyslexia. She was very understanding about time pressures with tests. At last, we had someone on board. We established rapport. Anna was comfortable talking with her independently. The Dean also gave us the name of an outside licensed clinical psychologist who went through a battery of tests with Anna. Those results were used to take the SAT with extended time.

In midterms and finals each semester, Anna asked for extended time. She got 80-90 percent cooperation from faculty. As early as her freshman year, I encouraged her to be her own advocate. Because of her active participation in team sports and drama, she seemed to have the confidence to do this. I reinforced that it wasn't a stigma to ask for special accommodations.

2 Select difficult classes early in the morning and choose teachers (where possible). Together with the Academic Dean, Anna tried to schedule the most challenging classes—math, biology, chemistry, and European History—for first, second and third periods. If there was a choice of teacher for a particular class, she tried to select the most compatible. It tended to be someone who was very experienced, someone who was empathetic to LD students, or someone very confident who wasn't challenged by a parent or student asking for minor modifications. I learned through experience that insecure teaches didn't feel comfortable making new rules.

There were several teachers who were new to the profession or who were seasoned teachers but were incapable of "understanding" LD students. Anna asked for extended time on tests and different methods of testing. She explained that certain types of tests just didn't reflect what she knew. But, some teachers wouldn't accept that, and she had to ride out the storm. Those years, we got outside tutors.

3 Become a success in the eyes of school peers. Anna was very involved in drama. Learning her lines, taking direction, being disciplined, having stage presence and gaining confidence in front of an audience helped her self-image. There's a certain attitude high school kids have toward the jocks, and there's a different attitude toward those involved in theater. (Anna also excelled in sports.) Anna had not only one asset; she had two.

4 Study efficiently for quizzes and tests. I would read a history chapter out loud while Anna took notes. Then, we'd discuss it. She also used index cards for algebra theorems, math facts, multiplication combinations, history dates, and vocabulary and foreign-language vocabulary. Anna would go through all the cards. The second time, she'd weed out the ones she didn't know. That way, she focused on those she didn't know. A simple strategy, but it worked.

5 Sports first, then homework. It was easier for Anna to write well or study well after she'd done some physical exercise. Anna is very athletic. She could swim before she could walk. She was doing gymnastics in pre-school and playing on a local soccer team at age 5. She loved sports and had a good athletic routine after school each day. One time, in 5th grade, she wasn't doing well, and I cut back on these activities. At the time, I didn't know she needed exercise to feed her intellect.

Once Anna got into high school, she spent 2-2$\frac{1}{2}$ hours on sports after school each day. She would get the important exercise—release the endorphins—and then be ready to come home and study. When soccer or volleyball practices were canceled, I noticed her studying was less focused and assignments were harder to complete. Then, the drudge of homework was obvious.

In her junior year, I attended a conference on learning disabilities. When the hypotheses was explained, suddenly the idea clicked. Anna needed to let off steam before she could concentrate on schoolwork. Anna knows what she has to do—a workout is a must before any term paper even can be attempted!

H

PEGGY AVERY

Peggy and Bill Avery attribute their daughter's success to school support and the technological age. Lacey is a junior at a parochial high school in Dallas. She reads at a 6th-grade level, her spelling matches 3rd-graders, but her comprehension is up there with college students. Peggy talks confidently about the family's central coping strategy—the use of a Mac computer.

Lacey loves her Mac. She isn't reading commands, just identifying icons. She started early with computers. In 2nd grade, she learned to touch type. I think, because of the severity of her dyslexia, she misspells many words when she touch types. But, she does type enough to get her by, about 21 words per minute.

Computers are part of Lacey's schoolwork. She creates documents, navigates the Internet and pulls in amazing graphics. It's an exciting time for her. The computer curriculum at her school is laid out very thoroughly. We always try to keep in step with the computer equipment being used at school. That way, Lacey isn't introduced to a different operating system.

Lacey definitely is computer literate. Some applications still are troubling to her, but others are just amazing. Let me explain.

1 The computer allows Lacey a great deal of freedom of thought. The only handwritten work she does involves in-class tests or short homework answers. She'll sit in front of the monitor looking at the keys, trying to organize her thoughts. She has her own way of approaching paper writing, and it seems to work. I proofread. I don't correct grammar. I don't make the sentences sound better. I'm there to be the spell checker.

2 CD ROM's are great for research. When CD ROM's first came out, I immediately recognized the importance of encyclopedias for doing research papers. Lacey cruises through Microsoft's Encarta or Collier's Encyclopedia. They are user-friendly. She uses them for book reports, a health course and history projects. There's a comfort zone for her. Heading to the library now is a major outing.

3 To this day, though, the spell checker on her computer might as well not be there. When you're severely dyslexic, have had years of remediation and have been through three different learning programs,

it's still difficult to tell which word is right. "Now" and "know" are confusing to Lacey; so are "their" and "there." To her, spell-checker options are like a list of Greek words. That's why I'm her spell checker.

Lacey has used Microsoft Word, the Mac version, for many years. Now, in her problem-solving class, she's been introduced to databases, spreadsheets and graphic programs—the PC version. She's having a difficult time because it's a new operating system. It's like a foreign language to her. She has her mind set on Mac. I'm trying to tell her IBM compatible machines are OK. But, after years and years of Mac usage, it's a tall order.

4 Being computer literate at a young age has made all the difference for Lacey. Computers are a normal part of college. Lacey will know how to look up information. She'll even learn to use speech-recognition programs. She'll be well-prepared. To me, that spells success. We owe a lot to our technological age.

FAYE AND HOWARD DIAMOND

Their three children, Beth, Adam and Nicole, all have dyslexia. Beth is a junior at the local high school. The Learning Center has played a central role in her education.

Beth is an over-achiever, and it drains her. Last week, she started crying because she was overwhelmed with so much work. She just works and works and works. She felt like she was going to burst. Thankfully, the Resource Center at school is very supportive. They have taught her how to study and budget her time. But, sometimes, all this help doesn't prevent her from sinking.

If Beth has trouble with a project, she asks for help at the Resource Center. She's fortunate enough to be outgoing. She also uses her Alpha Smart in class to take notes and has a friend who takes notes for her. She has study groups for history and science classes and she uses the spell checker, which has helped tremendously with papers.

It's written on her IEP that extra time is needed for tests. She's allowed up to three hours for her English exam. Other exams vary in time. It's never been an issue. She takes her tests in the Resource Center. A number of her friends are in the center, so there's no stigma attached. She is coping with test taking.

For the SAT, though, we got extra help. Beth started preparing nine months before the test. I hired a private tutor, and Beth and an LD student from school worked together. Beth took the SAT, with extended time, in the Learning Center at school. She spread it over two days. She felt she could do better in both the ACT and SAT, so she'll take them both again. She doesn't want to repeat her mistakes. She's very determined and wants to succeed.

At one point, our school system had an LD parent support group. It was a good group. I didn't feel alone with my daughter's struggles. It was kind of a release. Different speakers were invited to give talks on the college-search process or on coping strategies or the parents' role. About 20 people showed up once a month. But, nobody wanted to lead the group. Eventually, it fizzled out, but I've maintained contact with a few parents. Networking is very important in this narrow field.

Beth has been accepted at Lynn University, Boca Raton, FL. She'll be in TAP (The Advanced Program), a program for students with a learning difference.

ISABEL WESLEY

Isabel and Brett have two sons, Russ and Curt. Their younger son, Russ, is dyslexic. After dogged persistence in high school, he now is a freshman at the University of Oregon. Russ played varsity sports and also had time for his studies.

High school had its moments. First semester, junior year was hectic. It was the first time the amount of work surpassed Russ's free time. He was competing in varsity volleyball and was trying to get too many requirements out of the way. It definitely was a low point in his high-school experience.

Russ loves the sciences. Chemistry is his favorite, followed by physics. But, that class was difficult for him. He got a "C" or "C-." In my eyes, though, he got an "A+" for perseverance. Russ is able to memorize all the theorems, and he comprehends all the algebraic equations in advanced algebra. It's just those multiple-choice tests that cause the problem. If you sit down and talk to him about any subject, Russ fully comprehends the information. He's just not a fan of those tests.

Here's an outline of the special accommodations and strategies he incorporated in grades 9-12:

1 The Creative Learning Center (CLC) – Russ had a good attitude toward the Creative Learning Center in his sophomore and junior years. It was a one-period class, with a 5-unit semester credit. The center offered individualized help to groups of 4-5 LD students. He went there three times a week, for $1\frac{1}{2}$ sessions.

As a 12th-grader, Russ decided he no longer wanted to go to the Center. It was as if he wanted to see if he could do it alone. He was preparing himself for college. He also was reacting to a specific incident. Russ felt the CLC was treating him as a "dummy." He was asked to write letters to several colleges to gain sympathy as an LD student. The resource specialist suggested he appear helpless. LD doesn't mean he's a second-class citizen. Russ never returned to the Center.

2 Extended time on tests – The Creative Learning Specialist told Russ he could have extra time on any test, in any class. Most teachers were fine with this. In his sophomore and junior classes, Russ's teachers sent the test in an envelope to the CLC. Russ would complete it in the Center. But, one math teacher wanted him to take the test in class. The CLC was somewhat uncooperative. They insisted Russ take it in the Center. He was caught in the middle.

3 Note taking – Russ didn't like to take notes in class because he missed what was being said. His local public high school offers a note taker, but Russ declined it. He felt he would stand out. Instead, he thought up his own method of note taking. Russ went to his physics lecture at 8. Then, at noon, when it was repeated, he heard the lecture again. This time, he did his note taking.

Russ used this strategy when the class involved lecture or lab— mainly for physics and chemistry. He used this method instead of a tape recorder or a note taker. That way, it didn't raise any red flags.

4 Foreign language requirement – Russ took Spanish I and got a "C-." The school wouldn't allow him to go on to Spanish II. So, Russ went to night school for Spanish I, II & III and did it at his own pace. It was important that his transcript showed three years of Spanish. He didn't want to be turned down by a specific college. He also knew that, as an LD student, he could be exempt from the foreign-language

requirement. But, he didn't want to go that route. Spanish was a struggle for him.

Ironically enough, his conversational ability is excellent. Russ went to Costa Rica for a month to visit his older brother. He picked up the accent and everything. He wasn't inhibited at all in that setting.

5 SAT – Russ didn't take the test on Saturday, the regular day for SAT testing. Instead, the CLC set up a time during school hours, and he took it in the Center. He felt somewhat labeled because he was pulled out of class. He took the test with extra time.

The first time, he did quite poorly (440 & 520). Then, we got him a tutor, who made house calls. He showed Russ strategies for the verbal and math problems. The second time, Russ went up 100 points (540 & 580).

(Russ is a freshman at the University of Oregon and is managing successfully without help from Academic Advising and Student Services. But, he knows help always is there. He just has to ask.)

DIANE KAYE

Dyslexia runs in the family, on both sides. Diane, her daughter Laura, 15, and her sister-in-law all have been diagnosed with dyslexia. But, technology is Laura's friend. She is computer literate and is allowed to use her laptop in school for selected classes. She'll also be able to use it for three GCSE exams: English literature, history and religious studies.

I asked the principal if Laura could use her laptop in English and history classes. She said it was no problem, although a few teachers were concerned that her writing skills may deteriorate. The bottom line is that Laura's work has improved 100 percent since she started using a word processor. She's been freed from writing in exercise books and erasing her many spelling mistakes. Laura uses a Tandy computer with a five-line display. Thankfully, she learned to touch type five years ago at the special school for dyslexia in London, UK.

For projects and essays done at home, Laura uses our PC. She uses the computer not so much for speed, but for the collection of her thoughts, which, typically, are very jumbled. On the computer, she can shuffle paragraphs around, erase whole sentences and even print out a preview sheet.

Laura is a mainstream student at a girl's public—private in England—school. She doesn't get any allowances or extended time on tests or papers because we haven't asked for them. If I thought she needed them, I would ask. The only request we've made so far is the use of a laptop in certain classes. Actually, the day I spoke to the principal about this, I'd just been to a symposium on Special-Needs students at Westminster School in London. I learned from the seminar that Laura won't be the first to use a laptop in the GCSEs. But, she's definitely the first to use one in our school!

For her GCSEs, Laura will be taking nine subjects: English literature, English grammar, math, two sciences, history, art, religious education and French (a dictionary is permitted in the French exam). She's going to use her laptop for English literature, history and religious studies. She plans to use the spell checker in these exams.

This is a kid who only started to read fluently at the age of 10. I don't think you could call her a reader at any stage along the way, not even at 8 or 9 years. Academically, I made the right choices for her. First, she went to a school for dyslexia (elementary school), and now she's at a small public girl's school. Academically, she's accelerating, and I'm delighted with her progress. But, I must never take my eye off the goal post.

SUE & CHUCK HENDERSON

The Henderson children, Todd and Beth, have dyslexia. Todd is a sophomore at a community college in San Francisco, while his sister is a first-year doctoral student in developmental psychology at the University of Southern California. Sue and Chuck constantly were looking for answers to the LD puzzle.

When Beth was 2, I knew something was wrong. Easy puzzles were very frustrating to her. She had huge emotional outbursts when writing letters or numbers. Intellectually, she knew what to do; she just couldn't perform the task. As an infant, there were lots of milk spills. There was limited motor coordination. It was difficult for her to ride a bike or catch a ball. Yet at 18 months, she stood on the couch and said "airplane vanished but it will come back." She heard "Frere Jacque" once and could repeat it. These discrepancies were perplexing to us.

Our local school taught the Slingerland approach to reading in the LD gifted program, a big plus for Beth. Still, she didn't read until 3rd grade. All along the way, we brainstormed strategies that would help with her schoolwork. Here are some:

1 Visual imaging when reading a narrative story – {Chuck} I read some fairly sophisticated books to Beth and Todd. And I asked them questions. Why did the character do this? What's the plot? What does this sentence or word mean? What's the structure of the book? I did this with them at a fairly young age. I wanted them to listen with interest. I thought it would make the story richer for Beth. She wasn't reading at the time. I was providing important visual images for her.

2 Recorded chapters from history and biology textbooks – I wanted to know how Beth learned best. It was definitely auditory. I decided to record chapters from her history and biology books on to a tape recorder. The material came from textbooks where the size of the print was too small or the layout of chapters was confusing. Some nights, I'd be falling asleep as I taped the chapters. You could hear it in my voice on the tape.

3 Longhand writing; computer editing – Beth couldn't type very fast. She took typing twice in summer school and failed both times. When it came to doing papers in school, she wrote longhand first. Then I'd read the essay to her and ask what changes she wanted to make. She liked this form of editing. She'd give me synonyms for certain words. We'd go over her spelling. Then I made the editorial changes on the computer. At the time, it was the only way I could get her to formulate ideas on paper (she preferred this to dictating her thoughts to me). Of course, since those school days, she's developed competent touch-typing skills and college papers are turned out rapidly on her word processor.

4 Music, astronomy and math are like a foreign language to Beth. She is a talented flautist. She played for the San Francisco Junior Symphony Orchestra. Once she heard a piece of music—she's so gifted—she performed it without any mistakes (no sight-reading). Actually, it took her much longer to play a piece looking at the notes.

But as hard as she worked, music theory was very difficult. When Beth formalized her major (music) in college, she thought she had a good theory background. Then things started to crumble. She called one day and said, "I'm not going through another language in college." Midway through her junior year, she changed to a psychology major.

Astronomy also caused Beth problems in college. She couldn't untangle the mystique. She couldn't visualize the patterns. She's an auditory learner. She barely passed the class.

Then, for required math courses, she received very intense tutoring. They were able to teach her modality. All the learning was auditory. But Beth really didn't have the visual motor skills to grasp complicated math concepts.

JOSEPHINE ACCORDINO

Josephine and Tony have four children – Sal, 16, a 10th-grader, Frank, 14, an 8th-grader, Tina, 12, a 7th-grader, and Vince, 6, a 1st-grader. Sal is the only sibling diagnosed with dyslexia. He is a bright student, who is pragmatic about college. He just wants to get into the business world as soon as possible.

I'm lucky this kid is bright and knows what he wants to do. We'll go through the college application process just like other high-school students. But, we've already gone through some tough academic years.

Asking for extended time on tests bothers Sal. Last year was different. He was doing poorly in English and realized he had to be his own advocate for special accommodations. For tests on parts of speech, he asked for oral testing. Fortunately, his teacher was receptive. He also got extended time for the PSAT. That, he took at the end of 8th-grade. But, he did poorly on the written part. He also found the oral testing difficult. Test taking isn't one of his strengths.

A second area of weakness is Spanish. Sal knew he could be exempt from the foreign-language requirement, but he still insisted on taking Spanish I. Now, he's taking Spanish II. He has difficulty spelling and memorizing Spanish words. Reading English is difficult enough. Sal also is uncomfortable speaking out in his Spanish class. He doesn't have the confidence. At the fall conference, his teacher told me when Sal raises his hand, she doesn't call on him. But, later, when he doesn't have his hand up, she does. She says he's pouting when she calls on him at the wrong time. The Spanish teacher is in her late 20s and talks like she doesn't understand dyslexia. Maybe so.

Sal's Spanish project was to write a research paper and then give an oral presentation. The teacher was very impressed with his written work. But, he couldn't do the oral part. He'd practiced and practiced, but he got stage fright. Normally, he's very social and comfortable talking with people of all ages. I think it was just in Spanish that he froze.

He got an "O" grade on his research project. Sal decided to be his own advocate and meet with the principal, who knew his history. In the end, he negotiated a partial grade for his written work and backed off from doing the oral presentation. Sal still is determined to get a good grade in Spanish. He's planning to re-take Spanish II in summer school.

WHAT PARENTS SAY ON HOW-TO-COPE

Many of us supplement our diet with vitamins—vitamin A, vitamin C or a multi-vitamin. In the same way, we need to supplement our child's schooling with coping strategies. I'm talking about a modified homework plan, modified reading assignments, closed-caption viewing on TV sets, a Special-Ed tutor who can relate to your child, or just using past school experiences, as a dyslexic student, to better understand a child's frustrations.

Strategies come in different formats and for different reasons. Each grade, teacher, course, semester pose new challenges. What worked well last semester might need modifying this semester. Flexibility is the name of the game. Overall, parents say they need most help for homework strategies, followed by technology tips, Learning Resource Specialists and Special-Ed tutors.

Let's look initially at interviews where parents are considering a school for dyslexia or home schooling as an alternative to traditional mainstream schooling. This usually happens with elementary-school parents. As you've seen from their stories, it takes courage, uncertainty and a lot of "agonizing" to move out of the mainstream. But, if long-term benefits are there, whatever the risk, these parents feel that going out of the mainstream is their optimum choice.

The decision to move out-of-mainstream relates entirely to the child's self-esteem. If the child feels good about him/herself, whatever the degree of dyslexia, staying in mainstream will work, provided coping strategies are in place. But where a student's confidence is floundering, where dyslexia is not in a teacher's web of experiences, where a school's academic standards are foremost (as opposed to individual student support), a 12-month or longer stay at a school for dyslexia or home schooling, can turn a student around. Like any plan, though, closure on the project and the return to the mainstream, need to be addressed early on, even before the student starts on his/her new journey. Building or rebuilding a child's self esteem is a given in home schooling or a special school for dyslexia.

Now turning to parents with children in the mainstream, they come forth with practical suggestions. For elementary-school children, a software program for reading such as "Interactive Movie Book" by Sound Source Interactive Company and for writing, "Storybook Weaver" by the Learning Company is recommended. One parent suggests having a current spelling list at all times, allowing testing to be done while standing at the kitchen sink doing dishes, eating at the breakfast table or driving in the car. Another parent says taking a crash course in state law makes all the difference. She got her daughter into the school district's Special Education program, while still remaining in the private sector. She also felt more in control with the IEP (Individual Education Plan).

I expected touch typing and spell checker to be at the top of the how-to-cope list, but that didn't happen. My sentiments are that ALL dyslexic students should be typing competently by fourth grade, and starting as early as second or third grade. A successful software program that works well with elementary school children is "Mavis Beacon's Teaches Typing" and the use of a spell checker when typing up a story, ensures even more self-assurance. Pointing and clicking on the Internet (parental guidance necessary) and checking out different Web sites, too, can increase a child's knowledge immeasurably.

Families with middle-school kids say that being in a good school district with a proven Resource Center is a bonus; knowing that burnout is always in November and April provides valuable insight; implementing an incentive plan for report cards adds some excitement; and using headphones to listen to music while doing homework, makes work more pleasurable.

Another strategy I'd like to suggest is working on open communication with teachers and administrators. That means putting across a point of view and speaking with confidence about special accommodations, even minor ones. This takes time and practice, and it can't be learned in textbooks. Checking out what a teacher has previously allowed LD students will also help in the discussion. Checking out information on the Internet or in current periodicals will be additionally supportive. But, if a student can work on improving his/her communication skills with teachers sixth through eighth grades, then high school may become less daunting.

As for high school strategies, parents come up with pragmatic suggestions for time-management, organization, scheduling, American Sign Language (ASL) as a foreign language, last period for Study Hall to start on homework, and many more. From what parents say, high school flows much better when students speak out about their learning difference, make informal connections with teachers and become more informed about strategies that work and those that don't, in different classes.

Finally, let's look at coping strategies in a broader context. The Internet appears to be radically changing the teacher-student composition. Learning is no longer limited to the physical constraints of a classroom. Hence, many teachers are becoming more flexible with their teaching methods. The paradigm is shifting.

This new mode will most certainly benefit a student with a learning difference. Now is a good time to speak up about different learning styles, to ask for special accommodations, to self advocate. The Internet has erased global boundaries. It is also erasing teacher-student boundaries.

POINTERS FOR OUT OF MAINSTREAM SCHOOLING

About A School For Dyslexia

❑ Consider 1-2 years as a positive remedial plan—Orthodontic work takes the same amount of time! Don't wait until it's too late, for social reasons. First through fifth grades are the optimum years.

❑ Put closure on the plan. Let your child know this at the start. If there are no incentives, enthusiasm will wane. (If your child is more than 24 months below grade level, two years may not be enough.)

❑ Don't make neighborhood kids the excuse for not moving out of the mainstream—kids adapt. Some ways to stay connected are to encourage neighborhood kids to stop by, have plenty of food around, invite them to a local sporting event, for a sleepover, for a camping trip. It's OK for your kid to have friends from different social groups.

❑ Remember that when there's anxiety in the family about making "the decision", siblings pick up on this worrisome attitude. This only adds to the fuel.

❑ Look at the big picture. If this is short-term discomfort with long-term benefits, then there are no other choices.

On Legal And Financial Issues

❑ Don't let school fees, testing fees or hiring a private Special-Ed tutor prevent your child from getting the best possible education. Research your financing options—family contributions, local organizations, local school districts, attorneys' specializing in LD cases.

❑ If you feel your local school district is not providing your child with a complete education, and that one or two years at a special school for dyslexia is the way to go, try to work out an agreement with them on school fees. Bring in a mediator if that helps.

❑ If your child is at a private school and there's no Learning Resource Center in place, ask your local school district to include him/her in a resource class at your nearest public school.

□ If you've ended up paying school fees, find ways to balance the load. Don't take on two jobs—kids know when Mom and Dad are on overload. If family members want to pitch in, don't be proud.

For Home Schooling

□ Consider short term if your child's self-esteem is slipping in school. Work extra hard to keep your child socially active with his/her peers—baseball, basketball teams, church groups etc. Then, start to plan a smooth re-entry into the mainstream.

□ Sign up with an authorized local home-school group or find one on the Internet (www.homeschoolzone.com). Remember, a home-schooled child must keep up with grade level work in all subjects for a smooth transition into mainstream.

POINTERS FOR MAINSTREAM SCHOOLING

Kindergarten Through 8th Grades

□ Know that the school curriculum needs to be supplemented with a modified homework plan or a Special-Ed tutor or innovative software programs or an oral presentation instead of a written essay, etc.

□ Put your child's passion into out-of-school activities—arts, music, sports, technology, Boy/Girl Scouts, community service. See that smile on his or her face, see the enthusiasm.

□ Know that students do well in college because they communicate well with faculty, staff, students. Honing this skill starts early on.

For Homework

□ Set up a modified homework plan. Ask to reduce the number of math questions, spelling and vocabulary words, pages in an essay. It's quality, not quantity, that counts.

□ Same place, same time for homework. Then, there's still time for outside interests, which are essential.

❑ Suggest headphones for kids who enjoy listening to music. It often relaxes the child and helps them focus on the task. Then homework doesn't feel so threatening.

For Technology

❑ Check out new software programs for text to speech, speech to text (voice recognition), tape recording, and improved spell checkers (see college section, coping strategies). Technology will be your child's best friend. Maximize it!

❑ Use a touch-typing program (Mavis Beacon Teaches Typing) to familiarize your child with a keyboard. Start as early as third grade.

❑ Use closed-caption viewing on your TV to reinforce every day words. In this way, your child still enjoys a TV comedy show or movie.

❑ Work with your child on the Internet—it's click and point. S(he) will look good in the eyes of peers when quoting new Web sites. There are other ways than traditional reading to be smart.

For Special-Ed Tutoring

❑ Remember that personal chemistry between child and tutor is more important than the learning process. Often, the child looks to him/her as a role mode.

❑ Network with local LD organizations, LD parents, local graduate students in Education or place an advertisement in the local paper for a tutor.

❑ Check out Lindamood-Bell Learning Processes (LiPS) for after-school remediation in reading. Students identify with sounds while they're reading. Parents speak well of this reading program (http://www.lblp.com).

POINTERS FOR HIGH-SCHOOL STUDENTS

❏ Self advocate—most teachers respect students who speak up about their learning difference. There are always some, though, who don't, so tread carefully.

❏ Get retested in 10th or 11th grade—WAIS-R or WISC-111 tests[2] —by a licensed school psychologist, or a private licensed clinical psychologist who has been in practice 10+ years. Authenticity and longevity score here. Documentation is essential for extended time on the SAT; also College Admissions need testing within the last three years.

❏ Select the most challenging courses, some honors, but not neces- sarily AP courses.

❏ Remember extracurricular activities—varsity sports, drama, community service, leadership, unique summer experiences—gain brownie points. They're as important as the official transcript. It's the all-around picture College Admissions require.

❏ Work with the Learning Resource Center to get a notetaker, a scribe, tape recorder, books on tape or a software recording program.

Submit the following requests for papers, tests, assignments and projects:
- ❏ a project instead of a written paper
- ❏ an oral report instead of a written paper
- ❏ an oral test instead of a conventional written test
- ❏ short-essay questions instead of a multiple-choice test
- ❏ a paper instead of a multiple-choice test
- ❏ an oral test instead of a multiple-choice test
- ❏ reduction in the number of math problems on a test or exam
- ❏ extended time on quizzes, tests or exams
- ❏ extended time for reading assignments, papers and projects

For Scheduling

❏ Select difficult classes early in the morning, first through third periods. For example: European History, U.S. History, U.S. Government, chemistry, physics.

❏ Select teachers, where possible, who have taught LD students before.

❏ Select a last-period study hall to get a head start with homework.

For School Work

❏ Buy your own textbooks so you can write in the margins and highlight sections—textbooks on tape aren't as effective.

❏ Use a computer for homework, papers, filing previous work, spell checking and grammar checking. Minimize handwritten work!

❏ Use a wipe-off calendar to break down research papers/projects into smaller components.

❏ Take a time-management course at your local community college to help balance schoolwork and fun activities.

❏ Take an organizational-skills course at your local community college to help with scheduling and filing of schoolwork.

For A Foreign Language

❏ Know that American Sign Language (ASL) is an acceptable foreign language in high school. Don't struggle with Latin or German!

❏ Take ASL at your local community college. Remember to include the official transcript in your college application.

❏ If you are failing in a foreign language know that you can get exemption, provided you've studied that foreign language for at least one semester.

❏ Check out four colleges where you may want to apply, for status on their foreign-language requirements.

For The SAT

❏ Work with another LD student and start nine months before the test. Set up a semi-private lesson to share tutoring costs. Better still, try to find a tutor with Special-Ed experience.

❑ Know that the SAT is offered on the computer. Do a dress rehearsal to familiarize yourself with the format.

❑ Know you can get extended time and can take the test orally. BUT, you must get tested within the last three years to get these accommodations—critics smell a scam if testing is very recent!

❑ Do loads of prep work—get a bunch of past SAT test papers and practice, practice, practice.

❑ Remember . . . the SAT is a psychological test. Don't get psyched out!

For AP exams

❑ Know you can get extended time, and spread out your time, one exam per day. Ask to use a computer if that helps.

For Parents Of High-Schoolers

❑ Form an LD parent support group in your local high school. Commonality and networking with local parents for SAT preparation classes or tutoring and the college-search process are a bonus.

❑ Check out local college fairs. In a few major cities, some include specific LD programs.

---

[2] WAIS-R (Wechsler Adult Intelligence Scale-Revised) tests verbal and non-verbal intelligence of adults aged 16 and over. High schoolers between the ages of 16 and 18 should do this test, not the WISC-111. The WAIS-R test is used to identify areas of learning strengths, learning weaknesses, or disabilities.

WISC-111 (Weschsler Intelligence Scale for Children 111) is given to children ages 6 through 16, and measures general intelligence. It provides three IQ scores: verbal, performance, and full-scale, yielding information about strengths and weaknesses in language and performance areas.

3

THE COLLEGE SEARCH
PARENTS

THE COLLEGE-SEARCH PROCESS

John Bell, 18, is a senior in a public high school in Honolulu. Lacey Avery, 17, is a high-school junior at a special school for dyslexia in Dallas. They're both college bound. For students like John and Lacey, leaving high-school and moving on to bigger and better things is exciting, but also scary. For their parents, like most parents, though, it's the scariest. There are so many daunting questions. "Where will he /she get into college?" "How does College Admissions view students with a learning difference?" "Where do we even start with the college search process?" It's also the end of a passage and the beginning of a new one. Change and uncertainty are often uncomfortable.

During the *college-search,* the emphasis is on the PROCESS, not on the actual placement results. (Anyone can grab the *K&W Guide to Colleges for the Learning Disabled* or *Peterson's: Colleges with Programs for Students with Learning Disabilities* and gather information. I also list "Dyslexia Friendly Colleges" and pointers for the college-search, at the end of this chapter.) Most important, though, is reading the twenty plus parent inter-views, identifying with their strategies, disputing or agreeing with them, and then formulating—with your son/daughter—your own plan of action.

In interviews with 25 parents, I wanted to see how the college-search process affects family members. Is the student willingly part of the process or does he/she leave it up to the parent to do the research, or does he/she do it independently with a college counselor? And, do previous sibling placements influence college choices. I wanted to see if specific criteria were in place, if geographic location was an issue, if a strong LD program was important, and if exemption from specific courses—foreign language—even surfaced.

The results lead me to conclude that attitudes are dependent on the confidence or security level of the student and/or parent. Maturity and the severity of the learning disability are secondary. From talking with parents, the interviews fell into two groups: Strategic Planners and Sure Footed.

Strategic Planners
1 those with definitive criteria
2 those targeting colleges that had no math or foreign-language requirement

Here, parents and 12th graders formulate specific plans for the college search and try to remain focused throughout the daunting task. I say daunting because the amount of data out there—mainly college guides—can be overwhelming. And now, with college web sites producing more information,

I strongly suggest setting up criteria early in the process. In this way, the search is more manageable.

In this group, parents came forward with specific college choices that support their children. None of these interviews were alike. Paul Samo came up with eight requirements, Susan Smith had three. For Sadie Sheehan and Alex Mann, a strong varsity sports program was a priority.

Paul Samo wanted his daughter, Blake, to find her college "nirvana." He told her: "choosing a college is entirely about you, and not about us, your parents." He helped her identify her possibilities and then let her make the final decision. Isabel Wesley took a different route for her second son, Russ, but still focused on two definitive areas—a college setting where he'd be happy and one with less academic pressure. She incorporated realistic goals, all the while targeting a good school. For Susan Smith and her daughter, Anna, when it came down to decision time, Anna decided to modify her initial plan. What she discovered through the search process was that small liberal-arts colleges often don't have enough funding for specific Learning Resource programs. So, Anna zeroed in on a school that had a recognizable LD program, but was in a university setting.

Alex Mann targeted those schools that offered her daughter, Evette, an athletic scholarship in lacrosse and Kathryn Childers looked at strong drama departments for her daughter, Nicole. For Sadie Sheehan's son, Kevin, a champion sailor and racer, applications were narrowed down to those five with very strong sailing programs.

Parents in this group, pushed the envelope, looking for gaps in the "system." A few found what they were looking for. Marie Douglas went all out to find a school for her daughter, Francis, where a foreign-language requirement could be waived or substituted. Francis, an "A" student in a college preparatory high school, got her first and only "C" in Spanish I. Then in Spanish II, there was a "D." Marie was not going to let her daughter be pulled down. Betsy Wass combed the college guidebooks (east-west), to locate a school that had no math requirement and found Hampshire College near Amherst, MA and Pitzer College, CA. It wasn't an easy task. Her daughter, Ella, 26, got her bachelor's in psychology at Pitzer and now is a fourth-year doctoral student in Sociocultural Anthropology at the University of Washington. Betsy says "going that extra mile for Ella made all the difference."

For most *strategic planners*—with specific criteria—their college choices have been a good fit.

Sure-footed
1 geographically close and culturally like environments
2 LD programs with a track record

In this group of parents, it was OK to want security, "to play it safe," to opt for colleges within driving distance from home. Parents, too, feel safe if their son or daughter applies to schools with a viable LD resource center. For the most part, they don't want their child to chart unknown territory, risking failure after the first semester. They are aware of their child's limitations, and focus on getting help with their shortcomings.

In doing this, they ask the obvious questions: "Where can I find an emotional safe place for my son/daughter where he/she will grow?" "Where do I find faculty who are positive with learning-different students?" Stacey Parker found a safe place for her daughter, Tosha, in the S.A.L.T. program at the University of Arizona. It offers a comprehensive, nurturing program. The counselors are there to help at all times, and the program takes students by the hand before moving them on after two years. For Christina Peterson, she never dreamed her son, Allan, would make it to college. His senior year of high school, Allan refused to look at colleges and was dogged about "his" game plan. Then, a lucky break occurred when Allan met the faculty and staff at Marymount College in Palos Verdes, CA. They kindled something in him. In Christina's eyes, "that school was our saving grace."

Overall, more families opt for a near-to-home campus over a strong LD support system. This comes as somewhat of a surprise. In reality though, families with LD students (or without), value the closeness of family ties and this comes through loud and clear. Susan Olsen knew all three of her boys would stay in South Texas for college. Then again, there are SMU (Southern Methodist University) and Texas A &M, two fine schools. Both have comprehensive LD support programs. Sally Princeton's daughter, Sue, targeted schools in Ohio or neighboring states. All the schools she chose had a strong varsity track team and were within driving distance from home.

For Lisa Begley's son, Liam, going to the local community college and staying close to home was critical. Liam struggled in school. He wasn't ready to leave home and Lisa wasn't ready to send him away. It was a no-choice situation.

Parents and 12th graders, here, look for a comfort zone. They feel being close to family or having an in-place learning support system are more important than experiencing a new culture, new surroundings, new beaches or new mountains. Being sure-footed, they feel, is nice 'n comfortable.

The following interviews should show you how some families across America handle this search process and all its subjectivity. While LD college reference books list names and statistics, the process of your search—the elimination of certain criteria and the strategies you decide to include—will result in an even richer college placement for your student.

STRATEGIC PLANNERS

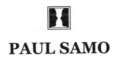

PAUL SAMO

Paul's daughter, Blake, 19, is a sophomore at the College of Wooster in Ohio. Her only sister, Brooke, 22, is LD (not dyslexic) and recently graduated from Whittier College in California. Paul reminded Blake to keep an open mind and explore all her options.

I wanted Blake to find her college "nirvana." I wanted her to be selfish. Blake took it all to heart. With help from her college counselor, she came up with a list of her own requirements. This is what Blake wanted in a college:

> A small liberal-arts school (between 1,000-2,000 students)
> An attractive campus
> A Midwest or East Coast school
> A colder climate than California
> A small student-teacher ratio
> Faculty, not TAs, teaching classes
> A school that accepts the Common Application Form
> Good-looking people on campus

Geographic location was perhaps the biggest factor. It's a huge advantage for Blake to be in a snow environment. There, most of the students are in the library, not surfing or sun tanning at the beach. We supported Blake completely. Many a wonderful paper has been written during a blizzard!

Blake wrote to 40 colleges. As she sorted through the return mail, she pulled out those schools that seemed attractive and had good-looking people on campus. Eventually, she applied to 11 schools. We visited five.

Blake probably was able to apply to so many colleges because of the Common Application Form. The form is an enormous plus for students with learning differences. It contains only one essay and it can be multiplied for other schools.

Although Kalamazoo College in Michigan and Beloit in Wisconsin are wonderful, small, liberal-arts schools, Blake decided on Wooster. Good choice. The school has about 1,900 students and a good Resource Center fully staffed with counselors and tutors.

Truthfully, she would have been happy at any of the 11 schools. They all had the same touch and feel. They were about the student, not the parents. I'm so thankful Blake saw the whole process as something positive. She let every college know she had a different learning style. And she never treated her learning disability as a disability.

Now at Wooster, my daughter has found her "nirvana." She's a pre-med student. She works her butt off, but still makes time to go to parties. She tries to get into as many study groups as she can and isn't afraid to ask for help. She's an individual: she speaks her mind and asks questions.

This is where her 11 applications went:

Wheaton, MA   Norton, MA
Colby, ME   Skidmore, NY
Drew, NY   Kalamazoo College, MI
Lake Forest College, IL   Beloit, WI
College of Wooster, OH   Kenyon, OH
University of the Redlands, CA

KARLA AND JACOB WOODS

Karla and Jacob's son, Brittan, 21, is an accomplished, All-American gymnast—winner of the Junior Olympic National Championships and the USA Gymnastics title. It was a given that he'd look at schools with a strong gymnastics program. There were several choices for him to consider.

{Karla} Brittan was a reluctant applicant. The whole college-search was frightening for him. I did most of the work and became very active in the search. I wrote away for specific information. Actually, I wrote the letter for him and had Brittan sign it. We sent off 14. When I got the mail, I'd go through the replies with him. We'd circle and highlight as we talked about the different schools. He was distant from the whole thing. I can understand. I just knew I had to do the search because, otherwise, it wouldn't be done.

{Jacob} I wanted Brittan to go to my alma mater—the University of Arizona. I was on a football scholarship there and thought it'd be a good match for him. I'd also heard good things about their SALT program. Brittan agreed, but then we found out there was no Division I gymnastics team.

{Karla} I had a printout of specific colleges that had Division I gymnastic programs. There were 24 total, but Brittan eliminated the 12 in California because of the distance from Missouri. He also eliminated schools west of the Rocky Mountains. He knew it was just too far away from home in St. Louis.

Our first preference was a strong gymnastics program, followed closely by a strong LD support system. Schools within driving distance from home were a third consideration.

I cross-checked those schools with Division I gymnastic teams with LD reference books—*Colleges with Programs or Services for Students with Learning Disabilities* by Midge Lipkin and *Peterson's: Colleges with Programs for Students with Learning Disabilities*. Initially, we looked at:

University of Minnesota	University of Michigan
University of Nebraska	Michigan State
University of Iowa	Ohio State, Columbus
University of Oklahoma	James Madison University
Penn State	Temple University
University of New Mexico	West Point, the Naval Academy
University of Illinois	William and Mary

The University of Nebraska had only partial services, and Michigan State and Temple University offered no extended time on tests/exams. The University of New Mexico didn't have much of a campus feel. We got down to the Final Four. We sent Brittan's video to those coaches and then followed up with a campus visit. The Final Four were: William and Mary; James Madison U; University of Oklahoma; and University of Iowa.

The coach at Brittan's high school was an alumnus of the University of Iowa. He gave Brittan a good pitch, but Brittan wasn't going to be persuaded. Despite being a reluctant applicant, in the end Brittan knew exactly what he wanted in a college. He wanted to go where he had a comfort level, where he could be a successful gymnast, enjoy himself, and not be overly pressured by schoolwork. Those were very important to him.

Brittan eliminated visits to some schools where he knew the coaches and didn't think it'd be a good match. He wanted a coach he could relate to and respect. He wanted to contribute to the team. The coach at James Madison was the right fit. The program was the right fit. Brittan was very comfortable with the gymnastics coaching level and he would make a contribution to the team. He wasn't interested in going to a high-level gymnastics program and end up sitting on the bench.

He made the decision for all the right reasons. Plus he's familiar with Virginia—for one, he was born there, we vacationed there, and there are touchstones there. The school is a 12-hour drive from St. Louis, and that works for us.

{Jacob} It's been a good placement for Brittan. Only the other day he told me "I don't think life can get better than it is." Now, he's looking at a new venture. He's taking a semester off to be part of a four-team kayak crew that is traveling the waterways of America. It'll take 100-120 days. It will start in the north, in Yellowstone National Park, work its way down the Missouri, then on to the Mississippi, and finally south to New Orleans. The team's sponsors are supplying equipment—most importantly, a satellite dish. This will allow them to hook up to the Internet, post daily entries and communicate via e-mail. Then anyone, anywhere in the world, will be able to get daily web site updates. The program is not sponsored by James Madison University, but his advisor in Environmental Science and his academic advisor, both agreed it's an opportunity that can't be missed.

That's what happens when you take Brittan on a three-day family kayak trip down the Mississippi!

JEAN LEE

Jean's son, Sam, 19, is on a 504 plan (students with a learning disability) and a National Merit student. This was confusing for the high-school college counselor, so Jean and Sam came up with their own plan. Sam is currently a freshman at Southern Methodist University.

Sam was open-minded about the whole thing. He went with the flow and let me gather the information. I started in seventh grade—I was afraid of the foreign-language (FL) requirement for him in college. I contacted three schools in Texas—Austin College in Sherman, the University of Texas and SMU—checking out what their policy was on foreign languages, and if they offered an alternative plan. What I found out was awesome—SMU had no foreign-language requirement. I realized, then, there must be other schools just like SMU. We had stumbled onto something good. It was an option.

Sam's college counselor at the local high school was not very helpful, and not informed about LD. To top it off, Adam was the first to chart new waters—the only 504 student and National Merit student the school had seen. We helped the counselor by educating her. But, in reality, we did the college search on our own. This was in 11th grade.

I have to say Sam's 504 coordinator guided us well—she helped with filling out the paperwork, and documenting his request for extended time on the SAT. She also suggested doing this for his AP's. That was yet another bonus. AP classes—physics, calculus, economics, English—were a real challenge, but by spreading the load over four days, one exam per day, and using the 504 coordinator's laptop, the task seemed less daunting. Sam wasn't allowed to use a spell checker—actually, the program wasn't loaded for this reason. But just being able to see the information on a screen helped him focus.

Sam will probably end up doing something with the Internet. It was natural for him then to look at schools with a strong computer science department. But then, he's also interested in engineering and loves music—playing the bass. By junior year, we'd talked about his preferences, and came up with this plan for the college search: major first—engineering—followed by computer science; an LD support system; and a smaller college, not a university setting.

Warren, my husband, and I felt strongly about visiting several schools. Sam needed to feel the character of the place, to see if the fit was right. We made visits in his junior and senior year, always when college was in session. Where possible, Adam would stay in a dorm. Before a trip, I'd set up two or three classes for him to audit. He needed to see how the teachers presented material, and what the makeup of the students were. Adam is very visual, and this was key to his school assessments.

Sam was keen on doing the campus visits. He'd received letters from several colleges—Vanderbilt, Carlton, Rhodes—because he's a National Merit student, with a 1460 SAT score. He was excited about seeing these schools. On some of the visits, he and his dad went alone because Warren, an engineer, kind of knew what questions to ask. In all, Sam visited four schools, four of them in Texas. They were also the schools he ended up applying to:

University of Texas	Texas A&M
Trinity, TX	SMU
Vanderbilt, TN	Carlton, MN
Oberlin, OH	Rhodes, TN

As luck would have it, Sam was accepted at ALL eight. That threw more confusion into the pot. Of the eight, Sam then eliminated five:

1 University of Texas – It was too big a campus, his sister went there, and the school just didn't do anything for him

2 Texas A&M – That's another big school. He spent a couple of days

there in a dorm. It's got a small-town feel in a large university setting, and it has a good LD support system. But, it didn't float his boat.

3 Vanderbilt, TN – The LD support didn't "knock his socks off."

4 Oberlin, OH – The college is accepting of everybody left of center. Adam is more church going, more conservative. It wasn't a good match.

5 Rhodes, TN – Sam actually didn't visit there. They offered him a $1/2$ tuition scholarship because of his National Merit status, but he decided to decline.

Then it was down to the last three: Carlton, Trinity, and SMU.

Sam really wanted to go out-of-state because he'd grown up in Dallas. He was ready to go north, to the frozen north, and Carlton, a liberal-arts school in Minnesota, became his first choice. It has a good computer science program, but not a strong engineering department. He knew his first choice was engineering. Then again, the LD program was wonderful, very supportive. But they didn't give any financial aid. Carlton had a lot going for it, but in the long run, Sam knew it wasn't the best placement for him.

Trinity was in the running, too, with a strong engineering department, and caring personnel in LD services. But then again, it meant staying in Texas.

SMU was actually the last choice on Sam's list. He sat in on SMU classes only after he'd visited several other schools. Student Life—the office for LD students and other students with disabilities—was welcoming, the engineering department was strong and the campus had a small, friendly feeling. He liked what he saw. When it came down to it, though, the two defining factors were: a math professor, an alumnus of Harvard who works closely with engineering students, immediately recognized Sam's talent. The chemistry was there, plus no foreign language requirement. The sale was over.

SMU is a good match. Sam got lucky; he fulfilled his college-search criteria. Before he started there, he took a studies skill course that summer so he'd be well prepared. Then, once on board, Sam was invited to apply for the President's Scholarship. He was chosen over 100 students. Only 21 were selected.

On reflection, Sam still used the LD support as a safety net in his final analysis. Even now, when there are nights when Sam doesn't understand something and the Learning Enhancement Center is closed on campus, he'll stop by or phone home. For me, there will always be an LD issue, even though he's so bright, so bright.

FAYE AND HOWARD DIAMOND

All three of Faye and Howard's kids have dyslexia. The oldest, Beth, 17, is a junior in the local high school. Faye, Howard and Beth were in the process of looking at colleges. To avoid becoming overwhelmed with the whole project, they came up with specific criteria.

Dyslexia runs in our family. My brother is dyslexic and so was my grandfather, who went on to become the founder and chairman of a Fortune 500 company. Beth has that same drive. She's very talented in the arts. And she's interested in merchandising, fashion and marketing. Knowing that will be essential in making a good school choice, as will our other criteria:

> Schools with an LD support program
> Schools with a small student population (not a university setting)
> Schools with a Jewish student Hillel House

Every college Beth is looking at has an LD program. I also used the *Hillel: Guide to Jewish Life on Campus* to locate student groups. It's important that she socialize with students of her own religion.

Beth definitely is involved in the college search. Actually, she's very relaxed about the whole process. Beth visits her guidance counselor weekly. And, next year, the counselor and Education Learning Specialist will give Beth all the information she needs to make a sensible college choice. I have every confidence in their work.

In addition, we'll stop by some local college fairs in downtown Cleveland. We'll visit the booths that offer a Learning Resource program. At the moment, though, Beth is going to apply to:

> Lynn University, Boca Raton, FL   Bradley, Peoria, IL
> Long Island College, NY   Denver University, CO
> New York Institute of Technology

We've come up with these college choices, really, through word of mouth and help from the school. I've asked those kids in our area with a learning difference where they've gone in the last few years. Several chose the S.A.L.T. program at the University of Arizona. Others went to Lynn University or Long Island College. If the University of Arizona offered a program in Fashion Management, Beth definitely would apply there. Right now, though, her first choice is Lynn.

Beth has been accepted at Lynn University. She'll either major in Fashion Design (College of Arts and Social Sciences) or Fashion Management (College of Business). She'll also be in T.A.P. (The Advancement Program)— a program for LD students.

SADIE SHEEHAN

Sadie's son, Kevin, 19, wanted only to go to Boston College in Massachusetts, where his older brother, Sean, 22, is a senior. Kevin didn't self-identify, didn't take the SAT with extended time and . . . Boston College didn't accept him. Recently, though, he transferred to BC after completing his freshman year at the University of Hawaii.

Kevin didn't particularly enjoy our New England "college tour." But one week with his brother at Boston College and one excursion with the sailing team, and he was hooked. He didn't want to look at any other school.

Kevin is a champion sailor and racer. In middle and high school, he sailed almost every day. As a senior, he went to the Olympic tryouts. Sailing cleared his mind. A top sailing program was imperative in his college choices. That narrowed his applications down to five:

Old Dominion College, VA	University of Rhode Island
Boston College, MA	University of Hawaii
University of Southern California	

I knew Boston College had an LD program. But Kevin was in denial during the application process. (He thinks he's outgrown it.) He didn't self-disclose. He refused to take the SAT with extended time. He got around an 1100. He's a solid "B" student. Imagine if he'd accepted help. Kevin is very dogged, but his pride affected his college acceptances. I guess, in the end, he'll come through.

The University of Hawaii was a bit too easy for him after a rigorous college preparatory school. He still wanted to have an East Coast experience.

Kevin transferred to Boston College as a sophomore and made the Dean's list his first semester. He didn't make the sailing team, but he'll try out again next year. He loves BC.

H

KATHRYN CHILDERS

Kathryn's daughter, Nichole, 22, graduated from the University of California at Santa Cruz with a bachelor's degree in Theater Arts. For her year abroad, she went to the University of Lancaster, England, where she specialized in Medieval Drama.

Nichole hated high school. Why would I spend money then to send her to college? So, she took a year off after high-school graduation to work and play. She still was very young, 16. After taking three years at the local, two-year, community college to get course work—her GE requirements—out of the way, she started talking to several people about college. She's very interested in theater and always has wanted to be an actress. As a family, we talked about several options. She came up with six schools:

The Juillard School, NY   New York University
University of California at Los Angeles   San Francisco State University
University of California at Santa Cruz   University of Southern California

All the schools had excellent drama departments. We weren't too worried about the LD programs because of Nichole's ability to advocate for herself and the protections guaranteed by the Americans with Disabilities Act. She did have to be retested, though, to qualify for assistance at UC Santa Cruz.

Nichole entered UC Santa Cruz as a junior. There, she created her own major —Dramatic Arts in Medieval Studies—and organized all the paperwork to get her to England. Actually, she organized her major so she HAD to go to England to get the courses. Old English as a second language was one of her requirements. I don't know how she did it. She still couldn't spell. But she was on her way to England.

We immediately were impressed by the University of Lancaster. They personally phoned Nichole to ask what accommodations she needed after noticing on her transcript that she'd self-identified. She uses extended test time and a note taker, but it turns out she didn't need a note taker in England. Instead, she got permission to tape lectures.

At Lancaster she took classes in Medieval Drama, Old English and English

History. Her college experience there was amazing. And there was no language barrier. When she started back up at UC Santa Cruz, she completed her senior project and took a few classes. Nichole graduated with her class.

SUSAN SMITH

Susan's daughter, Anna, 22, graduated from the University of California at Davis with a bachelor's in American Studies and a minor in Film Studies Anna and Susan carefully thought out the search process when it came time to apply to college.

We had a very definite strategy when it came to looking for schools—look at courses offered for a major; look for an LD support system; and find a small, liberal-arts school.

If a college met the first and second criteria, we looked deeper. Anna had completed the standard high-school courses—biology, U.S. History, European History, U.S. Government, etc. Now, in college, she was looking for less-traditional classes—marine biology, botany, archaeology, theater arts, film studies, American studies.

I also wanted our daughter to be in a small academic setting. But I discovered that most smaller, liberal-arts schools don't have enough funding for a specific Learning Resource program. We then decided to include a number of public universities with recognizable Learning Centers—i.e., the University of California at Davis, the University of Colorado at Boulder and the University of Arizona. It turned out that U of A had the most viable program.

All total, we researched 15 schools, east and west. Given our criteria, Anna decided to apply to 10:

Connecticut College for Women
Whitman College, OR
Occidental College, CA
Claremont McKenna, CA
Pomona College, CA
University of Colorado at Boulder
University of Arizona
University of California at Davis
Pitzer, CA
Scripps, CA

In the end, Anna chose a large school, close to home. We sensed she knew what she wanted. She used the Disability Resource Center to get her into a good dorm—being LD worked to her advantage for once!

■ ALEX MANN

Alex's daughter, Evette 20, is a sophomore at the University of Delaware. As early as ninth grade, Alex and Evette started looking at schools with good lacrosse programs.

It's complicated when there's schoolwork and adolescence. Evette was a key player on the hockey field, varsity lacrosse and soccer teams. But she cringed when she had to ask for extended time on tests. There, on file in the office, was confirmation of her official request. But still, she had to ask every individual teacher for every individual test, explaining why she needed extended time, over and over again. What ended up happening was that, after asking so many times—and being humiliated—she decided not to ask for extended time, period. This was a hard call for a teenager.

Then, in 10th grade, we hired a private SAT tutor, Sue. We thought, with her guidance, Evette could move up 100, maybe, 150 points. After only one session, Sue commented: "Evette's overall responses are well below average, and I've never tutored anyone of this level." This tutor had a master's in education, specializing in SAT preparation! I never followed up with her. I was somewhat outraged. After that, Evette did her own SAT preparation, as best as she could. She took the SAT with mainstream kids—no extended time —and scored 970 all three times. Evette saw the whole test as too painful, and didn't want to agonize through it—extended time just prolonged the agony. She wanted to just get done with it and move forward.

She had a few run-ins but that didn't put her off the college-search process. In high school, she already knew she would be recruited for an athletic scholarship. At first, she wanted to work with her college counselor, but the counselor's experience with LD students was minimal. After two sessions, Evette and I decided to do our own college search. We settled on four criteria, the first being the most important: a lacrosse scholarship; some LD support; a school close to home; and physical layout of the school.

We checked out four schools—all had good lacrosse programs and all were within driving distance from Baltimore—400 miles was the farthest. Although Evette was good in both hockey and lacrosse, I came to realize that more feminine girls are playing lacrosse. We decided then on the lacrosse route. In our preliminary research, we also looked at the physical layout of a campus and, finally, LD facilities, so support was there if needed.

In her junior year, Evette was offered a lacrosse scholarship at Harvard University. But she needed to score above 1050 in the SAT. This turned her off. Plus, Harvard is a private school. Evette had gone to a private college-prep high school for girls in Baltimore, and after the Harvard visit, felt she wanted to go to public school for college. She ended up applying to:

University of Virginia   University of North Carolina
Boston University   University of Delaware

Her first choice was the University of Delaware—she didn't want to be too far away from home. She also had played field hockey and lacrosse there as a high-school student, and that familiarity helped. The coach met with her the summer between her junior and senior years, and indirectly said she'd get in. She decided, then, to commit early and was 100 percent more relaxed in her senior year. That was a good call.

Evette didn't check the LD box on her application, didn't include any psycho-education tests with her application—not until she was accepted —and didn't write a cover letter to say that she had a different learning style. She just wanted to be accepted as a good athlete, period.

The University of Delaware won. Evette knew immediately "The campus, here, is very organized," she said. "I don't like places that are confusing." Intuitively, she knew Delaware would work for her. It had all the criteria.

It's a large school—14,000 students—but the campus is well laid out. They have a special learning center, in a separate complex, with a good program, and she takes all her tests in the resource center.

I think when it came to the college search, we had luck on our side. We found a school close to home that offered a lacrosse scholarship, and Evette would be with average students. It's turning out to be a good match.

ISABEL WESLEY

Isabel's son, Russ, 18, is a freshman at the University of Oregon. Russ' brother, Curt, 21, is a senior at the University of Colorado at Boulder. Russ worked with his school counselor and considered his dad's favorite schools to come up with a variety of college choices.

We took a different route for our second son. Russ' success in life won't be based entirely on academics. He has charm. He's very good-looking. And he's an All-County volleyball player. Our first criterion for a college setting was a place where he would be happy. A setting with less academic pressure, but still someplace that was a good school, was our second consideration.

After putting Curt through the college-search process, I was familiar with several potential choices. Russ' high-school counselor also had resources. Together, we came up with an extensive list:

University of Miami, FL	Boston University, MA
The American University, DC	Denver University, CO
Lewis & Clark, OR	Linfield, McMinnville, OR
University of Oregon	North Arizona State University
Arizona State University	University of Arizona
San Diego State, CA	University of San Diego

Initially, Russ was pretty casual about the whole process. But once he got accepted to the University of Oregon, he became very focused.

Russ used the Common Application Form for most of the schools. He wrote one essay and turned it into two or three essays wherever necessary. His essay was about Bob, his mentor. He reflected on their relationship. I made Russ take a Writer's Workshop to get rid of his writer's block for his college-application essay. Actually, we took the class together at our local community college. The course didn't grade on spelling, only on creativity. The focus was on spontaneous, in-class writing, with feedback from students of different ages. Russ' only concern was reading aloud.

Before the class, Russ would look at a blank monitor for hours. I'd ask him just to write any 10 words. Sometimes, I'd simply suggest he lie down on the floor, close his eyes and talk . . . about his summer in Costa Rica. He told me such incredible stories. He speaks much better than he writes.

Continuing, though, with the college-application process, Russ also got very strong personal recommendations and accentuated his personal skills on the application form. He did take the SAT with extended time and, in his personal statement, explained his different learning style. Russ didn't want to be part of an LD program. He wants to be accepted as a "regular" student. He needs to be in a place where he can be successful and not be labeled. Academic Advising and Student Services at the University of Oregon is there for him if he needs help, but, so far, he hasn't used their services.

◫

MARIE DOUGLAS

Marie's daughter, Francis, 23, graduated from Willamette University in Oregon with a bachelor's degree in English and a minor in art. Francis chose Willamette because there was no foreign-language requirement.

For the most part, Francis was an "A" student in high school at a parochial girls' school in Honolulu. But in Spanish I, she got her first and only "C." Then, in the last semester of Spanish II, there was a "D." Otherwise, she had a 3.5 GPA.

So, needless to say, when it came to the college-research process, we looked for a place where a foreign-language requirement could be waived or substituted. We researched about eight colleges, east and west. Francis then narrowed that down to West Coast schools. The "Final Four" looked like this:

Lewis & Clark, Portland, OR   Willamette University, Salem, OR
Denver University, Denver, CO   Colorado College, Colorado Springs, CO

Most of the schools we looked at didn't have a specific LD Department, but Francis was more concerned about the foreign-language requirement and the campus location.

Francis applied only through the regular Admissions Department at each school (not separately to the LD Department), but she included a letter of explanation about her dyslexia. Once she was accepted at Lewis & Clark, Denver and Willamette, we pursued the foreign-language waiver. She got a "conditional acceptance" to Colorado College. Colorado allows a student to design his/her own major. That way, the foreign-language requirement is excluded. But she decided to go with Willamette.

It was a safe place for her. It was traditional and small. It was a good place for her to grow. But, before accepting at Willamette, she talked with the Dean of Students, who suggested she pursue a Bachelor of Science (not a Bachelor of Arts) degree. Francis would be able to take three computer/scientific classes instead of a foreign language. If she pursued a Bachelor of Arts, she would need to petition for a foreign-language waiver. She didn't want to risk a refusal.

Francis also was fortunate to have an extremely supportive advisor—a Harvard Ph.D. graduate in the English Department. He understood her way of thinking. He liked her creativity and anticipated her occasional "C" or "D." But he always told her a different learning style was most refreshing. Francis graduated in four years.

BETSY WASS

Betsy's daughter, Ella, 26, is a doctoral student in Sociocultural Anthropology at the University of Washington. Ella got her bachelor's in psychology at Pitzer College in California and her master's in social work at the University of Washington. When Ella was looking at under-grad schools, she targeted those with no math requirement.

That wasn't an easy task, way back in 1990. But Hampshire College near Amherst fell into that category and so did Pitzer College. Actually, Ella's was the last class at Pitzer that didn't have a math requirement. Ella and I also looked at colleges that had very few GE requirements. We came up with these options:

Hampshire College, MA	The American University, DC
University of Arizona	University of Colorado at Boulder

Pitzer was a sensational school for Ella. She entered as a high-school kid and they made her into a "scholar."

SURE-FOOTED

PEGGY AVERY

Peggy's daughter, Lacey, 17, is a high-school junior at a special school for dyslexia. Peggy and her husband, Bill, are reviewing college options for Lacey, who reads at a 6th-grade level, spells at a 3rd-grade level, but comprehends at a college level. After months of research, Peggy has identified key elements that will make Lacey's college placement successful, one of which is finding a school close to home.

Most days, my teenage daughter didn't want to talk to me about the college-application process. Lacey has an underlying fear of performance and doesn't trust herself. She also doesn't know what college is about. She once said to me: "Mom, I have this much trouble performing in high school, with a great support system and teachers who know me, how will I ever cope in college?"

So, I just went ahead and did the preliminary college search myself. I networked with friends and other parents and listened to what happened to other college students. I'm also a member of a parent support group for children with learning disabilities. In addition, working in a school for dyslexia, we get calls from parents telling us about their child's college experiences. One alumnus of that school suggested visiting the University of Ozarks in Arkansas. A neighbor told me about Schreiner College in Texas.

I don't want to send Lacey someplace where she might fail. Her first year at college, in particular, needs to be successful. Lacey learns slowly and reads slowly. She needs to figure out what she can handle on her own. I hear too many stories about "Johnnie" going off to college and coming home after the first semester. In my heart, I know Lacey must have a learning support system wherever she goes.

I also have been looking ahead at career options for Lacey. She's good with little children and very familiar with a multisensory way of teaching. Elementary Education could be an option, although her deepest interest is in animals. But I think vet school may be too overwhelming for her.

This year, Lacey had to take a compulsory Career Curriculum course, requiring her to visit three college campuses and report back. She took the opportunity to look at possible choices. These are the colleges she chose and the ones we visited:

1 University of the Ozarks, Clarkesville, AR – This tops our list at the moment. With a student body of less than 600, this liberal-arts school can provide a personal touch. The Jones Learning Support Center on campus offers editors for papers and textbooks on tape. I told Lacey she'd instantly have a substitute mother on campus. The center also has DragonDictate, a voice-recognition program. That would be wonderful. For research papers, she would just speak into the computer. No spelling errors!

We'd have to pay extra, actually a lot extra, to use the Jones Learning Center—something like $4,750 a semester in addition to the $3,625 per semester tuition fee. But the additional charge only would be for one or two semesters.

2 Schreiner College, Kerrville, TX – We both felt comfortable with this choice. In the Learning Support Center, a resource specialist suggested a shopping list for Lacey—things she would need to succeed at college. We liked this approach. We were told by the Admissions Director they don't alter the curriculum for someone like Lacey, but would give her every means of support. That put us at ease.

3 Centenary College, Shreveport, LS – Lacey liked this campus. It's a small, Methodist, liberal-arts college with a student body of 800. But it doesn't have a specific Learning Center. The school relies on the students' advocacy with individual professors. There's a strict honor system, very strict. But, because it doesn't offer editing of papers and textbooks wouldn't necessarily be on tape, this might not be a good choice. Lacey needs that additional support.

4 Texas Lutheran College, Seguin, TX – Lacey liked this college a lot, but it doesn't have a specific Learning Resource Center. My concern is whether they really do give support to students like Lacey. Lacey is a good advocate for herself and she's a survivor. But she still needs an editor and textbooks on tape. I've got to be sure they're there for her.

Although we didn't visit them, there are three other schools where Lacey may apply—Arizona State University, the University of Arkansas at Little Rock and the University of Arkansas at Fayetteville.

They're all very large campuses. I think she'd be lost in such a setting. For 10 years, Lacey went to a small, elementary/middle school. The teachers knew her well. I don't think we should alter that formula.

Lacey was accepted to the University of the Ozarks.

ANN BELL

Ann's son, John, 18, is a senior in high school in Honolulu. He's heading to the mainland for college and is looking into schools with a strong science program.

Finances were a big factor in our decision. It was a toss-up between Cal Poly and Humboldt State University, both in California. My husband and I didn't want John to go where there was a huge cultural difference. California fit the bill.

All total, John applied to five colleges:

Humboldt State	Cal Poly
University of San Diego, CA	Oregon State University
University of Hawaii	

John applied ONLY to Admissions at these schools. He gave no LD indication on his form, yet he submitted SAT scores with extended time. His college counselor said he shouldn't self-disclose because he'd be classified. He's going to Cal Poly. We're delighted. It's a rural setting. That's more acceptable to our family. It might force him to stay on campus, although, we're sure he'll be tempted to surf!

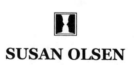

SUSAN OLSEN

Susan's son, Andrew, 19, wanted to follow in the footsteps of his older brother, Luke, 25, an alumni of Southern Methodist University in Texas. All three of Susan's boys looked only at schools in Texas.

I have to admit most Texas kids are parochial in their thinking. Most high-school students in Dallas stay in South Texas for college. My three boys, all dyslexic, were no different.

Luke is an alumni of SMU, which has an excellent LD support system; Jim is a senior at Texas A&M; and Andrew is a freshman at SMU.

SALLY PRINCETON

Sally's daughter, Sue, 27, is a 1st-grade teacher in a school for learning disabilities. She's a graduate of the University of Norwich in Vermont. Sally and Sue looked for colleges close to home in Ohio or neighboring states.

We also looked at schools with a track team and a learning support group. Sue applied to eight, mainly in Ohio:

Mt. St. Joseph, Cincinnati	Otterbein College, Columbus
Muskingum, New Concord	Wittenberg College, Springfield
College of Wooster, Wooster	West Virginia Wesleyan College
Bethany College, WV	Landmark College, VT

I suggested Curry College in Massachusetts and Landmark because of their superior LD programs, but Sue ended up at Bethany. She just didn't want to be labeled again.

KARI BROWN

Kari's daughter, Brenda, 22, graduated from the University of Arizona with a bachelor's in psychology with a minor in Spanish. Kari and Brenda wanted to look at colleges near home, but with good support systems. The S.A.L.T. program at the University of Arizona won, hands down.

I wanted Brenda to be in a place where she would be comfortable, somewhere close to home. She applied to four schools:

University of California at Davis	University of California at Santa Cruz
University of California at Irvine	University of Arizona

■
STACEY PARKER

Stacey's daughter, Tosha, 20, is a sophomore at the University of Arizona. Tosha's sister, Kimberley, 17, is a junior in a college preparatory high school. Tosha applied only on the West Coast and really wanted a small, liberal-arts school. Still, the University of Arizona, with its exceptional S.A.L.T. program became the favorite.

Tosha, a borderline dyslexic, was a "B" student in a parochial high school. The school started to get more kids with different learning styles. But, while this helped Tosha, she still ran into teachers who thought giving her special accommodations was unfair to other students. She was experiencing real-life problems. I couldn't go in to fight every battle for her. I advised her from the sideline. Meanwhile, I did a lot of research on the college-application process before she met with her college counselor.

Word of mouth was pretty powerful in my research. I networked with parents with similar or the same backgrounds; got very involved in a school for dyslexia in Monterey, CA (I knew older kids from that school who had gone on to college); and I talked with an education consultant who was a family friend. He'd compiled a booklet on how to find a good college for LD students. It was a great help.

After doing a thorough search, I came up with several college options for Tosha. She ended up applying to seven and we visited four.

University of Washington	University of Oregon
University of Colorado at Boulder	Denver University, CO
Dennison, OH	Arizona State University
University of Arizona	

Of the seven schools, Tosha really liked Dennison, a small school with a one-on-one touch. The people were so friendly and really bent over backward to help. In the end, though, it was a little too far from home. It also was $30,000 per year for school and board. The University of Washington and the University of Oregon were second choices. But they didn't seem as complete or as good as the S.A.L.T. (Strategic Alternative Learning Techniques) program. Tosha ended up going to the University of Arizona on a gut feeling. I give her credit. She's very intuitive.

The S.A.L.T. program provided emotional safety for her. Counselors were there to help. It's a comprehensive, nurturing setting but it does require an additional fee of around $1,500 per semester. The program takes students by the hand, then moves them on after two years. Actually, Tosha broke away the second semester of her sophomore year. She was ready to be her own advocate.

The University of Arizona is a huge place and, coming from a small high school, it seemed even bigger. Thankfully, the S.A.L.T. program made Tosha feel she was in a small community, within a very large setting.

H

GINGER LITLOVER

Ginger's son, David, 18, is a freshman at the University of Arkansas at Fayetteville. The family's research process involved extensive use of reference books, a private college counselor and David's school counselor in Dallas.

David did some of the searching independently. He researched the *K. & W. Handbook* for the LD College Student. I used it, too, and then we collaborated. David got a sense of where he wanted to go and ended up applying to four schools:

University of Arkansas at Fayetteville   Kansas University
Auburn University, AL   University of Arizona

David's desire was to be in a large university setting with plenty of LD support services. With the exception of Auburn, all his choices had support programs, but to varying degrees. The University of Arizona offered heavy support during the freshman year and then gradually began to taper off by sophomore year.

David self-disclosed on the application form and took the SAT with extra time. For the University of Arizona, we submitted an application to both the Admissions Department and their S.A.L.T. program. He had to be accepted by both. The other colleges didn't require this.

David was accepted at the University of Arkansas and the University of Arizona. He decided to go to Arizona, but transferred to Arkansas for the spring semester of his freshman year because, socially, he was unhappy. There is less academic support at Arkansas, but David is quite capable of fending for himself.

MURRAY CHILTON

Murray's son, Freddie, 20, is a sophomore at the University of Colorado in Boulder. He wanted a large school with an established Learning Resource Center. Boulder has been a good fit.

Freddie needs an active LD support center. It was important that we actually visited the LD programs because there are varying degrees of support. Freddie also is a social animal. He wanted to go to a larger school, preferably out-of-state, so he could experience a different living style. Freddie ended up applying to:

> University of South Carolina Montana State
> University of Oregon University of Colorado at Boulder
> Texas A&M

Boulder has an excellent Learning Resource Center, an Orton Society on campus and tons of outdoor activities. The campus probably is more liberal than Freddie anticipated, but he's found his own group. It's been good for him to experience life outside of Texas and to work and party with students from different states.

CHRISTINA PETERSON

Christina's son, Allan, 22, recently graduated from the University of Southern California with a bachelor's degree in Business Administration (Entrepreneurs Program). His senior year of high school, Allan refused to look at colleges and was dogged about "his" game plan. Christina was dying inside. A lucky break occurred, though, when Allan met the faculty and staff at Marymount College in Palos Verdes, CA. They kindled something in him. He completed his AA degree and transferred to USC.

I knew deep down he wanted to go to college, but he was frightened. I went with what was comfortable for him and our family. But it was tearing me up. At one point, I thought he'd end up working in a car body shop. He was into looking good and into cars. He really wasn't interested in college.

Allan and I had a very strenuous relationship through high school until, finally, in his senior year, I let go. I never discussed schoolwork with him. I let him do his own thing. But Allan didn't graduate with his senior class. He had to attend summer school because he hadn't turned in two English papers. He didn't even go to graduation. I think he couldn't quite believe it happened to him. I was shattered. But I put on a very nonchalant front. He told me: "I'm not going to college. I'm getting a GED certificate." "OK," I responded. "Well, this is what's available to you with no college degree. You get a job and an apartment. OK. This is real life now." He was amazed at my reaction.

That summer, his father, David, suggested we go down to L.A. to look at Marymount. No commitment; just a fact-finding adventure. He listened to his father. He had interviews with Admissions and the Learning Center. Immediately, they said they'd love to have him. With a 94 percent success rate of getting into good schools (i.e., USC, UCLA) after Marymount, Allan was impressed. The sale had been made.

The school has a wonderful Learning Center. His advisor constantly told him how bright he was. Faculty were so positive. This was the first time in his life that he blossomed. His grades were coming up. That school was our saving grace.

Allan now was an adult. I let him tell me how he was doing. The pressure was off me. He started to believe in himself and, for the first time, he even told people he was dyslexic. That was his freshman year. He also took all the help he could get from his profs and the Resource Learning Center. He decided there was no shame asking for help.

Allan got his AA degree at Marymount and then transferred to USC, the Entrepreneurs Program, for his junior year. He's thrilled with his courses. He's very positive and self-assured. I asked him why he's so different now. He said: "You know, Mom, in high school you were always on my back. In college, I do my classes when I want to do them." He's developed into his own person. He's taken on responsibility. He's become independent.

I remember when Allan left for college I felt as if a 50-pound weight had been lifted off my shoulders. I told David we'd better enjoy ourselves because Allan would be back at Christmas, permanently. I was apprehensive. David thought otherwise. He was right. The most difficult thing for me all through this process was to let go. Just let go. I thought my son had disappeared down a drainpipe. As a parent, I cared so much. But Allan is a real success story. Now, I'm very proud of him.

WHAT PARENTS SAY ABOUT THE COLLEGE-SEARCH

While listening to what parents said about the college-search, some other interesting factors surface relating to the maturity of the 12th grader, the severity of the learning disability, financial concerns and the parents' attitude. Let's first look at the parents' responses within the framework of attitude.

Attitude

The confidence or security level of the 12th grader and his/her parents, absolutely alters the way families approach the college-search process. Those who want to embrace the process—take it on as a new adventure, incorporate specific criteria, and handle the process like any other search—represent the strategic planners. Those who feel more comfortable with a "secure" setting, look for a place of familiarity—familiar learning, people, culture and climate—I refer to them as sure-footed. Of the 26 parent interviews 52 percent represent strategic planners, 48 percent are sure-footed. (The maturity of the 12th grader, the severity of dyslexia, financial issues and the parents' attitude toward the college experience may have contributed to the interview results. I'll address these later in this section.)

Without a doubt, families who are sure-footed have an easier time with the college-search. They look at schools within their state or neighboring states and schools with an in-place LD support system. In doing this, they simplify the search. In their eyes, close family ties and a supportive LD system are essential to a smooth college transition from high school.

For strategic planners, they target schools with specific criteria—a small student-teacher ratio, a particular major, varsity athletics, a different culture, a religious campus etc. Geographic location and/or a strong LD program are also important but are not critical. Some parents search out colleges where a foreign-language or math requirement can be waived or substituted. They find several schools offering American Sign Language as a foreign language(FL) option—Brigham Young University and Stanford, to name a couple. A few that don't require an FL are Southern Methodist University, Colorado College, Boston University—School of General Studies, School of Management, School of Drama and Sergent College of Health & Rehabilitation Sciences. And, some schools substitute a cultural course, a Reading Sequence, for a specific language, and others offer a Bachelor of Science instead of a Bachelor of Arts (Williamette University, OR). The University of Oregon offers a foreign language or math option as part of the

General Education package. Then, in grad school, substituting a math class for a "like" class sometimes happens.

Degree of Learning Disability

Here, past school experiences seem to influence the way families approach the college search. If a student has difficulties in 9-12th grades, and his/her self-esteem is unsteady, parents go the sure-footed route. If the student requires extensive help with school work, parents focus on selecting colleges with comprehensive LD services, those that offer voice-recognition software, a reader, a scribe, individually recorded books on tape, advisors, etc.

Most students are considered to be moderately affected by dyslexia. At the other end of the scale, there is a small percentage who are slightly affected and a small percentage who are severely affected. Those with the most severity have no option but to apply to schools that provide the most comprehensive learning programs such as the American University DC, Landmark College VT, University of Arizona, AZ, University of Colorado at Boulder, CO and the University of Ozarks, AR.

Maturity

It seems that high-schoolers—in most instances, boys—who are not ready to do college, need to be handled cautiously. Staying local and attending a two-year community college is a sensible short-term measure. For those who have unpleasant high-school experiences, staying local is probably also a good idea. But, at some point, the apron strings need to be cut. In the final analysis, it still came down to how confident the student is about the next chapter in his/her life.

Financial Commitment

Only one parent, Ann Bell, said finances are a big factor in the decision process. But I think this is an underlying concern in most families. The low tuition at state schools definitely is more acceptable and accounted for $2/3$ of the interviews.

Some students choose to take a fifth year to graduate from college, while others find it "necessary" because they can't get all their required credits within four years. Whichever way, the additional costs need to be calculated.

Parents Views and Influences

From what parents told me, the home atmosphere overflows into students' attitudes toward college. When there is calmness in the family, the student approaches the process as a new experience, one to explore. Where there is anxiety—concerns about who will replace mom or dad as "house-editors" or the driving distance between home and college—then the sure-footed approach prevails.

I was left with a feeling that, if parents can inject more objectivity into the search—this is especially difficult with a personal commodity—there is less strain on the relationship with their son or daughter and less tension in the home. It is important to remember that 12th graders still soldier on with their daily studies, despite the college-search. So, timing becomes essential in all of this. Setting aside 30 minutes per week for discussing college issues, usually after a good meal, is a good way to go. Definitely, don't toss around important college questions just as your 12th grader is leaving for school or going on a date. Timing is crucial.

Most families I interviewed, do their own college search and don't rely on the college counselor. Many counselors may not be aware of comprehensive LD programs or colleges with special services. (They have enough to do with mainstream student placements.) This is not a criticism, more a suggestion that they need to become more up-to-date on LD college programs.

In talking with parents across the country, there is no right or wrong way to do the college-search process. It's like choosing a vacation. Both formats can work; one produces security—returning to familiar territory, selecting a place similar to the previous one, or only targeting English-speaking countries; the other offers new horizons—new cultures, cuisine, transportation modes, languages.

Never forget that, less than 20 years ago, students with a learning difference had a hard time convincing Admissions to accept them into an under-grad program, let alone grad school. Now new standards have been set across America. We have the Americans with Disabilities Act of 1990, Learning Resource Centers, special accommodations, state-of-the-art equipment and software. The stage has been set.

POINTERS BEFORE APPLYING TO COLLEGE

❑　Get tested early—K-8th grade. Critics smell a scam if testing is done as late as 11th grade because more juniors are requesting extended time on the SAT with recent testing results. For your college application, admissions asks for testing done within the past 3 years.

❑　Network with teachers, professionals and personal friends for college references, even as early as the summer of your senior year, or before. Select individuals who can best describe your attributes (with specific examples) and NOT your grades!!!

❑　Get involved in out-of-school activities you enjoy such as sports, drama, music, computers and, especially, community-service projects. This will show Admissions that there's more to your application than just "B's" and "C's." Commitment in specific activities will highlight your skills and character traits.

❑　Show you have a track record of part-time work, and that you've taken on responsibility and, in some instances, leadership.

❑　Understand how you learn best—visually, auditorily or kines-thetically—so that you are well prepared to include a cover letter about your different learning style and your strengths and weaknesses.

❑　Ask for extended time, oral testing or a reader for the SAT, well in advance of the test dates (telephone and fax numbers are listed in the SAT handout). In past years, students with special accommodations take the test on a different day, at a different time and in a different location than mainstream students.

POINTERS FOR THE COLLEGE-SEARCH

❑ Talk with your college counselor, alumni, teachers, high-school coach, neighbors, friends, friends parents, etc. Gather as much information as you can so you'll be better informed when you start to work on your college-search.

❑ Get a copy of *Choosing the Right College*, by Georgeann duChossois and Elissa Stein, a step-by-step system to assist students with learning differences. It is published by the Access to Learning Program, NYU (New York University), New York, NY 10012.

❑ Set up 3 criteria. Decide on one that ranks first and then keep focused. Keep second and third choices not too far behind. Consider the following:

for school work
      effective Learning Resource Center
      comprehensive LD program
      exemption from a foreign language (FL)
      availability of American Sign Language as FL requirement
      Bachelor of Science degree with no FL requirement
      courses offered for your major
      acceptance of Common Application Form in admissions process
      scholarships in the athletics, academics, fine arts, music etc.
about the college
      large or small (>2,000 students) student population
      physical layout of campus
      type of school—conservative or progressive, private or public, religious or non-denominational, university or liberal-arts college
      geographic location—close to home or neighboring states, or "across-country", inner-city, uban or rural setting

❑ Check out 2 College Guide Books (more than two gets confusing). Try to get acquainted with what's available and where your specific criteria fit into the puzzle. *K&W Guide to Colleges for the Learning Disabled* is reader friendly and lists colleges by states, not alphabetically. Two additional choices are *Peterson's: Colleges with Programs for Students with Learning Disabilities* and *Colleges for Students with Learning Disabilities, by Midge Lipkin*

(Schoolsearch). Both offer a more traditional format but are equally useful. Remember to locate current issues, within the last two years.

❑ If you're feeling confident about the college experience, spread your options wide, explore different areas. At first it's scary, but then you handle it.

❑ If you want to be within driving distance from home, apply to colleges in your state, or neighboring state. That's totally OK. Go with your gut feeling and don't look back.

❑ If you feel you're in a "vacuum" and want to take a year off, postpone the college-application process. But, DO something worthwhile that will make college Admissions go "Wow!" Spend a year abroad in an English-speaking country or if you're in the Boy or Girl Scouts of America, volunteer at their worldwide campuses, or work on a community project. Make a difference. Remember, "time out" means you can include a unique experience on your college-application form!

❑ Look for colleges offering a Bachelor of Science degree in your major, with no foreign-language requirement. Look for colleges offering American Sign Language as your FL requirement. And look for a few colleges, usually liberal arts that have no foreign-language requirement. GE (general education) exemptions, are rarer. I only know of one place—Colorado College, CO—where a student designs his or her own major.

For A Campus Visit

❑ Where possible, check out the physical layout of the campus. If a visit is not possible, ask to see a campus map. Physical layout is important when navigating classrooms, resource centers, etc. The more modular the system, the less confusing it is.

❑ Check out the Learning Resource Center, talk with advisors, tutors and LD students. Try to get a feel for the center and assess what is offered to the student—i.e., advisors, note takers, proof readers, scribes, readers, extended time on tests and exams, books on tape, a quiet room to take an exam, pre-registration for classes, dorm preferences, one-on-one tutoring and software programs, those with voice recognition, in particular. Find out if there is an additional cost for these facilities above tuition.

POINTERS FOR
THE COLLEGE APPLICATION FORM

❏ Use the *Common Application Form*—one size fits ALL colleges. One application, one essay. It saves so much time. It's difficult enough to keep up with senior-year classes and then to fill out college application forms at the same time. Find ways to simplify the process.

❏ Send two sets of your application form to each college—one to Admissions, the other to the Director of the Disability Resource Center. You want to keep both parties in the loop so an informed decision can be made about your acceptance or rejection.

❏ Check off the LD box on the college application form. Please self disclose. Red flags fly when inconsistency occurs. When 11th graders take the SAT with extended time but don't self-disclose on the application form, Admissions suspect something.

❏ Include a cover letter in your application discussing your learning difference, your strengths and weakness and your preferred learning style (auditory, visual, kinesthetic). Make sure that they know how you learn best (give specifics) and what services (a note taker, proof-reader, etc.) you would require on campus. Don't use a "poor-me" approach. Rather, show you can handle the situation.

❏ Include personal references from people who know you for your attributes, not just for your grades.

❏ Include a photograph of yourself. Admissions can then see who you are.

❏ The college-search process involves self-reflection as well as an evaluation of colleges. The process is about you, the student, not about mom or dad. You are looking to achieve your college "nirvana" —a place where you are safe, where you won't fall through the cracks and, most importantly, where you'll be happy.

DYSLEXIA FRIENDLY COLLEGES

East Coast

American University, DC
Bates, ME
Bethany College, WV
Boston College, Boston, MA
Boston University, Boston MA
Bowdon, ME
Brown University, RI
Clarke, MA
Colby, ME
Connecticut College for Women, CT
Drew, NJ
Hampshire College, MA
Landmark College, VT
Long Island College, NY

Mitchell College, PA
Norwich University, VT
Norton, MA
NY Institute of Technology, NY
NYU (New York University), NY
Old Dominion College, VA
Syracuse University, NY
The George Washington University, DC
Vassar College, Poukeepsie, NY
West Virginia Wesleyan College, WV
Wheaton, MA
University of Maryland @ College Park, MD
University of Massachusetts, Amherst, MA
University of Rhode Island, RI

Midwest

Beloit, WI.
Bradley, Peoria, IL
College of Wooster, Wooster, OH
Dennison, OH
Kalamazoo College, MI
Kenyon, OH
Kansas University, Kansas City, KS
Lake Forest College, IL
Mt. St Joseph, Cincinnati, OH

Michigan State University, MI
Montana State, MT
Otterbein College, Columbus, OH
University of Indiana, Bloomington, IN
University of Indianapolis, IN
University of Michigan, Ann Arbor, MI
Washington University, MO
Wittenberg College, Springfield, OH

South/Southeast and West Coast - see page 228

DYSLEXIA FRIENDLY COLLEGES

South /Southeast
Auburn University, Auburn, AL
Centenary College, Shreveport, LS
Lynn College, Boca Rotan, FL
Prairie View A & M, TX
Schreiner College, Kerrville, TX
SMU (Southern Methodist University), TX
Texas A & M, Corpus Christi, TX
Texas Lutheran College, Seguin, TX
University of Arkansas @ Little Rock, AR
University of Arkansas @ Fayetteville, AR
University of Miami, FL
University of the Ozarks, Clarkesville, AR

West Coast
Arizona State, AZ
Brigham Young University) UT
Cal Poly (California Polytechnic State University) CA
Cal State @ Northridge, CA
Colorado College, Colorado Springs, CO
Denver University, CO
Lewis & Clark, Portland, OR
Marymount College, Palos Verdes, CA
North Arizona State University, AZ
Occidental College, CA
Pitzer (Claremont Colleges), CA
Scripps (Claremont Colleges), CA
SFSU (San Francisco State University, CA
University of Arizona, AZ
University of California @ Berkeley, CA
University of California @ Davis, CA
University of California @ Los Angeles, CA
University of California @ Santa Cruz, CA
University of Redlands, Los Angeles, CA
University of Colorado, Boulder, CO
University of Hawaii, HI
University of Oregon. OR
University of Washington, WA
University of Southern California, CA
Williamette University, Salem OR
Whitman college, OR

4

THE COLLEGE EXPERIENCE
STUDENTS

COLLEGE STUDENT INTERVIEWS

College students with dyslexia, here, offer unique stories. Some humorous, others sad, and many with creative coping strategies. It is refreshing to see how most of them have "blossomed" in college.

For these students, like most, college is a whole new ball game. The umbilical cord is cut—Mom and Dad are no longer local. New terrain is being traversed. The question is how students cope in this new setting and what tools and strategies, if any, they use.

In 47 interviews, I pose the question "Are you asking for special accommodations in college?" That included extended time on tests or exams, extended time on reading assignments, readers, scribes, note takers, books on tape etc. I also ask if they add their own coping strategies, if Dragon NaturallySpeaking (a voice-recognition program) or MicNote Pad (a Mac shareware recording software program) are working as enhancement tools, and if ASL (American Sign Language) is being substituted for a Romance language? Are papers e-mailed home for editing or is the Learning Resource Center replacing mom or dad's proofreading skills?

It turns out most students are asking for special accommodations and many are incorporating their own coping strategies. Attitudes about accommodations and strategies, however, are dependent upon individual character traits, such as how they handle a situation or get through life.

The themes that best categorize their responses are as follows:

1. *Conventionalist*   3. *Independents*
2. *Low Profilers*   4. *Pragmatists*

Special accommodations go with *conventionalists*. They work closely with the Learning Resource Center on campus and with academic counselors and tutors, and work less on creating personal strategies. *Conventionalists* go with the flow, become situated in a zone, and really have no reason—and often no time—to look beyond what is offered, to come up with personalized strategies. *Conventionalists,* in general, prefer structure and stability.

Low profilers want to lie low. They are light on both special accommodations and coping strategies. These students don't disclose their learning disability, don't associate with the Learning Resource Center, don't ask for special accommodations, and let as few people as possible know about their different learning style. Getting papers edited from home often still is the norm. *Low profilers* don't want to muddy the waters or raise red flags. Some have been burned, others are scared to show their LD, a few just want to be left to do college as they prefer.

Independents are heavy on personalized coping strategies and light on special accommodations. They don't officially hook up with the Learning Resource Center, but ask for special accommodations on an informal basis, working directly with a professor. Independents tend to be individualistic, prefer flexibility, and are somewhat visionary about the college scene. They prefer to do it their way, and in doing so, utilize their personalized strategies over conventional accommodations on campus.

Pragmatists try to strike a balance between special accommodations and personalized coping strategies (and they do a good job!) The bulk of student responses are here. I refer to them as *pragmatists* because their attitudes range from "I'll take what's out there at college and then top it with my own strategies," or "I'm on cruise control. I'm comfortable with what's out there, but I like my own way, too." *Pragmatists* work closely with counselors, proofreaders, note takers, etc., in the Learning Resource Center. They also work on their own strategies. Periodically, they fine-tune their plan, balancing the scales.

Overall, students talk openly about their college experience and their self esteem. Some interviews are analytical, some emotional, and some just plain factual. Others include risky strategies from gutsy students. I'm sure you will embrace them all and learn from their experiences and anecdotes. Tips from some of the students are at the end of their interviews; these are directed at K-12 students and college students. And, at the end of this section the pointers touch on strategies for test taking, researching papers and reading assignments, dealing with math and foreign-language classes, and developing computer strategies.

College students have some strong opinions about special accommodations, the Learning Resource Centers and faculty. They also speak frankly about multiple-choice testing, foreign-language classes, and standardized testing for grad school (GRE, GMAT, LSAT, etc.) In some ways, they are a direct contrast to the sibling respondents (young ones).

I hope you will read these interviews with the understanding that they don't represent one particular university or college. More, they're an indicator of where young people with dyslexia are going to school today. I also hope you will see reflections of yourself or young adults you know, in their stories.

CONVENTIONALISTS

Special accommodations go hand-in-hand with athletic and academic scholarships. For some students, though, special accommodations simply keep them afloat. *Conventionalists* tend to be heavy on special accommodations and light on personalized coping strategies. Let me explain further.

Jon Roberts and Sara Rogers tap into the Learning Resource Center on a regular basis. When Jon starts out at the University of the Ozarks, AR, classes are tough and it takes him a full semester just to learn how to study for tests. His coordinator and tutors meet with him daily, and, subsequently, become his "life-line." Sara, too, takes extended time on tests at the B.U.I.L.D. (Baccalaureate for the University of Indianapolis Learning Disabled) center for all classes, and also requests a reader. Sara, a junior, is in the Early Childhood Education program and wants this "additional" support to get her through college.

Just when Nicole Childers has her special needs in place at the University of California at Santa Cruz, CA, she decides to spend her junior year abroad at the University of Lancaster, England. She has to check out the learning resources, once again. Before she leaves, she makes sure she takes documentation of her dyslexia. The UK school offers a note taker, tape-recorder, editor and PC. They also point her in the direction of a dyslexia support group on campus. She is armed.

Jazmine Wilkins, Brittan Woods and Evette Mann focus on weight training, practices, match play and NCAA achievements. Special accommodations and personalized strategies aren't in their vocabulary. For Brittan, having an athletic advisor on board to help organize classes and get early registration is a major plus. His advisor steers him through all the chaos of trying to balance schoolwork and represent James Madison University in gymnastics. Jazmine's situation is similar. Her personal tutor at Indiana State University works weekday nights with her after track practice. Sometimes, Jazmine phones her to look over a paper. Jazmine knows her tutor is her security blanket. For Evette, on a lacrosse scholarship at the University of Delaware, free tutoring is offered whenever she needs help, usually when she's organizing a paper and proofreading it. Evette also asks for tutoring if the lacrosse season—during spring semester—takes her out of class too often. College is made comfortable for these athletes.

Sam Lee, a President's Scholar (academic scholarship) at Southern Methodist University, TX is failing in fiction and rhetoric (both honor classes). Sam is an engineer major. Fortunately, the Director of the Writing Center steps in to help and becomes his mentor. The rest is history.

A downside to these *conventionalists* is that they get situated and then have no desire or time to create personal coping strategies. These students take what they can get and run with it.

CONVENTIONALISTS

JAZMINE WILKINS, recent graduate, Indiana State Univ

Jazmine, 27, didn't have any "low times" in college. Being on an athletic track scholarship with special accommodations meant Jazmine was pampered. There was no time and no necessity for her to come up with her own coping strategies.

How did I become involved in track? I was 15 at the time, a freshman in high school. One of my friends suggested I try out for the team. She said I was an exceptional sprinter. Together with the track coach, they gave me so much encouragement, I ended up on the varsity team three straight years.

I found out about my dyslexia in 11th grade. I would study long hours for tests, well into the night, but only pull "C's." My mother realized something wasn't right and connected with the Partners Center for Education in downtown Indianapolis, where she got advice on how I might best take the SAT. I ended up getting a reader, extended time and took the test outside class, in a quiet room.

I wasn't planning to go to college, though. In reality, I really didn't think I could make it. But I'd heard Indiana State had a strong LD program and a great track team. My parents suggested I talk to the track coach. The rest is history. I got offers from Purdue University, Ohio State, Ball State, Monsee, IN and Alabama A&M. Indiana State won hands down. It was close to home, had a solid LD program and the coach wanted me on the varsity track team.

Help was always there in college. I had a personal tutor and we worked weekday nights after track practice. Other times, I'd just phone her to look over a paper. My tutor was my security blanket. I was also required to do study hall—20 hours per week—and there I got help from more tutors, in any subject!

I was pretty well-known around campus for track—I won the NCAA 200 meters indoor title and seven NCAA titles, 100 and 200 meter outdoor event —and my tutor sent notes to all my profs, so I had an easy time with special accommodations. I got extra time on tests, used a tape recorder for lectures but took my own notes, got preparation tests to study before a test, and was allowed a reader. The reader, a paid grad student from the Learning Center, worked miracles with me. I needed to hear the words out loud. For more complex work, I'd ask the reader to read paragraph by paragraph, paraphrasing everything so I could understand. She and my one-on-one tutor definitely made college doable.

I know there's so much more required reading material at grad school, but I know I can handle it. I eventually want to own my own recreation center, so I'll need a master's in Sport Finance & Business. I'll probably end up at Indiana U/Purdue University because my tutor lives in Indianapolis. I need my whole support system to pull me through. Then, I know I can do it.

Jazmine suggests:

❑ Remember Philippians 4:13: "I can do everything through him who gives me strength."

❑ Keep your head up because there's always a light at the end of the tunnel.

JON ROBERTS, freshman, University of the Ozarks

Jon, 18, is in his second semester and uses the Jones Learning Center on a daily basis for maximum support with his learning disability.

The first few weeks at college were overwhelming. Classes were tough and it took me a full semester just to learn how to study for tests. My coordinator and tutors helped me make it. Actually, my coordinator is my lifeline. She's part of the Jones Learning Center, where I get my textbooks taped and get specialized help in math, reading and writing. I also have peer tutors and get copies of lecture notes for all my classes. Most importantly, though, I see my coordinator on a daily basis.

She helps me with my tests, which are given to me on a one-to-one basis. If there are short-essay questions, she writes my answers. For longer essays, I dictate my thoughts while she types them on the computer. I either use this method or use the voice-recognition program on the computer. She taught me how to use flash cards to help me match facts and discussion in my "New Testament" class. She also wants me to take more time preparing for tests. And, yes, my test results have improved. With her help, and the faculty support here, college definitely is doable.

I was determined to get my high-school diploma, but I wondered whether I was college-bound material. After all, I have cerebral palsy and I'm dyslexic. But my mom kept telling me: "Hang in there. You can do it." My friends were supportive and everyone in my small country-school class of 13 treated me like a regular student. Then, I was accepted at the University of the Ozarks.

There have been some drawbacks, though. Studying longer hours has cut down on the amount of time I spend with my friends. There are times I miss going out with them. But I know after I graduate, it will pay off. I'm in college for a purpose—to get an education. I know I'll make it.

Jon suggests:

❑ Research the LD programs, like the Jones Learning Center, where you can get accommodations and support *without having to fight for it!* I didn't think I could make it to college, but I'm lucky enough to be here. I don't think I would have succeeded otherwise.

BRITTAN WOODS, sophomore, James Madison University

Brittan, 20, believes being on a gymnastics scholarship takes all the hassle out of asking for special accommodations. His athletic advisor helps plan out his classes and register early for them. Brittan gets one-on-one tutoring, in any subject, whenever he needs help. Personalized coping strategies aren't necessary.

My love for gymnastics keeps me going. I've been competing since the age of 6. I forget about schoolwork when I'm performing under the bright lights (I've won the Junior Olympic National Championships, the USA Gymnastics title and I've made All-American.) My family and a special school for dyslexia from 7th to 9th grade, helped, too. My dad is a CEO of a manufacturing company and he has dyslexia. I had a great role model. Still, it seemed like I had to climb Mt. St. Helen's.

I remember in 6th grade being taken out of most classes and placed in the Resource Center—a confined room with a resource teacher and LD students—at the local public school. From then on, I knew I was different. On my transcript, it indicated that I'd passed every class, but there were no grades. There was nothing. OK, I was slower than my classmates, but wasn't I worthy of grades?

It was really scary in class when I had to read out aloud. I'd start to cough, stumble and just try to get the words out as quickly as possible. I don't think it was really an option to ask not to read. My best friend was exceptionally smart and he understood my dilemma. My parents understood, too, and, eventually, I asked to go to a different school, somewhere other than our local neighborhood school.

Moving ahead a few years, I've completed all my GE requirements except for math at James Madison. I'm required to take two math classes for my degree in Environmental Science—one in statistics, the other in algebra. I also have the option to take these classes at a community college and then transfer the credits. Bottom line, math is really difficulty for me. I understand the work. I'm just years behind everyone else. I also read very slowly and have a lot of trouble spelling and writing papers. I've had no serious trouble with academics so far, though, shooting straight "A's" and "B's."

I have to say my athletic advisors have steered me through the chaos. They've been a great help in organizing my classes and getting early registration. Sometimes, I'm in classes I shouldn't be in just because of early registration. I've decided now that 12 units per semester is most comfortable.

I haven't asked for books on tape. I haven't really needed them. But I always take advantage of extended time on tests. I'm a little uncomfortable cutting into the prof's time when I take extended time in the regular exam slot, so I prefer to take the test in the prof's office or in a room next to the office so they can continue their work. There's a handful of teachers who raise their eyebrows about special needs, but most of the time, the profs don't mind. I just set up a different day and time.

Most days, I use practice time in the gym as a nice contrast to schoolwork. Sometimes, though, I have so much work our coach lets me miss practice.

Brittan suggests:

❑ Know you have a problem, then get help.

❑ You have to work for "it."

SAM LEE, freshman, Southern Methodist University

Sam, 19, has the kind of charisma and outgoing personality that get him where he wants to be in college, with faculty and staff. Everything else is secondary.

I have a lot of internal motivation. I just want to do well. I also want to prove to people that I'm smart. But, no matter how hard I try, I can never do as well as I want to. My older sister, 29, is an alumna of the University of Texas and, in some ways, I try to mirror her.

I have my successes too, though. At SMU, I'm on a full-tuition scholarship. I'm a President's Scholar—someone who demonstrates all-around excellence. I'm also an Eagle Scout and very active in our church.

I don't think I could have made it this far without my family. They've been extremely supportive and advocated for me several times in grade school. My dad, who has a Ph.D. degree in physics from the University of Pennsylvania and was first in his class, shows me systems to improve work output.

A low time for me was when I got diagnosed. My pediatrician suggested testing very early because my disability had manifested itself in speech. In kindergarten through 2nd grade, only my godmother and my mother could understand me. After the testing, I was put into speech therapy. I tested above average in IQ (135) and my reading disability didn't unfold until much later. It was in high school and college when telltale discrepancies surfaced.

Most frustrating was my first semester at college. My schedule included rhetoric (honors) and fiction (honors), two heavy reading classes, two heavy literature classes, all in one semester.

Well, I'm an engineer major, so let's just say humanities isn't my forte. But, I made my fiction class a priority, followed by rhetoric. That first semester, I was required to read 150+ pages a week and write a critical essay, at the same time. I soon realized I didn't have to read the entire book to get a good grade. Still, it was overwhelming. And I thought I had an excellent English prep class in high school. I seemed to go from bad to worse. Plus, it was kind of complicated because I'm a President Scholar.

Thankfully, someone stepped in and awarded me a mentor—the Director of the Writing Center. She was interested in how I process information and how

I deliver. We talked about the book or the paper and she helped me organize my thoughts. The fiction course was exceptionally hard for me. I'm more a factual guy. My prof's criticism on papers sometimes was sensitive and sometimes was harsh. I landed a "C," never anything higher. He really liked my analysis. He just couldn't handle my use of the English language.

Even though I was carrying 18 hours, 50 percent of my time that first semester was taken up by rhetoric and fiction. At least, I could relax in Calculus 1, Mechanical Engineering and Computer Science. Spring semester was a breeze, only 16 units, with an emphasis on my major instead of General Education.

I might audit a foreign language. It's so nice to feel relaxed about that here—there's no FL requirement. I don't have fond memories of those two years in a row of high-school French. I can't spell in English, let alone in French. I'll probably complete my junior year abroad in England because my engineering major requires me to study at University College in London.

I haven't asked Student Life—the office for LD students and students with other disabilities—for books on tape because listening to lectures isn't my style. If a book was on tape, I'd probably tune it out. I don't like to learn by listening. I'm more a visual and kinesthetic learner.

For writing papers, it's been a huge plus getting help from the director. For reading assignments, I rarely ask for extended time because I start to go into a downward spiral and it becomes never-ending. Then, psychologically, the load gets even heavier.

Time management still isn't one of my best suits. But it's a lot better than it was. I understand the importance of it now. Until I'm really motivated to include it in my daily routine, though, it always will haunt me. I've finally managed to write down a "to-do" list and that's helped considerably. But, in reality, all the planning goes by the wayside if I don't put it into practice. I'm working on it.

I'm having a lot better social life at college than I did in high school. I've made an effort to get to know more people and, spring semester, I joined a fraternity. (I deferred "rush" because I wanted to feel settled.) There are some extremely nice guys in the fraternity. They understand when I have to stay in and do a paper or study for a test. Differences are respected, be they religious or learning.

I definitely see myself going on to grad school because I like to be recognized as the expert in my field. Looking down the road, I'll probably end up doing something with the Internet.

Sam suggests:

❑ Try to keep in mind that K-12 is the least important part of your education.

❑ There are better times ahead.

NICOLE CHILDERS, senior,
University of California at Santa Cruz

Nicole, 21, spent her junior year abroad at the University of Lancaster, England UK studying Medieval Drama. She grew up in San Diego and has a sister, 19, who doesn't have dyslexia.

Just when I had my special needs in place at UC Santa Cruz, I decided to apply for my junior year abroad at the University of Lancaster, England. I would have to leave behind all the things I had come to know.

At UC Santa Cruz, I'm taking advantage of the DRC (Disability Resource Center). They know I'm dyslexic, so I get extended time on tests for certain classes and math tutoring when needed. Tests, whether essay, short-answer or multiple-choice, aren't easy for me. But I'm comfortable telling my professors I'm registered with the DRC. Once I tell them, they're really quite understanding. Some aren't that knowledgeable about dyslexia, so making time to talk with them is necessary.

Then, it was off to England. First, I had to check out learning resources, once again. I knew they had a Disabled Students Services department. (Before I left for the year, I made sure to copy documentation on my dyslexia.) They offered me note taking, a tape recorder for classes, assistance with my writing and a computer for my personal use. They also pointed me in the direction of a support group for dyslexia. That group had a newsletter of events and important happenings, both on and off-campus.

There were a large percentage of students with visible disabilities at this school. They were either in wheelchairs or had walkers and usually were accompanied by a "buddy" in the most severe cases, and friends, in the less-severe cases. All in all, I was impressed with the steps the university took toward accommodating students with disabilities.

I'm not ashamed of my dyslexia. It's just another part of me. I happen to be female, left-handed and dyslexic. It's no more or less than any other part of me. Most of the time, I really don't think about being dyslexic. It isn't an excuse to do poorly in school or to act out. Everyone has a different brain and a different way of processing things. Mine just happens to be more different.

Nicole suggests:

❑ Remember, dyslexia isn't a handicap! Just because you look at the world differently and process information unconventionally, it doesn't mean you're unintelligent.

❑ People may not understand you and why you need extra time and attention. Don't let it get to you. Some of the most brilliant people in history were dyslexic. If they had believed what others thought of them, we would never have had the marvelous contributions of people like Albert Einstein and Winston Churchill.

❑ As for college, it will take care of itself as you take care of yourself. Don't let anyone or anything limit you in what you want to do with your life.

CAROLYN FARMER,
master's student, University of Michigan

Carolyn, 32, is studying Psychiatric-Mental Health Nursing. She completed her under-grad degree in nursing at Michigan. Carolyn says she wasted several years before returning to college.

Thank goodness for the concert and marching bands. They kept me going. They gave me a sense of belonging. They were my creative and physical outlets.

High school was the most difficult for me. I didn't know I had dyslexia. I just thought I was stupid. My grades didn't meet my parents' expectations. They criticized me for not doing my homework, even though I studied for hours without accomplishing much. I think my teachers would have been more supportive if I'd opened up to them, but I felt so much shame.

The first time I went to college, at Stephens College in Columbia, MO, I didn't know how to cope. Again, I "studied" for hours and hours without accomplishing much. I just knew I couldn't read like the others. Again, I thought I was stupid. I failed some of my classes. After one semester, I flunked out.

It took me several years to try again, but my desire to learn never left. I felt compelled to get a college degree, but I continued to believe I was stupid. I went through serious depression. Then, as I got treated for my depression, I gradually began to notice others around me who had college degrees. I started to compare myself. I decided they didn't seem any smarter than I was. Maybe I could graduate from college, too.

I enrolled in the University of Michigan, School of Nursing. There, I recognized I had a "unique" learning style, I created many strategies and I did well the first year. But the second year was the lowest of times. I couldn't keep up with the reading. I also would read the questions incorrectly on exams. I never finished in time. I also had trouble coordinating the different tasks I was trying to learn in the hospital. I had an unforgiving instructor and I became extremely anxious. That's when I knew I needed an assessment.

I got a neuro-psych test and discovered I had dyslexia. It was the most wonderful news because it validated a lifetime of struggles. It also gave me evidence to support my requests for special accommodations. Confident that I was really intelligent, I realized I could learn. I just had to do it a little differently than most of the students.

After I was diagnosed, the Center for Students with Disabilities gave me lots of ideas. They gave me the backbone to request extended time on tests and to be allowed to take tests in a separate room without distractions. I also arrange for books on tape and a tape recorder through the Center. Taping lectures and listening to them while I take thorough notes has been helpful. I never was good at taking notes in class because I couldn't really keep up. I also couldn't really listen to lectures if I was concentrating on writing at the same time. Everything took me more time. So, I decided to take $4^{1}/2$ years for under-grad school and $2^{1}/2$ to complete my master's. The pressure was off.

The exams in the School of Nursing are probably most challenging. They're multiple-choice, but the questions are based on a description of a scenario. We're asked to choose which answer is the "best intervention." The questions are designed to test one's critical thinking. It was common for me to read either the scenario or the intervention incorrectly. Now what I do is rewrite many of the questions, to clarify what really is being asked, before choosing the correct answer.

Carolyn suggests:

❑ Get diagnosed. Find out about your rights and resources. Remember, you're smart and dyslexia has nothing to do with intelligence.

❑ I wasted years of my life believing I wasn't college material. Don't let this happen to you. If you want to graduate from college, you just have to apply yourself. Don't be embarrassed to ask for accommodations.

T.J. BLANC, master's student, Auburn University

T.J., 31, will graduate with a master's in Community Counseling. She completed her under-grad degree, also at Auburn. T.J. is totally enjoying her college days. The Center for Special Services offers a very supportive program and her professors have been accommodating.

I quit public school by my 16th birthday. But my sister, Kate, and my dad encouraged me to go to adult GED (General Education Diploma) study classes at night. Two years later, I received my GED. I thank God every day for my family's unwavering support. Not only did they love me, they respected me. (My mother died when I was 9.)

I can't say the same for some of my elementary-school teachers. The preferred method of teaching for my 3rd-grade and 5th-grade teachers was humility. The 3rd-grade teacher, Miss A., regularly asked me to stand up and read aloud. Then she would say: "Oh, I forgot. You can't read. You can sit down." The 5th-grade teacher, Mrs. D., was cut from the same cloth. She told me: "You're a retard" because I still couldn't read fluently. Yes, that's right, a retard.

Well, now I have my master's. I owe a lot to the Center for Special Services at Auburn. Some of the things they offered:

1 Textbooks on tape – I took a lot of Criminal Justice and Abnormal Psychology classes in my under-graduate days. If the Recording For the Blind & Dyslexia didn't have the book, then a reader would record it for me. The Center provided the reader.

2 Tape recorder with counter – I would write down the number when the professor said something important.

3 Speech-recording programs – "Dragon NaturallySpeaking" is the main one I use. I also use "Jaws," "IBM Via Voice," "Kurzweil VoicePad for Windows: Platinum Edition," "Autotext in Word 97," and "Hot Keyboard." With "Dragon Naturally Speaking," I've had to train it to recognize my voice. This has taken many, many hours. (It's a pain in the butt, actually.)

4 A note taker – I get a note taker for all classes, someone with good handwriting.

5 Extended time on tests – I had no hassle with any profs, this was the norm.

AUM has been wonderful. I couldn't have asked for a better campus setting. Once I demonstrated a desire and dedication to learn, my professors were supportive. I really enjoyed my undergraduate days. I never missed a class, studied at least 3-4 hours a day, paid attention in class and did all my homework and reading assignments. The myth about LD students being social outcasts or having terminal melancholy is totally wrong. I love studying and love most of my classes. I plan to get my doctoral degree in Information Technology.

T.J. suggests:

❑ Be proactive, not reactive. Take responsibility for your own services. Don't let other people advocate for you. It's just as important to know your responsibilities as it is to know your rights.

❑ Educators should be respectful of their students. Using humiliation or verbal abuse as a teaching technique isn't only bad form, it's cruel. Moreover, that memory may stay with the child the rest of their life. Teachers are role models!

❑ Dream the Impossible Dream. Remember, LD stands for "learning differently," but we do learn.

HELEN FARR, junior, Syracuse University

Helen, 21, is in the School of Nursing. Eventually, she will take the Nursing State Board Exam to become an RN.

The awful years were in middle school. I hated being in "special" classrooms with kids who couldn't sit still or complete simple tasks. It was hard to tell my classmates why I didn't take tests with them or didn't do the same type of work. I became known as the "dumb kid."

On top of that, I had a disease called ulcerative colitis. I was diagnosed when I was 8 and had five surgeries during my middle-school years. It kept me out of school for several weeks at a time. I think if I hadn't had this disease, my dyslexia might have been diagnosed sooner.

I was finally diagnosed with dyslexia my sophomore year in high school. After the evaluation, I got tutoring. But my family had to pay for it. My mother kept me going. She did whatever it took to make sure I got what I needed to learn. My church friends also were a major support system.

I've always been up-front with my professors about my dyslexia. They know ahead of time about my special needs. Most of the time, they're very under-standing and willing to help. The special accommodations are: extended time on exams and a reader to read the exams. I usually run into problems with professors who aren't teaching in the nursing program and who teach large classes, like 50 or 100 students. Any time I've needed to use the Resource Center, I've been able to get the material and pass the class.

Sometimes, I need professors to make up special exams for me. All the nursing tests are multiple-choice, though, so I usually don't need a special one. For the most part, multiple-choice works for me because I know the answer is written down there somewhere. It doesn't confuse me unless there are similar words like hyperkinesia and hyperlipemia.

At Syracuse, I use all my resources to help me study—books on tape, taped lectures, tutoring, a note taker, and a computer to take written exams and type up written assignments. I have a counselor at the Resource Center who has helped me since my freshman year. She's a friend and an advocate. I'm very fortunate.

In nursing, we're required to write 5-6 page plans for the patients we take care of at the hospital. This has been a huge challenge because my spelling and grammar are so bad. I usually only have one patient a week because I only work in the hospital one day a week. The assessment covers everything, from head to toe. In the care plan, I have to explain the treatment and drug the patient is receiving and why. I also need to know any adverse reactions of the treatment and drugs. And, I need to state why the test and lab values are the way they are and how I, as a nurse, can improve the patient's health.

I usually start writing my care plan early and do several drafts so I can weed out most of the spelling and grammar mistakes. I write the assessments at least three times before I let anyone look at them. Then, a writing consultant or a friend reads over my work. I'd rather not ask a friend, though, because it's embarrassing to have them see how bad my writing skills are, now that I'm in college. Usually, only one person reads the care plans. But if it could work out, I'd rather have about three people look at it.

The workload definitely is a lot harder now that I'm a junior. But I'm coping. I get most overloaded when I haven't gotten my reading assignments on tape in time for a test. It's hard to read and study at the same time. The Learning Center has improved, but I still don't usually get the tapes until the week before the test. But some of it might be my fault because I usually leave reading until the last minute.

Time management is a big deal for me. As a freshman and sophomore, it was hard to do anything but go to church on Sundays. Now that I'm a junior, I have my own room and have learned better time-management skills. But, I still think it was important to have a roommate when I was a freshman because I came from Massachusetts and I didn't know anyone.

Helen suggests:

❏ Read: *Word Book: Based on the American Heritage Dictionary*, Kaethe Ellis, published by Houghton Mifflin Company, Boston (1976); and *Spelling Dictionary,* published by Lyons & Carnahan, Inc. (1967).

❏ Don't let anyone tell you that you can't do something. Somebody once said I wouldn't make it to a four-year college or become a nurse. If you put your mind to it, nothing can stop you.

❏ If you feel your teachers are teaching you in a way you can't understand, get outside help. It's out there and it doesn't cost a lot. It's also a law that, if a public-school teacher doesn't know how to teach a student, they have to find someone who does.

❑ College isn't easy. You can't fool around. But, in the end, it will be worth all the late-nighters and the pain and suffering.

❑ Finally, a great book to read is: *Oh, The Places You'll Go,* by Dr. Seuss.

LOW PROFILERS

Low Profilers are in the minority when it comes to college-interview categories. They are light on both special accommodations and personalized coping strategies. They continue with the task at hand (schoolwork), make little or no connection with the Learning Resource Center, and, in some instances, don't connect with faculty on the LD issue.

Madison Kendell doesn't use the Learning Resource Center and won't ask for special accommodations. She refuses to repeat her elementary-school feelings. She won't tell anyone at Prairie View A&M she has a learning disability. Instead, she relies heavily on her mom, dad or sister to proofread papers.

Jerry O'Brien and Paul Young are from the same mold. They don't want to raise any red flags; they want to be mainstream students. Jerry doesn't ask for extended time on tests, books on tape, etc., at Landmark College. He sees no need because he isn't having difficulty in any particular class. Paul doesn't ask for special accommodations either. He wants to see if he can do it alone at the University of Kansas. Paul feels getting books on tape will make him rely on them more, and getting a note taker may make him forget how to take notes himself. So far, he hasn't called the Student Assistance Center (SAC).

Kendall Henderson takes on too much as a freshman. He doesn't ask for help, doesn't self disclose, takes 17 units a semester, has the lead role in a play, and works 30 hours a week as stage manager. The end result is burnout. Kendall drops out of Theater Arts at the Cornish College of the Arts in Seattle and transfers to a community college. Kendall's story is not unique. Freshman, across the country sometimes follow a similar pattern. Then, it's too late in the semester to get formal help.

Maria Wolfe offers a different twist. For four years, Maria hides behind her screen door, fearing discrimination. Then, Maria sees a need to disclose her learning disability to more professors, those in the French department. She establishes herself as a dedicated intelligent student during the first few weeks of class, then has Academic Advising & Student Services send out the LD letter. For Maria, it's a tossup being known as an LD student or lying low. It's a discussion she has with herself at the start of each semester, at the start of each school year.

For various reasons, Maria and her counterparts don't want to surface above the crowd. They know their own character best and must do what feels best for them at college.

LOW PROFILERS

MADISON KENDELL, senior, Prairie View A & M

Madison, 30, will graduate with a bachelor's in Early Childhood Education. Although Prairie View A&M historically is a black university, and Madison isn't African American, she chose this school because it offers hands-on learning with project-based courses.

At 28, I finally had the courage to pursue a college degree. It's always been one of my secret desires, but I didn't attend college right out of high school because I didn't think I could make it. Neither did my teachers. Now, thanks in large part to computers, I only have nine hours of student teaching to finish my degree. But, it's been a long road. My past is filled with special reading classes, summer school and low-to-average grades.

Elementary school was the hardest thing I've ever gone through. I thought I was normal up until the 1st grade. Then, because I was a Special-Ed student, I was sent to another school for part of the day. I missed the regular school day and the other children in my class. As luck would have it, even though we moved cross-country between 2nd and 3rd grades, the next school had the same policy. There, I was bussed to a different school, where there were Special-Ed classes, different schedules and no class friends. I felt so bad for not being perfect. And, during this time, I also missed every Vacation Bible School at my church because of summer school. It was horrible.

Once I got to high school, though, I really stopped thinking about dyslexia. I accepted that I wasn't going to get wonderful grades and I wouldn't be going on to college. Ironically, years later, when I ran into school friends, they all said how smart I was in high school. Please . . . I wasn't even in honors or AP classes. I thought my friends knew I was dyslexic, but they didn't have a clue.

Still, I was advised against going to college. Instead, I worked full-time as a loan processor in a busy bank lobby. The company was understaffed and behind the times. Although I rarely tell anyone I'm dyslexic, I told my supervisor. I kind of had to because she was concerned about my error rate, even though it wasn't any different than anyone else's. I told her I wanted to be removed from the lobby so I could concentrate better. But, by telling her this, I ruined my credibility. I had to make some changes in my life. That's when

I decided to return to college full-time.

I'm so thankful to be in college. But I still don't tell anyone I have a learning disability. Except, one time, in a freshman paper. And now, every time I see that instructor, I'm ashamed. So, I end up working harder in class. I haven't used the Resource Learning Center and I don't ask for accommodations. I would rather not repeat my elementary-school feelings. But our campus has many deaf students and they have been well integrated into our classes with note takers and interpreters.

Instead of using the Resource Learning Center, I rely heavily on my mom, dad or my sister to proofread my papers. I don't catch errors like I should. Sometimes, I conjugate verbs wrong. Their/there, know/now, and s, 's, s' are my most common problems. But foreign language is my biggest fear. My advisor wants me to take Spanish as an elective. I keep talking her out of it. So far, so good. When I took Spanish in the 11th grade, if the girl next to me hadn't been so cooperative, I would have failed.

All in all, I think dyslexia has driven me to succeed. I didn't stop until I realized I was a very productive member of society. Tom Cruise, Whoopie Goldberg, Bruce Jenner and many successful people are dyslexic. When I feel low, I think of these celebrities. But the guy I admire the most is the Yale law student who can't read. But he made it because his mother helped him on his life-long journey.

Madison suggests:
- ❑ Get involved with people outside the school circle.
- ❑ Find a hobby, something, anything, you're good at.
- ❑ Use highlighters, make lists, get a note taker.
- ❑ You must have a computer to use "SpellCheck."
- ❑ Most importantly, relax . . . it can make a world of difference!

JERRY O'BRIEN, former sophomore, Landmark College

Jerry, 20, left after the first semester of his sophomore year. He didn't think Landmark, a private two-year college specializing in students with learning differences, was a good placement for him. He returned to the San Francisco Bay area where he is writing his first fiction novel.

What a great combination. I'm considered gifted and I have dyslexia. I'm caught in the balance of what I'm capable of doing and what I want to do. I gravitate to high-achieving students, yet I have a different learning style. Economics comes easy to me and I love history and English. Drama also is one of my favorites. But math and science are killers. And, with limited math skills, I was excluded from chemistry and found physics really tough. Then, when it came to foreign languages, people said I had an ear for French (my accent was superior to my classmates). But, conjugating French verbs took all the fun out of it. So I took Latin for a semester, but I failed miserably. Because of an inquiring mind, I want to take as many courses for interest and I want to dialogue with the "intellectual" group.

Still, I have a love for learning and, in my senior year, I was elected class president and got a reputation for being a fine spokesman. Everyone assumed I was smart.

I got caught up in the high-school frenzy of going to an East Coast college. Actually, a better plan would have been to go to the local community college. But, I wanted to go to a small liberal-arts school not one of the UCs (University of California) or the University of Arizona. Regrettably, I didn't get accepted at McAlister, MN or Kenyon, OH. So, Plan B was to go to Landmark College for two years and then transfer to a top four-year college like Harvard or Duke. Both my parents are Stanford alumni and I know I was expected to get a great college education. But that didn't work out either. I've since dropped out of college for a while.

College just wasn't like high school. My wit and loud mouth that were well received in California weren't accepted on the East Coast. Maybe it was a cultural difference, but I felt like the lid had been put on my vacuum. You see, I'm fine being the combination of dyslexic and gifted. I just want to get on with learning.

But at Landmark, I wasn't intellectually stimulated. There wasn't much diversity and, with so many LD students, it made me more self-conscious of my dyslexia. I felt I had a real problem and the school highlighted it. They also have a clinical view of dyslexia. They believe students with dyslexia have trouble picking up music. So, no hands-on music courses are offered. Instead, emphasis is on music theory and the history of music. There is also no language requirement. But, recently, the college started to offer Spanish. Landmark did have a required tutorial, one-on-one. We compiled a master notebook system. For the first semester, I found it helpful. I was happy to try any new organizational help. That's where Landmark shines. Still, my academic growth was being stifled. With the absence of intellectual stimulation, I partied and I went skiing in Vermont and took trips to New York City.

I didn't really have difficulty with classes. Sometimes, I asked for extra reading materials. I became known as the intellectual snob. By the third semester, I was ready to leave. It's a great idea to have a place for students with a learning difference, but it's not for everyone. Landmark just didn't work out for me.

Now I'm at a crossroads. Without a college degree in this country, I'm regarded as McDonald's material. But I still want to try my own path. I know Steve Wasnick and Steve Jobs are college dropouts! It's not an easy road to take now that I've stepped out of line, but I still want to try.

Jerry suggests:

❏   Plan a different course if you're not fitting in with the norm. It's OK.

❏   Find other ways to get to where you want to go.

❏   If college is going to be a satisfying situation for you, do it. I wouldn't say college is a necessary exercise. It has its time and its place.

MARIA WOLFE, senior, University of Oregon

Maria, 22, is studying Romance Languages, with a minor in Special Education. She says by taking five years to complete her undergraduate course work, college has become manageable.

I wanted to graduate in four years, take 15 credits a term and let as few professors as possible know about my LD. In hindsight, I realize I was being foolish and unfair to myself. Still, after doing well in my freshman year, I was on a roll. I began to place tremendous pressure on myself. (I've always had a tendency to compare my academic abilities to my non-LD friends and, often, it's been detrimental to my psyche.) For two years, I struggled. My lowest points definitely came in my sophomore and junior years. A critical turning point came at the beginning of my senior year. I needed to make important decisions about graduation. I decided to make them based on my own learning needs and remove the peer pressure I had created. I also saw the need to disclose my learning disability to more professors and educate them about the help I needed.

Up to then, I'd never identified my LD to any of my French professors. I took the plunge and went before the Romance Language Department with a presentation on dyslexia. This was in conjunction with Disability Awareness Week. It was a scary thing for me to do. I risked being misunderstood. My own department also could have discriminated against me. I took a chance. At the same time, I was confident that, if I went about it in the right way, I would be able to educate them and help them understand learning differences. This was important to me, not only because of my own vested interest, but because I've always seen myself as a trailblazer for future LD students. The presentation was a great success and I've continued to receive thanks and support from people who were in attendance. I needed to do this. I was hiding behind a screen door for too long!

I convinced myself it was unnecessary to self-disclose my learning disability to any French professors. Big mistake! My LD does affect my foreign-language abilities, yet my learning differences have given me advantages over other foreign language students. I compensate for what I lack in visual skills by using auditory skills. For example, if I'm writing a paper in French or Spanish and I get stuck on a grammar question, I'll figure it out by what SOUNDS best, as opposed to how it should look. A lot of the compensatory mechanisms I use are based on the fact that I'm an auditory learner. This, I think, explains why my speaking abilities in foreign languages often are better than my peers. When I was an exchange student in France, I often got dragged along because I could speak and translate better than my peers. I chose to major in RL (Romance Languages) because it gave me the opportunity to study Spanish and, at the same time, continue with the French I love. U of O doesn't offer an undergraduate degree in Special Education, so I've taken it as a minor. I realized my education/experience in Spanish would benefit my long-term goal in Special Ed.

I can safely say multiple-choice tests and I do not get along! Primarily, I dislike them because of their format. After narrowing the answer down, by decoding both the question and the option, I must make transference from test to scantron. It's just too much! I hate processing all my thoughts, studies and knowledge of a particular subject into someone else's broad question and pointed options. Give me an open-ended essay question any day. I also struggle with the large amount of college reading I have to get through. In hindsight, I wish I had requested books on tape and perhaps an alternative to multiple-choice tests.

As for the balance between schoolwork and social activities, I pretty much knew from my freshman year that, if I sacrificed things I hold near and dear (theater, ballet, religion), I'd be unhappy. I've tried to keep pursuing activities I enjoy, while still dedicating enough time to my studies. It hasn't always been easy, and, sometimes, the scale gets tipped pretty heavy in one direction. But that's life.

In some classroom situations, I've chosen not to identify my disability. I fear discrimination. I realize the law is on my side, but, sometimes, I feel I make better headway if I first establish myself as a dedicated, intelligent student, and THEN have the LD letter sent. (The protocol here is for me to request a letter from Academic Advising & Student Services to be sent to my professors. The letter states the strengths and weaknesses of my disability and lists the typical accommodations I will need.)

The way I handle special accommodations is this: at the start of each term, I sit down with all of my syllabi and decide which profs need a letter about my LD and which don't. If there's a mid-term or final, I pretty much have no choice because I need the extended time.

Next year, I plan to apply to grad school to pursue a master's in Learning Disabilities & Literacy or in Educational Administration.

Since I struggle with the workload at the undergraduate level, I do worry about grad school. But, I've found a solution. This past summer, I took three classes, one at a time. I LOVED it. I felt like I had plenty of time to accomplish what was being asked of me, learn from it and excel. I learned a big lesson this summer—I never want to be in school full-time again. I don't care how long it takes to get my master's and I don't care how many grants I'll have to write to cover the expenses. Frankly, sacrificing my soul to academia is not worth the price.

Maria suggests:
> ❑ Prepare for college to the best of your ability while still in high school. Follow the honors or AP track. (The skills I learned in those classes saved me my first year here at U of O.)

❑ Don't listen to professionals who try to get in the way of your aspirations. If you want to apply to a certain school, do it. Determination builds character.

❑ Learn to advocate for yourself. Mom and Dad may pay for college, but they won't be around.

❑ Learn from your mistakes and don't punish yourself for them.

❑ Listen to yourself. Stress doesn't help most LD situations. If you get in over your head, prioritize and eliminate.

❑ Pursue non-school activities you love—sports, arts, your faith, hobbies—whatever floats your boat!

INDEPENDENTS

Independents tend to be individualistic, problem solvers and, often, forward thinkers. They are heavy on personalized coping strategies and go light on special accommodations. They choose to do college "their way." They find out what's offered at the Learning Resource Center, then follow their own blueprint.

Freddie Chilton comes up with this formula—he takes only 12-15 units per semester at the University of Colorado at Boulder, plans to complete his under-grad degree in Business Administration in five years, and buys lecture notes ($10.00) for GE classes from Class Notes, a company specializing in note taking off-campus. His journalism friends proofread his papers and his teacher's assistants explain concepts he doesn't grasp in class or give him outlines of what is expected. Freddie's outgoing personality is his strong suit. His dad says he gets away with a lot!

Hope Stone and Patrick Karstens prefer to work independently. Unless Hope feels pressure, she functions like any other student at BU and doesn't use the services at the Learning Disabilities Support Services (LDSS). She does, however, surround herself with classmates who are willing to help explain questions. She hustles to form study groups, and keeps an electronic organizer with her at all times. Patrick also doesn't work through the official channels— the Academic Advising and Student Services at the University of Oregon. Instead, he approaches his profs independently without a formal letter. He gives them his spiel, they give him extended time on tests/ exams, and both parties work it out amicably.

Jason Brown, a visual learner, works on using flash cards, charts and diagrams to help memorize chemistry, biology and history facts. He also taps into the latest software programs in the learning center at Texas A&M. Jason uses "DragonDictate," a software program that lets him speak into the computer, and then writes what he says. He also uses "Text Help for Windows 98," a program that reads what he types and then gives him different options when he misspells a word. Jason knows how lucky he is to be in college now, rather than 20 years ago when personal computers were just coming off the drawing board.

Most *independents* work on improving schoolwork strategies. Alice Wonderwater, a master's student at Brown, tries to improve her attitude and the attitude of others. She's given up being a normal student and doesn't care if she never learns to spell. But she does care about knowing as much as possible on a particular subject. If she takes longer to do it, so be it. As a seasoned student, she tries to educate faculty on how she functions. She challenges professors to really teach her, to present mathematical equations in word-oriented language, to make her love economics, to help her understand numbers. She initiates dialogue, sets the scene. The professors take the lead from her. Alice goes that extra mile.

Independents are not going to be trampled. They value their personalized coping strategies over anything else offered on campus. They meet roadblocks, resistance, and failure along the way. The more experienced *independents*, though, come to expect this and often implement new strategies on a trial-and-error basis. In reality, they use college as a testing ground for the real world. Strategies that help increase work output, create more understanding of the material, increase speed and make their workplace less overwhelming, are central to them. *Independents* get a head start on the real world, the work place, the next chapter in their life.

INDEPENDENTS

ELLA WASS, fourth-year Ph.D. student, University of Washington

Ella, 26, is studying anthropology after getting her under-grad degree in psychology at Pitzer College, CA and her master's in social work at the University of Washington. To survive college, Ella says, she had to contin- ually think up individualized coping strategies e.g. searching out a college with no math requirement, writing an accompanying letter about her LD when applying to grad school, and petitioning to retake statistics for a third time.

In 2nd grade, I started to panic. My self-esteem was low and I was having trouble reading and writing. My parents, the school psychologist and several teachers were trying to figure out what was wrong. Finally, at an annual check-up with my pediatrician, we discovered I had dyslexia. Coming from a highly academic home setting, this was a curse. My brother was a gifted student—he's since graduated from Yale, and Stanford Business School—and my father was unable to deal with any learning differences.

But even though I knew I had dyslexia, the mystery wasn't over. I also had behavioral problems in elementary school. None of the teachers understood. I was constantly being punished. I didn't fit in. I became defensive. I wasn't unintelligent. It's just that, when I was given less-taxing work, I was bored. And every school report said I talked too much. I didn't find out there was joy in learning until my junior year at Pitzer College.

Mine was the last Pitzer class that didn't have a math requirement. (They've since changed the rules.) Plus, Pitzer wanted very few GE requirements. Luck was on my side. I chose the college. They had a learning center, but I didn't use any of the resources on a regular basis. If I did get poor grades in a class, I would talk to my professor or then get help at the center. I worked very hard and played very hard. I was involved in political engagements, too, (Native American issues), music and film, backpacking and hiking. I'm such an intensely social person, I need the stimulation. When it came to studying, I used something I call the laser technique. That is, I waited until the last possible minute to do everything, then I would hone in the laser until I could pull off writing a paper. I pulled many all-nighters.

There were low times at Pitzer, too. I was getting a bachelor's in psychology, and part of the course requirement was statistics. I needed daily tutoring, literally 4-5 hours a day. Pitzer didn't have the resources. I went to my advisor and asked if I could petition. She suggested that, before I embarrass myself in front of the entire Psychology Department, I should take a statistics class in summer school at the local college. I knew I couldn't do statistics, but I enrolled anyway. I failed. Well, to keep redoing statistics and taking five hours of daily tutoring seemed nonsensical. So, I petitioned the panel. I had a 3.8 GPA. They conceded. I graduated with a bachelor's in psychology.

I did run into problems, though, my first year of the Ph.D. program. I had to take a class in Physical Anthropology and Populations. That involved a lot of math. I was getting "A's" in the other classes. I was getting a "D" in that class. My professor had never met anyone with dyslexia and was astounded that I'd been accepted into the Ph.D. program and been able to get so far in college without a math background. But I became more a victim than a success. I remember going back and forth with him about his class requirement. He wanted me to take the course again, one-on-one. Welcome to the world of the Americans with Disabilities Act. Then the head of the Anthropology Department got involved. We worked out an alternate plan. At the same time, I suggested we talk about accommodations for the foreign-language requirement. I told him I was paying for my education, so I wanted some action. I was 25 and it was the first time I had to get tough. I had to negotiate. We settled on an alternate way of testing me in Spanish—translations only; no multiple-choice or essay tests.

Actually, the faculty were surprised I needed help because I write so well. But the Ph.D. program was all about reading. Many of the doctoral students were depressed, but I wasn't. Hey, I was dealing with that in 3rd grade. I just figured out at an early age how to skim a book. It became my survival skill. By the time I got to grad school, I could have bottled and sold my technique. I also learned very quickly in grad school to form reading groups. Why read all the material if you can share duties?

The faculty members and other students knew I was skilled and intelligent. But my best coping strategy was definitely my sense of humor. Without it, I'm sunk. It's what keeps me going on bad days, when things hit the fan. I've also learned to take one course per semester that I shine in—creative writing, sports, drama. As long as I play to my strengths of visual and verbal skills, I know I can survive.

Now I want to become a successful anthropologist and clinician. I plan to finish my thesis work next year and graduate with a Ph.D. in Sociocultural

Anthropology. I've come a long way since elementary-school days.

Ella suggests:

❑ Place yourself in a position that maximizes your strengths.

❑ Even when things are difficult, don't believe people when they try to pull you down.

❑ Passion rules all. Don't take NO for an answer.
FOLLOW YOUR PASSION.

PATRICK KARSTENS, recent graduate, University of Oregon

Patrick, 23, got his degree in Marketing Communications (advertising). He thought it was better to work out his accommodations on a one-on-one basis with his professors than to be documented at the Academic Advising & Student Services office. He utilized the "footnote" system (private note taker), as well as previous tests filed in his fraternity, and scheduled writing assignments one or two weeks before the due date.

I work around my learning disability instead of confronting it head-on. I don't let it affect my life. Instead, I work on my pluses, not my minuses. Presentations, projects and papers aren't a problem. I excel in these areas. Math and foreign languages are a no-no. I need a lot of help.

I have to say that, all along the way (K-12), my "survival kit" was paramount to me. It included:

1 Parental support – My parents made me focus on my strengths. They told me to shine, to stand out in athletics instead of letting the LD crumble me. I was never ashamed of having a different learning style. They taught me to be realistic with my grades. I never aspired to a 4.0 GPA. I was happy with myself. My father has wonderful work ethics that rubbed off on me. My parents also encouraged me to read what was within my realm. I didn't like to read. I wouldn't pick up a book and I still don't. But, I love to read short articles in newspapers, periodicals and on the Internet.

2 Competitive sports – I'm an over-achiever in sports. Our whole family is sports mad. I was incredibly popular in grade school because I was out there dunking baskets or scoring a goal. Even on

swim team, I brought home 1st-place ribbons. I was on the varsity track team and we won the CCS (Central Coast Section) my senior year. I also played basketball and swam on the local swim team through high school. I focused 80 percent of my time on studies, but still allowed track and basketball to let me soar.

3 Part-time jobs – Lifeguarding and a maintenance job at the local swim club were crucial in maintaining my self-esteem. I've always liked kids. The ability to rescue them made me feel self-worthy. Then, when I was promoted to head lifeguard, lifeguard instructor and maintenance manager, I gained so much confidence. I was in charge of pool activities and had to see that the operations of the club ran smoothly. This was the real world. And, I excelled in it.

4 Sense of humor – I don't have a problem laughing at myself, this has been a key component. It just doesn't bother me. My sense of humor got me through some uncomfortable situations in school. Thank goodness it came with my "package."

Once I embarked on the college-application process, I pretty much narrowed it down to three schools. I looked as USC (University of Southern California), the University of Oregon and the University of Pacific. When I visited U of O and stayed overnight in a fraternity, I fell in love with the school. I wanted to get in. I pretty much knew when I started there that I'd go for 5 years. That would include a semester in London, England. It was my parents' idea for me to learn about a different culture. Most importantly, I knew my parents had put away college funds for me when I was an infant. There was no pressure. I'm so thankful.

All freshman year, I was trying to find my niche. It was a difficult time for me. Core classes were a challenge with so many multiple-choice tests. I had to take math and foreign-language requirements. But, once I decided to change my major at the end of sophomore year—BINGO, I was focused. I started out as a business major, but, because of so many required math classes, I changed to advertising. My junior and senior years, I was rockin' and rollin'. I loved what I was doing. College definitely got easier as I matured because I was in a major I really enjoyed and I learned the system.

I didn't self-disclose when I applied to the U of O. I became familiar with the learning center   because of a study class I took my freshman year. Unfortunately, I had to get documented again to be put in their program full-time. I decided not to go that route. I only needed some help. I didn't need books on tape, a reader or a scribe. I got help on a drop-in basis. I ended up getting a math tutor at the center twice a week. I had to pay for it. Then, once I changed to advertising, I faxed all my papers to my father for proofreading. It made sense for him to check my papers because he's in the account side of advertising. It was important to get feedback, too.

For special accommodations, I decided to approach my profs independently. That is, they didn't receive a formal letter from Academic Advising & Student Services highlighting my special needs. Instead, I gave them my "spiel" and it worked out fine. Depending on the class, I had profs give me extended time on tests. Usually, I went with them to their office to take the test. Other teachers arranged for me to write essays instead of taking the multiple-choice tests. In a few GE classes, I had to read 400 pages and then answer 50 short questions. It was only in science and history that I needed these accommodations. Fortunately, once I declared my major, I was able to do more project-related exams and take computer courses instead of math and language classes.

But the best coping strategy I had was the test files at my fraternity. I felt very prepared for tests. A second benefit was the footnotes system. For $20 a term, a note taker took the lecture notes for the larger, core classes. This was incredibly helpful because I was able to concentrate only on the lecture. A third strategy was to start papers right when I got the assignment, without question. I started my assignments early, usually a week before they were due, and finished a day before the deadline. I know this discipline is going to help me in life. I formed a good habit.

Actually, my parents drilled into me, at an early age, to be organized. At college, I map out my week. I know where I'm going and what I'm doing. Class presentations are never a problem provided I organize my thoughts in advance and then practice, practice, practice the info. Everything is written out on note cards. I practice 50 times, imagining I'm performing on stage. I ask the prof to use the classroom a day before, rehearsing the question-and-answer stuff and running through the final presentation. It all comes back to getting into something I enjoy and being organized.

Things were a bit different, though, when I did my junior year abroad at the American College in London, UK. The main run-in I had came in theater class. We saw one play a week. I did the first assignment which included writing two papers on four plays. When the test/paper was handed back, I waited until the end of class to speak to my prof about my LD. She immediately told me I wasn't dyslexic. She's seen people who had dyslexia. Based on my paper and my written test, she decided I wasn't dyslexic. Dyslexia, she told me, was when people wrote words backwards. She didn't back down. I never discussed that subject with her again. I ended up getting a "C+" in the class. I decided I wasn't in London for the theater; I was there to learn about European advertising practices. I did well in that class!

Looking ahead, I don't think I want to go to grad school. Now that I'm going into advertising production, I have to learn hands-on. For my animation training, I need to attend workshops and seminars on a regular basis. I'm better off taking two and three-day courses that offer state-of-the-art information, than trying to achieve this through a grad program.

ALICE WONDERWATER, master's student, Brown Univ

Alice, 30, is pursuing a master's in environmental studies. She also completed her under-grad degree at Brown. She's changing faculty attitudes along the way.

Brown was the first place I ever questioned my ability to write. When it comes to making an outline for a paper or putting my thoughts into a topic sentence, I freeze. When I was an under-grad student, teachers always were amazed at the high quality of information in my papers, but the low-quality writing skills. I spend days and days on a five-page paper and often find myself delivering papers to profs at their homes hours after exams are over. One professor even said to me: "Alice, sometimes I feel like you are a star and we are shoving you in a box and knocking off all your points."

Finally, I spoke to the Dean of Students who helps LD students. Yes, I found out I had dyslexia. Since then, Brown has been so much better. Having a coach is the best thing I can imagine. Wearing headphones in the computer center so I can't hear what other people say really helps, too. But the best coping mechanism has been to find ways to really push my strengths. I've given up on being a "normal" student. I really don't care if I never learn to spell. But I do care about knowing as much as I can about something. If it takes me longer, that is going to be OK.

Actually, I only find success in classes where I can do projects with other students. When I select classes, I usually look for project work in the course outline. I try to avoid an overload of term papers. I've also trained myself to be a very organized person. And I've taught myself to remember things in a pattern.

I've found that most professors really are unaware and uneducated about different learning styles. But, as a teaching assistant myself, I now realize how hard it is to catch students who are scraping by because of dyslexia. (It's fairly easy to catch those who are in serious trouble.) Professors usually have such a stressful lifestyle that taking extra time for students who need help puts them on overload.

Luckily, when I took an economics course, the professor was willing to teach me in a separate language, more word-oriented. He gave us options on the final to present mathematical equations in words or numbers. He made me feel it was possible to learn to love math and economics. That professor and a few other rare pearls make all the difference. Their style is to teach instead of loading material onto students. These teachers somehow have the ability to alter the class to the understanding of the students.

I firmly believe I've taught as much as I've learned here at Brown. I think many of the professors I've challenged to really teach me are better educators because of it. It seems like I've become a warrior. It's the only way to survive.

Still, don't let anyone or anything convince you to go to grad school. If you don't really want to learn in the academic world, then don't be pushed. Going to grad school has been the hardest thing I've ever done. It seems that by the time you get to graduate school, you're expected to have figured out your learning style. The reality is that it may be the first time you even start to realize you learn in a different way.

Alice suggests:
   ❑ Find out all you can about your own learning style and educate others. It may seem like an interruption in your studies but you're not only making it possible for yourself, you're making it better for future students with different learning styles.

HOPE STONE, recent graduate, Boston University

Hope, 23, got her degree in advertising. She self-disclosed on her application but didn't utilize the Learning Disabilities Support Services (LDSS). Instead, Hope took advantage of tutorials, one-on-one tutoring and the extended test time offered at the College of General Studies. After her sophomore year, with a mandatory +3.0 GPA, she transferred to the School of Communications.

My family was the most influential in building and maintaining my self-esteem. They gave me constant support and always believed in my abilities. They focused on my positive attributes. I, in turn, focused my energy on helping others. In high school, I got involved in peer counseling and community-service projects. I also gained confidence from swimming competitively and pursuing photography as a hobby. Keeping an organizer was a key coping strategy for me. It helped me allocate time for studying, school activities and social events. I always surrounded myself with positive people, both family and friends.

Despite all the support, though, one of the most challenging times was taking the SAT and AP tests in my junior year. I was in a college-prep school. Most of my classmates were extremely advanced in multiple subjects. Although there was no official ranking, it was evident I was ranked in the lower part of the class. That became even clearer once I completed the SAT. Having to hide my true score was one of my hardest battles.

Another difficult time was during the college-application process. It seemed like most of my class was applying to four/five-star Ivy League schools. I found myself in another league. I was targeting schools with a learning disability resource center. Dealing with rejection letters and telling my friends the news also was difficult. No one likes to talk about rejection. I did do a smart thing, though. I applied early to the University of Arizona. They have a rolling admissions policy. So, by December of my senior year, I'd already been accepted somewhere.

To be honest, I experienced more low times in high school than in college because the pressure was more intense. In high school, I was in a class of 60 where everyone knew their skills and abilities. In college, we were more dispersed, so people knew less about my academic skills. In high school, I had trouble processing the information and struggled with learning new ways to retain data. It took several years to resolve. Initially, flash cards worked well. Later, writing out all the questions on a single sheet of paper worked. In college, I moved toward highlighting in textbooks. I also rewrote my notes, memorizing where they were placed on the paper. This would help me recall/visualize where the information/answer was on the paper and help me recall it during the test.

By the time I got to college, I had learned within myself how I processed information, so I didn't use the services at the LDSS. But, had this type of resource been available in my high school, I would have spent many hours there. At college, I found that, unless I really felt pressured, I tried to function like any other college student. Math was by far the most challenging course. To me, it was like trying to dissect a foreign organ. I surrounded myself with classmates who were willing to help explain the questions. Our math professor would run through the information and leave me in a "fog." Although I never improved my math grade, I didn't fail the class. Just passing a math class became my personal goal. If I could excel in other classes and only do poorly in math, that was good enough for me.

Sadly, though, there are many "old-style" professors who don't believe in learning differences. They feel if you're seriously impaired, you should be at a special school, out of mainstream classes. They don't comprehend you can learn differently, yet still achieve high academic standards. Some think you can't read, write, spell, speak, etc.

At BU, though, I ran into professors with a limited knowledge of dyslexia, but they were open-minded. It was up to me to sell my story. I never used dyslexia as an excuse. Instead, I used it as a last resort when I was unable to handle a situation. I only occasionally asked for extended time on a test because many professors looked down on this so-called "privilege." Most faculty members, though, after explaining where I was coming from, were willing to make exceptions. It wasn't a problem. But on some occasions, I was told "no" and felt extremely frustrated. That's when I found myself drawn to LD student activities. If you don't educate yourself, you can't expect to change.

I'm strongly considering getting my MBA within the next few years. I'm concerned I won't be able to get into a good school because I do so poorly on standardized tests. The GMAT focuses a large portion on math concepts and computation. But if I don't try, I'll never know. I think, initially, the workload of an MBA program could be intimidating. But, after being in the "real world" (workplace), you learn to balance multiple tasks and obstacles. I view being dyslexic as a mission, a mission that was handed to me by a higher source who believes I can make a difference in the world.

Hope suggests:

❑ Go and find out what makes you happy. Learn by experiencing different classes, activities and people. The more you learn about yourself, the easier it becomes to deal with this learning challenge.

❑ Surround yourself with people who believe in you. Being positive is so important. You'll take a lot of blows from individuals who don't understand your position. If you have a support system, you'll rise above whatever comes your way.

❑ Try helping others who are less fortunate. You'll find this puts everything into perspective.

CLEO AMANDA, master's student, Monterey Institute of International Studies

Cleo, 25, is concentrating on International Policy Studies. She completed her under-grad degree at Goucher College, MD, a small, four-year liberal arts school. Her senior year in high school, she spent in Heidelburg, Germany, while her junior year abroad was at the University of Tubegin, also in Germany. Cleo likes coming up with better ways to gather and present material. She doesn't ask for special accommodations in grad school. She just utilizes her own coping strategies.

Kindergarten through 3rd grade was a tricky time for me. My teachers wanted to hold me back. They put me in the Difficult Education Curriculum. That totally confused my parents. They'd recently emigrated from Jamaica and still were adjusting to the U.S. school system. I was considered slow and put in a class full of students with behavioral problems. At that point, I was memorizing everything because I definitely couldn't read.

In high school, though, I began to find my passion—writing. My 11th-grade English teacher kept telling me to write the way I spoke. "Don't do anything tricky," he'd say. "Keep it simple. Your concepts are beyond your years. Your writing is below grade level." Then I had one high-school teacher who yelled: "You're nothing like your sister. You're lazy." (My sister, Lisa, was a straight-A student.)

Halfway through my junior year, I decided to apply for a scholarship in Germany. My French teacher told me I was crazy. She said it was geared to accelerated students with foreign-language capabilities. Well, I was one of four students picked out of a field of 4,000.

Still, at that point in my life, my self-esteem was very low, extremely low. My grades were down. I was tired of being black and I had issues with being female in the 90s. I wanted to see "life" in Germany. I wanted to see the parallelism between the German people and African Americans. And, I wanted to return to the U.S. with a better understanding of my position in society. I needed to find myself.

I ended up in a village in southern Germany, near Heidelburg. One sister in my family spoke English. I used a lot of body language, listened attentively and tried to remember what to say. I attended the local gymnasium, where I took English, German, Russian, calculus (in German), biology and art. I asked to take my exams orally and the school agreed. By the end of the year, I was amazed how much my German had improved. I even had an accent.

Overall, I had an amazing experience in Germany. I found myself. I found I had guts I didn't know I had. I could sing. I was creative. I worked out a plan for when I returned home.

While I was in Germany, I sent off my college applications and also took the SAT test. My U.S. college counselor was very helpful. She sent me brochures and any information for me to review. Goucher made me a great offer, one I couldn't refuse. They agreed to pay a large sum of money for me to attend. I was walking on air in Heidelburg, Germany.

But that high feeling soon disappeared. Goucher is heavy on writing, even in physical education class. I had some problems. Because of my low SAT scores, admissions had me on probation the first semester. They took me off probation the next semester, once I proved I could be a 3.5 student. I ended up taking my papers to the Writing Center to be edited. My writing improved.

I still didn't know, though, that I had an identifiable learning disability. It surfaced in a psychology class on feminist writers. I found myself explaining concepts to the class. They were complex readings. But when I submitted my paper, my prof was shocked. "Did you do this on your own, because your other papers aren't in the same light?" she asked. She humiliated me, but, really, she was testing me. She realized I do better writing stories and giving anecdotes than I do writing non-fiction. She figured out I was dyslexic.

Now that I'm a seasoned student, I've come to know what works best for me. My list includes a tape recorder, oral testing, skimming reading assignments, alternative visual presentations and knowing my strengths and weaknesses.

1 Tape recorder – I read my ideas into a tape recorder before I go to

sleep. As I type my thoughts, I listen to the tape and it all seems to come together. I format the essay, put it into organizational context and then, it's Systems Go!

2 Oral testing – I asked for oral testing in Germany and this played right into my hand. I memorized all the info and then was confident at testing time. I seemed to come out of my shell. I no longer was inhibited.

3 Skimming for reading assignments – I always jump to the first chapter to give me an idea how the author writes. Then I look for the major themes and highlight them. I learned quickly I couldn't sit down and read every assignment.

4 Visual presentations with a difference – I stay away from Power Point. Every presentation is very Power-Point oriented now at grad school. I feared if I read aloud, I might mispronounce a word. I had to come up with an alternate way to present—like slides, music and poetry.

5 Knowing my strengths and weaknesses – I started at MIIS in the Commercial Diplomacy program, but soon learned I had to turn around papers in 24 hours, like five days a week. It was all writing. Total stress for me. I talked with faculty and we concluded I'm more humanities than business. I transferred to the International Relations master's program. I never looked back.

There is a big place in my schedule, too, for my social life. I'm president of the German Club at MIIS. Every Christmas, we help needy students on the Monterey Peninsula. I'm also the founder and VP of the Caribbean Club on campus. And I'm in a jazz ensemble and sing professionally.

Cleo suggests:

❑ Never believe you're worthless.

❑ If you know you're different, then do things differently. (I went to Germany). Being different is beautiful.

❑ It's OK to ask for help.

❑ There's no harm in trying.

❑ Feel the fear and do it anyway.

LEE ANTHONY, junior, University of Maryland

Lee, 24, is studying anthropology. He transferred from Montgomery Community College in Maryland, where he was a part-time student. He works as a research assistant for an archaeologist in the Anthropology Department. After graduation, Lee plans to work for the Peace Corps.

With my father being in the Navy, I always felt like I would be leaving and that none of this would really matter. My family moved all the time. But, in 9th grade, we moved to Maryland and I've been here since. Before that, I had been in the Aleutian Islands in Alaska, Japan, Florida and Virginia.

It's hard to remember my most difficult years in school. They all seem to blend together. I always was just a "passing" student. That probably had some effect on my self-esteem. So did not being able to read and write. They always seemed to get harder and harder. I never finished reading the assignments and I didn't remember what I'd read. I thought I was creative, but I couldn't get it out. I spent so many hours laying in bed reading fantasy stories. But I did do well with computers.

The main thing I can think of that really helped me through high school was a close friendship I had. My buddy and I spent many hours talking and writing. He helped me with my work and respected my creativity. I've always believed that, no matter how difficult things get, at least I'm still alive. And there's always been a drive inside me. I've always thought I'm going to do something great, something wonderful for humanity.

I didn't know I had any kind of learning difficulty until the summer of my junior year in college. I also learned I was socially phobic and depressed. I haven't done anything specific about my LD. I just ask for accommodations in certain classes. Just realizing there was an explanation for my problems really made the difference.

Still, at college, every semester follows this pattern: I begin in the mood for school and all the new learning, I start to feel overwhelmed, I get discouraged, then I feel useless, I realize my grades are committing suicide and then I try to concentrate and throw myself into the work. After all that, I basically just do OK— "B's" and "C's."

I take a reduced course load (less than 12 units a semester) and work part-time as a research assistant to an archaeologist in the Anthropology Department.

I'm also a TA for a bio-anthropology class. That takes several hours a week. And, I've been named the first vice president of U of M's ASA (Anthropological Students' Association). I spend at least four hours a week working on that.

I also have a job at a physical security company, but I'm not working right now. I'm a technician/installer/assembler there. My dad taught me a lot about electrical stuff when I was growing up, so that's probably why I got the job.

Most definitely, I feel pressure from school. But I'm not discouraged. I believe you need to be your own advocate at college. Though I haven't done that yet, a friend and I both decided to try the recorded-book idea. I drive 40+ minutes to and from campus, so I have a lot of listening time. This could make a big difference in my workload.

This is my fifth year in college and I've always understood one thing about my learning. I can learn and understand anything, as long as it doesn't include reading and writing. I don't spell very well. Words that have combinations like these really confuse me—lly/ly, ley/ly, sion/tion, there/their. I have avoided the foreign-language requirement, but I have dreams of learning French, Greek and Cantonese. Fortunately, my experience with the faculty has been quite exceptional. I have a feeling one of my instructors is dyslexic, so she's fine with my special needs.

I'm considering graduate work, just not yet. I want to work for the Peace Corps after earning my bachelor's in anthropology. I need some hands-on experience first. Once I do get to grad school, I'll look at majoring in Human Ecology, Sustainable Development or Environmental Geology. Of course, I'm worried about the standardized tests. I'll do my best and explain my life to the necessary people. I'll also explain my leanings toward hands-on learning, my extreme eagerness to learn as much as possible, and my plans to save the world.

In closing, though, there's something I need to say. It's about the word "dyslexic." There's a difference between saying: "John is dyslexic," and "John is a dyslexic." Dyslexia doesn't make us stupid (rather, the contrary). It just means we need to work harder on our goals than mainstream students.

Lee suggests:

❑ Be persistent.

❑ Become involved with student organizations and faculty research.

❑ Try to understand that others don't understand. Then help them with that.

MICHAEL JOHN, medical student, UC system

Michael, 29, tapped into the services offered at the Learning Resource Center in undergrad school—a note taker, editors, spell checkers and extended time on tests. But now he works independently of them and likes it that way.

I'm living proof that even someone who almost is a high-school dropout can graduate from college with the highest honors, and be in medical school. I did very poorly in high school. I knew I wanted to be a doctor and I felt I was smart enough to be in medical school, so I stayed in. I didn't know I could have gone straight to a junior college and bypassed all the high-school shenanigans.

I had one 10th-grade teacher tell me I was border-line illiterate and to shape up, without offering any help, without even suggesting I get tested for a learning disability. I had to write an in-class book report, but I never bothered to read the book because I hated reading. I put the assignment to one side, telling myself I was just a lazy student. On the day of the in-class report, I made up the author's name, the story, the characters, plot and climax. What else was there to do? I figured out I could make up the whole thing and the teacher would never be the wiser. Actually, back then, I felt clever to outsmart the teacher. I learned early on though to understand the "system." That's how I got through high school.

On the flip side, I was a varsity swimmer. But, just as I was in peak shape the last semester of 12th grade, I was disqualified from the team. Why? I was failing French and the policy was that, if a student was failing a class he or she was dropped from varsity sports. I hated the class. I could speak fine, but I just couldn't master the spelling or grammar. I didn't know I had dyslexia. I just thought I was a "bad" student.

I was definitely a "C" student in high school. I was a bit of a jock, a bit of a nerd, a surf bum and I had some friends. The college counselor didn't really understand me. I was never part of the college-preparatory scene. I didn't take the SAT because I had no chance of going to a good school with my grades. Family support kept me going. My dad, a clinical psychologist, always had confidence in me and that's what made the difference.

The first few years at community college were the worst for me. But I got through them somehow. I wasn't diagnosed at the time and, having large loads of material to read, weighed me down. A few years later in grad school, it wasn't even the spelling of medical terms that was baffling (I love to spell those words). It was more that I couldn't spell common English words.

I finally was diagnosed with dyslexia at the age of 22 at a community college in Los Angeles. It happened when I went to see the English tutor. It was the first time she'd seen my original work, without the help of a word processor, so I wasn't able to spell check my work. Immediately, she said, "We need to get you tested." It's so important I found out because, at medical school, the workload is very intense. There are copious amounts of reading material. But outside school, I'm running into a slight roadblock. The national board of medical examiners refuses to give me accommodations for the medical licensing exam, even with elaborate documentation of my disability. Without extended time, the exam simply will be a measure of my reading speed and not my knowledge.

I reconnected with some fellow students at my 10-year, high school reunion. Some guys were working in Target, others in investment banking. Then there I was, a medical-school student.

Michael suggests:

❑ Just get through "it" (kindergarten through 12th or college)

❑ It is not a measure of your intelligence. It is only a measure of your ability to hold on and go for your dreams later.

PRAGMATISTS

Students take a realistic approach to college, they strike a balance between special accommodations and personalized coping strategies. I call them the *pragmatists*. Their attitudes range from: "I'll take what's offered and then add my own strategies" to "I'm comfortable with the plan in place but ready to make changes as I move forward." Several one-of-a kind strategies surface, a few gutsy ones, and a few common-sense approaches. Over 40 percent of responses land here, so it was natural to further categorize interviews into: under-grad students and grad students. Some interesting stories unfold.

Alex Black starts off at Stanford going it alone but by the second quarter of her freshman year, she's sinking. Then her life turns around. She gets a formal letter from the DRC (Disability Resource Center) to give to her profs and works on putting more passion into her outside activities and community service. Jack Peters talks openly with the dean in charge of LD students and gets extended time on papers. Spelling is not counted against him during in-class exams, and some professors even express personal concern for his different learning style. He works with an English tutor—trained in the Orton Method—off-campus. He has that tutor, or a friend, review his papers. With this combination, Brown definitely is manageable.

To fine-tune their college plans, Elizabeth Ball and Brenda Brown tap into formal services and personal strategies. Elizabeth, a final-year law student, takes advantage of all the accommodations available to her by law. She takes her exams with double time, takes a reduced course load and spreads out her exams over the exam period. When she's in class at Boston University, she sits in the very front row, in the middle, follows every word and tries to write everything down. If not, she has an official note taker for the gaps. For Brenda, working out at the gym on a bike and memorizing note cards at the same time, makes her feel less pressure about preparing for a quiz or test. Then with help from S.A.L.T. counselors at the University of Arizona, she learns to select specific classes on the basis of difficulty and faculty approach-ability.

On the other hand, Marty Monk is a graduate student who has picked up new strategies along the way. Marty uses Academic Support & Disability Services for reading and proofreading and has a learning assistant for his master's project in music education. He also petitions for a master's project instead of a written thesis and doesn't take the GRE for acceptance at the University of Southern California. Rather, he negotiates with the dean and is put on probation his first semester.

What can we say of these *pragmatists?* They alternate between "formal" help and their way of doing college, and they do a good job. They're like tourists choosing the all-inclusive package; they eat in designated restaurants but supplement that with own-choice restaurants; they take guided tours but supplement them with personal day trips. Striking a balance in anything we do, seems to work well. These college students, the *pragmatists,* are no different.

PRAGMATISTS
under-graduate students

JACK PETERS, junior, Brown University

Jack, 25, is studying political science after working for several years before entering the university. For his junior year, he is studying abroad at the London School of Economics.

I felt like I was walking in the dark in high school. I'm a poor speller and writer and a slow reader. I would get a "D" in English, then an "A" in math and science. I was bright, but I had dyslexia. I was confused. I found ways, though, to keep going . . .

I listened when my teachers, counselors and family told me I was very smart. I avoided any work that involved a lot of reading or writing. I learned by listening and took advantage of being a good talker. But after high school, I wasn't living up to my potential. I was working in L.A. I went from job to job. Then I decided to take classes at a community college, part-time at first. After a year, I went full-time. That was the start of my college experience.

There wasn't anything easy about college. The sheer volume alone of reading and writing was unbelievable. But I tell myself it's more fear than reality that I'm a slow reader. And I've learned to break down the projects into small bites. How do you eat a box of chocolate? One piece at a time. How do you read a book? One page at a time. That's how I've managed to get through the mounds of reading. Also, to keep me on-target, I use some coping strategies:

> I remind myself constantly that I have the ability to get better at English. It's just that I need the information presented to me in a different manner.

> I work with a tutor who is trained in the Orton Method. Sometimes, just having the tutor or a friend review my papers is encouraging.

> I talk with my professors about special accommodations at the beginning of each semester.

The dean in charge of LD students at Brown has been great. The college policy on reasonable accommodations for LD students is excellent. All my professors have complied. Some have even expressed personal concern. They wanted to make sure I was getting the help I needed. Others were curious and wanted to know more about dyslexia. I get extra time on tests, spelling isn't counted against me during in-class exams and I get extended time on papers. Plus, I talk openly with the dean if I have any worries. And now, I've become an advocate for other students with dyslexia.

Of course, I've had low times at college. I tend to sit in my room and procrastinate. On some level, I'm still afraid. So, the time I should be studying, I'm watching TV. And the time I should be spending with my friends, I'm studying. I tell myself I have to jump in the pool and start to swim. It's sink or swim. Sometimes, it works and I get rolling with the assignment. Sometimes, I hide under my sheets. A good nap is always appropriate.

It's too early to tell if I'm going to sink or swim in my new setting in London. I still have fear about reading and writing. But I have worked with a private tutor in Providence who practices the Orton Method. The tutor gave me lots of tools to help me with reading and writing. Now, I understand language. I can see new problems I have and ask the right questions to solve them.

But the London School of Economics doesn't seem to have the same type of accommodations for LD students as they do in the United States. I would say they're about 10 years behind. But, they're very willing to help. I just have to ask.

Once I reach grad school, I'm going to handle it like everything else. I'm going to walk through my fear and jump in the pool and start swimming.

Jack suggests:

❑ Realize dyslexia is a learning style, not a disability in the classic sense of the word. Find someone who can teach you in the style that best fits your learning.

❑ Work with a tutor who specializes in dyslexia, preferably one who teaches the Orton Method.

❑ Work on maintaining your self esteem.

ALEX BLACK, freshman, Stanford University

Alex, 18, says she needs to find somewhere, besides academics, to put her passion. She's active in NOW (National Organization for Women) and SHPRC (Sexual Health Peer Resource Center). As for the DRC (Disability Resource Center), she avoided it the first two quarters of her freshman year. But, by the third quarter, she was sinking. She now aligns herself with the center.

In 4th grade, it stopped being OK that I wasn't reading. There was concern. I call it the "What's Wrong With Alex?" game. I could talk. I had a large vocabulary. And there was evidence of intelligence. But I couldn't read or write. My mom, a high-school English teacher, was worried. She dragged me to an eye-and-ear specialist. The final stop was a psychiatrist. At 10, I actually started reading a 20-page book. That's when I had the lowest self-esteem. I saw myself as smart, yet I was held back in reading and spelling. My frustration showed up in problems with my friends—social problems. But, as soon as I was diagnosed with dyslexia—in the 4th grade—and got remedial help, my anger disappeared.

Fast forward to middle school and foreign languages. In 7th grade, I struggled with Japanese and failed with intensity. Then, in 9th grade, I took Spanish for a semester, but I couldn't finish the course. (Once I got out of the foreign-language requirement, I was fine. But I had to take them first to get it documented in my LD file.) Fortunately, my Spanish teacher also was the LD coordinator. She was on my side. She suggested I take more computer classes. I wanted to take sign language because I had learned a song in sign language at camp. It intrigued me. My college counselor agreed I should take a sign language course at the local community college. I took it after school at three different community colleges and then at San Francisco State University.

I got good at it. I worked at an after-school center for deaf children in San Francisco. It's more a social thing for the kids. Some of them can't talk to their parents because their parents never learned sign language. That certainly put my learning disability into perspective. I became so interested in these kids; I worked in a summer camp for deaf children my junior year.

By the time I hit 11th grade, I never felt left out because I was an LD student. Instead, I wanted a healthy place to focus my energy and frustration. I started a NOW group at my high school. We had weekly meetings. We marched to protest. And we worked in battered women's shelters. I was the main organizer. I found a place to put my energy.

As you can probably tell, I'm an action person. In my senior year, I thought we needed a sex-education program. I started the program and helped plan what they would talk about. A teacher and I gave seminars to juniors and seniors. It was a healthy place for students to talk about issues they had with sex. It was also a healthy place for me to put my energy. All of this helped distract people from my dyslexia.

Now, at Stanford, I feel like the one student with dyslexia. It's not easy when you have an "invisible disability." I spend a lot of time explaining what it means. Even the guy tutoring me in calculus asks how it affects my learning. He's the teaching assistant and he's clueless. He doesn't realize that, every time I write or spell, it has an impact on my life. Before I came to Stanford, mom used to edit all my papers. That doesn't work now. For the first quarter, my boyfriend helped me. Then, when we broke up in December, my papers were a mess. That middle quarter, I turned in really poor work. I was sinking. I was embarrassed to ask my resident assistant for help, my roommate wasn't very good at editing and I didn't know if the DRC did any of that. (I've since learned they do.)

Spelling is one of my biggest challenges, especially in my history lecture section. I had to turn in weekly reading responses, my thoughts on the readings. The TA said my spelling errors were so distracting and that I kept repeating them. She doesn't know I'm dyslexic. She doesn't know I check it over the best I can. Sometimes, it's done late at night, but she thinks I'm lazy and can't use the spell checker. I didn't talk to her because I didn't think she'd be receptive. In any case, the course is nearly over. This is what I face on a daily basis.

There was another problem during my spring-quarter calculus class. I have a different prof for each quarter of calculus. My dream is to become an OB-GYN. But, to finish pre-med requirements, I have to take these classes. So, this was my last calculus class. The previous two quarters I got accommodations with no problem. But, I ran into trouble with my third-quarter teacher when I asked him about extra time on my mid-term. He was mad that I hadn't talked to him at the beginning of the quarter. He took me into his office and said I was taking my learning disability lightly. As a freshman, I didn't know all the procedures. I'm supposed to take a letter from the DRC to the prof to indicate I'm an LD student. Just my luck, this prof already had been through this with another LD student. He seemed to resent the university telling him how to run his class. Then he told me he wouldn't give me extra time because

I hadn't requested it at the beginning of the quarter. Fortunately, the LD specialist told him that, as a freshman, I was new to this and he could be sued if he didn't give me the accommodations. He agreed. The most frustrating thing about all of that was that, before I approached him, I thought he was an excellent math teacher. But now, I feel uncomfortable in his class.

Up until the altercation with my math teacher, just being honest with my professors worked well for me. I don't think that's true now. I've learned my lesson the hard way. Just being punctual and handing in the letter from the DRC at the beginning of the quarter saves a lot of tears. In short, I need to conform.

For the most part, the DRC gives me a lot of emotional support. They let me cry. I ask for a note taker, but I don't ask for books on tape. The main thing I need from the DRC is support and their letter to faculty explaining my learning disability.

Actually, once I was accepted to Stanford, I phoned the DRC twice to ask about my foreign-language exemption. Both times, they said it would be no problem. This is important to find out because six quarters of a foreign language would end me. Now, I definitely want to do sign language instead.

When I came to Stanford, I promised myself I wouldn't get involved in group activities. I'd give myself some time to adjust to my new setting. But now that freshman year is nearly over, I've already planned for next year. I'm going to take on more responsibilities in the SHPRC and not just be satisfied with counseling one hour a week. I'll get involved in planning events. I'll spend more time in the center. I'm also definitely going back to NOW after being on sabbatical this year. Without these extra activities, my life is missing something. And, because I'm doing mediocre in school, I need other stimuli.

Looking down the road, I definitely want to go to medical school. I'm worried about the workload, especially memorizing all those technical words. First, though, I need to cope with pre-med classes and then see if my dream to be an OB-GYN is still there.

Alex suggests:
    ❏ Find somewhere else, besides strictly academics, to put your passion. Then, go to it and excel.

**NOAH ANDREWS, sophomore,
Southern Methodist University**

Noah, 21, takes what is offered in special accommodations and then supplements it with his own strategies.

I kind of waited to be the last to read, and then prayed time would run out. Teachers knew I preferred not to read out loud. I talked with them outside of class. Most understood my dilemma. But in the frenzy of high school chemistry and physics, sometimes they forgot. I always was into competitive sports—football—so it countered the challenges of school.

As for college, I'd have to say my savvy personal skills made all the difference. For example, my chemistry teacher and I are really good friends. We even go fishing together. He knows I hate to read out loud in class and he respects that. He also helps me out with class work and before tests.

I now have home phone numbers for my teachers' assistants and my profs. I don't abuse the privilege, but I feel more in control. The first week of school my sophomore year, I sat down with my chemistry TA and had a conversation about my different learning style. I got his e-mail address and copies of last year's tests. We got along great and I ended up meeting with him three days a week, one-on-one for extra help. Another time, in macroeconomics, I mentioned to the TA that the required textbook wasn't making much sense to me. She gave me another reference book, a more approachable one. I ended up with an 89.6 percent on the final. I was the only person in class to get an A- (90 percent).

I've already declared my major—business with a minor in chemistry. I'm also a pre-med student, so I'm taking classes that will lead me into dentistry. Some faculty are helpful; others are not. One or two don't believe in dyslexia. But, overall, it's never a problem because I just talk to them and try to make them understand where I'm coming from.

I use the Learning Enhancement Center on campus for tutoring. Then through Student Life—the office for LD students and students with other disabilities—I get extended time on tests and books on tape. The office sends out a letter to my professors requesting extended time.

A couple of things work really well for me at SMU. I share notes with my fraternity brothers. I also join study groups with the same people, semester after semester, when possible.

As for test questions, I totally dislike true/false, even though there's a 50-50 chance of getting the right answer. Actually, I'm OK with multiple-choice because I enjoy the elimination process.

Grad school still is a question. I want to go on to dental school, but it seems like I've already been in school forever. Every summer, I've taken extra classes. I think grad school needs to be put on hold while I work for a few years.

Noah suggests:

❏ Know your teachers/profs personally. From my experience, they love it and definitely will make time to give you additional help.

❏ Don't listen to anyone's negativity. Prove them wrong!

JERRIE RAMBO, junior, University of Maryland

Jerrie, 26, is studying sociology. She dropped out of school in the 9th grade, struggled at community college, and was first diagnosed with dyslexia at the age of 22 at the University of Maryland. Now, she's heading to law school.

Drugs and alcohol got me through middle school. Teachers didn't know where to place me. I went from being in the English honors class to the skills class. Without a doubt, 8th grade was my worst year. Between 7th and 8th grades, I made friends in the honors classes. Then, when they switched me to the average classes, I made friends there. Then, when I was switched to the skills—"dumb-dumb"—classes, I didn't want to be there. My friends couldn't understand why I was in "those" classes. I medicated myself with drugs and alcohol. It was a very tough time. By the time I got into high school, still undiagnosed, I dropped out of 9th grade after three months. No one understood me!

Not even at home. My mom didn't want me to quit school, so I moved out. I lied about my age and I took a job as a waitress. It was a crazy time. But, through it all, I managed to get a GED (General Education Diploma). And then I went on to Montgomery Community College in Maryland to get an AA degree. For five years, I took classes on a part-time basis. Then I transferred to the University of Maryland at College Park. Then, my life turned around.

I was diagnosed with dyslexia. I was 22. It was like someone pulled up the shade in a very dark room that had never seen light. Before that, I remember being terribly lost. One time, after fleeing from a math tutor session in tears, I prayed. I actually went into the bathroom stall and prayed I could get an explanation about what was wrong with me. Even if I had a brain tumor, like my father did before he died, I just needed to know what the problem was. Two weeks later, I was diagnosed. It all made sense.

Foreign languages and math are especially hard. I took pre-algebra in 7th grade (yuck, mixing letters and numbers) and was placed in it again in 8th grade, and again in 9th grade. Then, when I took the math placement test for community college, I took the same class, passed again and was tested years later for the university and was placed in it and passed it again! Obviously, there was a problem there, wouldn't ya' think? Undiagnosed dyslexia!

Now that I'm at U of M, I cope by advocating for myself. Actually, it's not just for me, but for others who will come after me. I'm a very determined and strong person. Not everyone has that. And, with a law degree . . .

When I have low times here, I reach out. I have a network of friends and professionals, from the Justice Department to the university counselors. I use Disability Support Services and seek out counselors at the Health Center. I use the DSS to take tests. I get time-and-a-half, a calculator, extra scrap paper and a separate, quiet room for test taking. DSS recently got a learning disability specialist to help the 400+ LD students. Time and attention is limited, but it will make a big difference. I also use the DSS to get through to stubborn professors who don't want to give me special accommodations.

I don't want "exceptions" from the professors, just accommodations. Sometimes, there seems to be a fine line. I've heard a few professors say: "I don't want any excuses." Well, I'm sorry, but, "my dog ate my homework" is an excuse; dyslexia is a disability. Our school also has a Legal Aid office for students, and those with disabilities have free access to an attorney. I've also gone to the Equity Officer, the school's attorney, to get things resolved. Our school has a human relations code prohibiting discrimination.

As for learning, books don't really do it for me. Now that I understand more about dyslexia, I definitely need a two-way interaction between the teacher or tutor and me. Off the top of my head, it's important for me to show up in class every day. Actually, though, one of the best ways to overcome my different learning style is to have a "coach," someone to help me stay focused and get organized. I use my counselor.

Social life? What social life? Life is school. School is life. For now. I wanted to join the theater. I also thought about joining Mock Trial. I've looked into legal internships. I was president of the Honors Pre-Law Society my first semester at U of M. But, it was all too time-consuming. To get into law school, I need to keep up my grades, and being dyslexic slows me down. So, I have no life outside school.

I'm determined to fully understand dyslexia. I do research in the library on the laws of access to an education. I need to know all my rights. I've worked hard to get here and I'm not going to just disappear like I did in high school. I deserve an education just like everyone else.

Jerrie suggests:

❏ Choose your battles wisely. You may not get through school in a "traditional" manner—full-time, on-campus, in a fraternity or sorority. But, if what you really want is to get through college, with focus, you can do it!

❏ Get a lot of sleep. My dyslexia gets worse with less sleep and I retain much less.

LEA BROWN, freshman, Stanford University

Lea, 19, has tapped into what is offered in special accommodations and is holding his own.

I never leave messages on the white boards around the dorm and I never pass notes in school. I can't always count on words. They come out differently than I expect. But when it comes to math and science, I'm right up there. I'm an engineering major and hope to co-term (stay for a 5th year) to get my master's in electrical engineering.

As a child, my mother and father read to me nightly, sometimes even twice a day. When I first learned to read, I read upside down because they were reading to me upside down. It took me awhile to undo that one. Despite my reading limitations, every day, my parents told me how smart I was. And, I have a photographic memory. I never doubted myself.

Still, 2nd grade was a disaster. I vividly remember a class project where I had to cut out shapes, then paste them on to paper. I couldn't do it. The teacher thought I was stupid. I hadn't mastered reading. Spelling was a big problem and so were grammar, punctuation and handwriting. And, now, shapes. Still, I always raised my hand in class, but the teacher never called on me. I was kind of pushed aside. She'd be shocked to know I'm at Stanford now.

I hit another roadblock in 5th grade. My papers came back with red all over them. It was humiliating. Plus, the teacher used my work as an example of the wrong way to use grammar. I'd come home crying. The teacher tried to fail me and the school tried to place me in lower classes. But that didn't work either because I'm accelerated in the sciences and math. I had to read my essays to teachers because they couldn't understand my handwriting. At recess, the kids asked why I was in the classroom so long. They never knew the whole truth.

Finally, at a parent-teacher conference the spring of that year, someone suggested I go to Dallas for psycho-education testing. For three days, professionals asked me questions. Then the pieces of the puzzle began to fit. I had dyslexia. The testing indicated I had an IQ of 137 and was in the top-two percentile for math and science. From then on, I got a tutor every day for an hour.

But high school was difficult for personal reasons. My peers didn't believe I had dyslexia because I got good grades. They didn't know I was paddling fast. After school, I would stay behind and talk to teachers. A lot of my friends would study together. I couldn't do that. That part hurt. I always felt different.

In class, I took tests during the regular test time, but typed up my test at home later that night, stapled it to the original test and then handed it in the next day. For note taking, I asked really good friends if I could copy their notes. I told them: "I'm not lazy. I just can't write as fast as you can." But even my teachers didn't understand.

For the SAT test, I had an option to take it with extended time, but decided not to go that route. I worked really hard to prepare. Over and over again, I did practice tests. It became my life in my junior year. I was so proud of myself. I got a 1410 on the test. I did self-identify to Stanford and had my tutor write a supporting reference.

The biggest problem at Stanford is writing papers because it takes me a long time, often 12 hours. Luckily, several friends in the dorm, and the resident assistant, enjoy editing. Although it's hard depending on my friends, I've found I can get by with their help.

Besides writing papers, Spanish is a major challenge. I took two years of it in high school but I still struggle. I'm considering doing a semester abroad in Spain, for total cultural immersion. I'm more an auditory learner, so that could work well for me.

Through the Disability Resource Center, I get a note taker, time and a half on tests and the use of a voice-recognition software program—"Dragon NaturallySpeaking." Faculty has been very accommodating as long as I have the DRC letter at the beginning of each quarter. I haven't tried to talk to them. Some are interested and some just don't have the time.

Lea suggests:

❑   Have a good attitude. Don't think of yourself as stupid. Don't see dyslexia as a disability, just a difference.

❑ You can do anything when you work hard enough and get the right help. Remember, it can be frustrating working harder than others, but it's worth it.

❑ There's no reason you can't do as well or better than others. You see things in a different light and you're often more perceptive. That's one heck of a bonus.

MAUREEN BARDEY, freshman,
Oxford College at Emory University

Maureen, 24, gets frustrated trying to pull together all her special accommo-dations and personalized strategies. Still, she has several things that work well for her.

Sometimes I wonder if I was adopted. My siblings all are gifted. I joke about it, but it hurts. It hurts a lot. My older sister, 26, graduated from Georgia Tech in electrical engineering. My brother, 20, signed up for the Navy and his test scores were so high he immediately was accepted into the Nuclear Power Program. My other sister, 14, is in 8th grade. Next year, she'll be in all honors classes and currently is in 10th-grade honors geometry. My other sibling is in the 6th grade. He, too, is a year ahead of himself in math. Both my parents have college degrees, my mother a Ph.D. in education and my dad a bachelor's in art. And here I am, a struggling college freshman.

But my family has been my rock. I never liked school and never felt I fit in. In high school, I was separated into honors classes and found many friends.

But, after I was diagnosed, the honors classes became AP classes and I couldn't keep up with the fast pace, the amount of reading and paper writing. I missed my friends. It was frustrating being smart and fitting in with those at the top of the class, but not being up there with them academically. Only my best friend knew what was going on.

I wasn't sure what I wanted to do after high school. I worked in paid jobs, in between going to a commuter college, all the while trying to find out what I really wanted to do in life. I tried several entry-level jobs. I thought if I worked hard, a boss would notice and maybe I could move up. I never felt I did well at any of the jobs. Often times, I felt extremely stupid. I was sobbing hysterically in the clinical psychologist's office one morning, after being fired from the easiest waitressing job, when I learned a very important lesson. She smiled at me and calmly said: "Don't you get it? You'll never be good at those jobs. The easy, no-brainer, redundant jobs play directly into your weak areas. What you have is the higher thinking that most college graduates have. The jobs you will do best in are the jobs graduates get." I'd never looked at life like that before. It was a new beginning. I decided then that college wasn't going to be easy, but I was going.

Now that I'm here, just about everything is a challenge. Most classes consist of reading, writing and lectures. English has been especially hard because of all the required papers. I'm planning to get a Bachelor of Science instead of a Bachelor of Arts so the amount of papers required will be reduced.

Here at Emory, there's a small pool of learning-disabled students and the Office of Disability Services handles all my requests. The Office has offered to get me books on tape, extended time on tests, a quiet room for testing and a note taker. Ah yes, a note taker. I try to talk to the prof before the first class starts or after the first class. I'm asking for someone to take notes in the class (it's a paid job). This turned out odd. A prof agrees to make an announcement in the next session and, usually, he'll say "Jennifer, how do you want to play this one?" Undiluted humiliation. This took me by surprise. Don't they know about anonymity? Finally, I got a note taker, but often it was difficult to read their notes. They were written on a carbon pad, with one copy for me and one for them. Most times, I feel like I'm fighting alone.

For extended time on tests, I hand my professors a standard letter from the Office. It covers my documented disability and outlines legal rights. I try to meet with individual profs to discuss what would be best in their class. But, in reality, I'm asking to take a test differently. I'm asking to be different. Most of the time, their response is "yes, we can work this out." Then comes the actual first test. Some profs start to wriggle. They feel uncomfortable about the whole thing. Now they're saying: "I'll have to check with the Disability Office." Suddenly, it's all a problem. They're worried if they're being fair, if it's legal, if I'm cheating.

School is hard enough without fighting "the system." I don't need the social battle between the faculty and the Office. The Office is flooded with requests. If I were in a school where all this was in place—no fighting, no hassling—I would be 50 percent better off. Then I could concentrate on schoolwork.

There's something else that has more to do with the system than the office. A GPA list gets posted at the end of each term. So far, I have a 3.0 GPA for two English writing classes, algebra, Sociology 300, The Health Care System and P.E. But I didn't see my name on the list. Why? Because administration has classified me as a part-time student (I was taking 10 units) and my grades were lost somewhere in the computer. Talk about being different and feeling different!

Because LD students are a minority here, the profs aren't used to our requests. One of my strong suits is my analytical mind. But it plays against me when I evaluate special-needs facilities on campus. On the other hand, it's a bonus when I come up with my own coping strategies. Here are some of them:

Maureen suggests:

❑ Advocate for yourself. It's usually darn uncomfortable, sometimes humiliating, but it has to be done.

❑ Establish a support system right off the bat—before the start of the semester—instead of waiting for problems to occur. See a counselor, meet with the Academic Dean or the LD office, talk to an advisor, and identify yourself to each professor before classes starts.

❑ Take difficult courses daily or three times a week, not as all-day classes. Spreading out the difficult information into smaller pieces helps. Consider taking a difficult class at other institutions—just make sure the credits transfer equally.

❑ Don't ever think you're less worthy than someone else. Try not to compare yourself with others, especially siblings.

❑ Be prepared to work hard and have a list of fun-activities when you feel frustrated or "stuck."

Maureen has since left Oxford College at Emory and is working as a marketing associate in Atlanta.

ANA SINTO, senior, Brown University

Ana, 22, plans to go on to medical school. Faculty members are not encouraging her to do this. Science courses and statistics classes are very difficult for her. She's determined to be a doctor.

It's like not noticing the fat at a health spa. Then again, maybe it's not that obvious here at Brown. But dyslexia is obvious to me. This is a highly academic environment. The first three years were extremely difficult because I didn't know what my problem was, why I couldn't do well, why I was struggling. Then I got tested and my life seemed to turn around.

All along the way, my family was very supportive, especially since we didn't know exactly what my problem was until my junior year in college. I think they thought I was just kind of slow. Or that I was still trying to adjust to college life. That wasn't it. I needed help.

I think that accomplishments, despite the dyslexia, are something to be proud of. But, I wouldn't go around waving a banner announcing it to everyone. Special accommodations are very important. It's not going to get you the "A" or, in some cases, the "B." You have to do that on your own. But, you don't need anything else working against you. For instance, noise and too little time. Fortunately, the faculty has been fine so far. I think they understand. I also believe if you go to a faculty member saying you have ADD, and not dyslexia, they still accommodate you, but they may seem hesitant.

After graduation, I plan to go to medical school. No one else thinks I can do it. Most of the faculty here aren't encouraging me because science classes are really difficult for me. But I know I can be a great doctor. Statistics also is very hard. I admit, I'm a little worried about the workload at medical school. But it's something I really want to do. I'm not going to be put off because grad school is challenging.

I don't think anyone should shy away from something because they're not as good as someone else or because it's too challenging. If you want to do well, get help with your disability. I can't really tell you the magic words for maintaining good self-esteem. To this day, I struggle with my own. It's just a day-to-day battle.

Ana suggests:
   ❏ Find out when you work best and always work during that time.

Also, you can't afford to procrastinate. It will kill you academically.

- ❑ Stay away from pill-pushers.
- ❑ Don't listen to the pessimists.

MICHAEL LEVINE, senior,
University of Southern California

Michael, 27, is studying communications. He transferred from Los Angeles Community College, where he earned his Associate degree. Michael plans to go on to grad school to major in film and television production. He was born in Israel, came to study in the U.S. when he was 21, and is severely dyslexic.

Sometimes, I think I'm like a blind student. Thank goodness I'm not. I just need so much help—a scribe, a reader, books on tape, taped lecture notes. The hard part about transferring from Los Angeles Community College to a four-year college was finding a system that worked for me. USC didn't know me and I had to tell them what I needed. Thankfully, they responded to my special needs.

But let me backspace. I always was a bright student. I participated in classroom discussions and understood the material. I managed to get "B's." The teachers knew I had a lot of potential. But, I made the most horrific spelling mistakes. Actually, I was the one in high school who took the initiative—not my parents or my teachers—to find out why I was struggling. The school psychologist tested me and I had dyslexia. I managed to get extra time on the matriculation exam. I passed and was offered a place at Tel Aviv University.

I was upholding a tradition. My whole family went to college. It was expected of me, too. I started in the theater directing program at Tel Aviv, but I didn't like the classes. I left after my sophomore year and went to Los Angeles to study drama or photography. (I was looking for ways to study without having to read and write.) I took a bunch of film and television courses through the UCLA extension program. It wasn't a degree program, so I felt more comfortable, less threatened. I figured, with a degree program, I probably wouldn't be able to read all the textbooks. Then, I wouldn't be able to pass the exams. I was frustrated. I never thought I didn't have the intellect to go to college.

I really got interested in television production while I was studying film and

TV through the UCLA extension program. I heard Los Angeles Community College was a good school for that. I signed up for three classes—television production, psychology and speech communication. But, after the second week, I dropped psychology when the first paper was due. I also dropped speech. I just wasn't able to write the papers or read the books. The speech teacher said I should contact the Learning Resource Center. This is where I began to become a mainstream student. As soon as I met with the counselors, I felt relaxed. They tested me and offered me all the accommodations I needed. That's where I found a learning assistant who really helped me. I finally felt I had a chance to get a formal education like anyone else.

Another turning point came when I was encouraged to take the English Placement Test at the community college. I scored high enough to get into English 101. The day of the first in-class essay, I came in late. The teacher asked me why. I told her I couldn't spell words in a way that wouldn't insult my intelligence. The paper wouldn't reflect my abilities or my understanding of the material. She immediately suggested I go to the Resource Learning Center and get someone to scribe it. That's when a bell started to ring—I could dictate my thoughts. I wrote a paper on "The Invisible Man." I got an "A." The Center gave me the tools to make it possible to write a paper. I owe a lot to them.

I'm the one responsible for getting accommodations at USC, not anyone else. I have to let the office of Academic Support and Disability Services know what I need. So, at the beginning of every semester, I tell my professors I'm dyslexic and show them a letter from the center explaining my special needs. If I'm lucky, they have most of my GE classes on tape. They're a great resource for English literature books. And, there's no charge. They also gave me a four-track tape player to use. Plus, I have readers who will record a book for me if that's what I need. I'm allowed to choose my readers, so the sound is reliable. They record handouts, journal articles and some chapter book readings. It's going very well. For lectures, I use a tape recorder. That's how I read and learn, by listening to everything. I follow the book and highlight while I'm listening to the tape.

When I have to write something like a 20-page paper, though, it's tough. Usually, I think about the topic, sketch out an outline and then discuss it with my professor. Once I've selected the library books, I get together with my reader, who reads to me and writes down my thoughts. I also get shortcuts off the "Web."

I have to schedule all my work very carefully with my readers and scribes. I'm taking 18 units a semester, plus doing my job on campus as stage manager. That's a 20-hour-a-week commitment. I really like the work, though. I'm also in the honors communications program, so I'm required to do an internship. Mine is with ABC's "Politically Incorrect" and it takes me 18 hours a week. I help writers with their research. I'm definitely thinking of applying to grad school to get a master's in television production.

Michael suggests:

❏ Find out the technical reasons why you're not succeeding.

❏ After understanding your needs, find a college that will accommodate you.

ALICIA VARGAS, senior, Brown University

Alicia, 22, is focusing on American Civilization. Alicia, who is Latino, grew up in the inner city of Hartford, CT. She was diagnosed with dyslexia during her sophomore year at Brown. It was a difficult time for her. She no longer was the Wonder Woman she'd been in high school. She uses any accommodations she can get.

I got labeled before I even reached adolescence. I was Latino. The people around me in school said I was going to "mess up." They had it all scripted. I was going to drop out of high school, meet some guy and get pregnant. Some of my relatives believed this, too, and so did some of my teachers. I wanted to prove them wrong. Not only was I going to college, I was going to an Ivy-League college. Funny, at that time—I was only 10—I didn't even know what that meant. All I knew was that I was going to become one of the best.

I graduated as the valedictorian from my junior-high school. But, when I got to high school, the faculty told me I couldn't get into honors classes. I became enraged. I knew legally I had the right to be in those classes. With my parents' help, we managed to persuade the principal. My personal WAR had begun. I was Latino, but I was college bound. I already was looking into college scholarships in the 9th grade. This was the only way for me. No matter what I had to achieve, I'd do it. I took the most challenging courses, played soccer, ran track, joined clubs and was a member of the National Honor Society. I would stay up until 3 or 4 a.m. every night reading, note taking and writing papers. No one but my parents knew how hard I worked. I did everything I had to do to get into a good college.

At first, I thought everyone had to work that hard to get "A's." I didn't know I had dyslexia. And, sorry to say, no one in my school ever noticed it either. It wasn't until I won a Connecticut Youth Math and Science scholarship and attended summer classes at a private school, that someone realized. The teachers and dorm advisors noticed that I would study all the time and never socialize. They were the first to recommend I be tested. But, my high school had no facilities and it was too expensive for my parents to pay for testing. I didn't get tested. Instead, I learned to work twice and four times as hard as everyone else. I just figured that was the only way to be successful. And, it worked. With determination, good grades and my parents' emotional support, I got into Brown.

Then, I reached the second semester of my sophomore year. I started to get anxiety attacks and even an ulcer. I took on too much. My limits were tested. I became human. I became destructible. I failed a class. Not because I didn't have the ability to pass it or to understand the material. It was because I ran out of time. I couldn't re-read the material. I decided to talk to the Dean of Students and he suggested I get tested. When I found out what I'd suspected was true all along, my world came crashing down. I had run myself into an unhealthy state. I was staying up until all hours of the night, studying, re-reading notes and drinking lots of coffee. I couldn't sleep, and I had horrible nightmares.

After the diagnosis, I wanted to run and hide from myself. Why wasn't I normal? I felt dumb. Why couldn't I be like everyone else? I hated being me. I felt like I could never accomplish or go beyond what I'd already done. This had never happened to me before. It was at this low point when I was awarded a Carnegie Mellon Fellowship. It jolted me, made me see the light. Throughout my self-evaluation, I told myself I had proven I could make it at Brown. It didn't matter if I was special; I had what it took to succeed. This seemed to free me.

I used the summer between my sophomore and junior years to figure out how I was going to work with this learning difference. It took all of my junior year and several deans to help me do it. Multiple-choice tests still are my nightmare. So, I've avoided taking classes with that type of testing. Writing long papers is terrifying, too. Every time I write a term paper, I usually revise it six times. I have a writing tutor and I try to take as many English classes as possible. It all helps.

Organization is one of my strong points. I carefully allot time for my social activities. I work out daily and I spend time at meetings and with friends. I set up a schedule to do my assignments ahead of time and only use additional time to hand in papers if I'm really pushed. I take the regular amount of classes and I'm concentrating on graduating with honors. If you look in the dictionary under "organization," you'll find my name.

I now know how to work with my dyslexia. That makes a big difference. So, I'm not concerned about coping with the workload at grad school. I know it will be harder than at Brown, but I can do it. I am concerned, though, about taking the GRE and LSAT tests. I know I can take them with extended time, but it's still scary. I'll most likely try to get a history or law degree. After I graduate, I'm going to get a research fellowship. Then I'll probably apply to grad school the following year.

Alicia suggests:

❑ Concentrate on what you've already achieved, not on what you haven't. It will give you the strength to go on.

❑ The worst trap you can fall into is questioning yourself, questioning your intelligence, questioning your self-worth. Dyslexia isn't going to stop you from doing what you want to do. The only thing that can stop you is who you are deep inside—your fear of trying, your fear of fighting, your fear of succeeding.

❑ Find an organizational pattern that works for you. But never model yours after someone else.

❑ And, above all, carry a pen and paper with you at all times.

SCOTT JESSER, senior, private liberal arts college, NH

Scott, 22, tapped into the Academic Development Center for accommodations and talked openly with faculty about how they could better understand and help him. In Scott's eyes, having determination brought everything together for him in college.

I was in the 7th and 8th grade when I started feeling so different from everyone else. I was in the Special Ed class in a local public middle school in Connecticut. I was so ashamed. I would sneak into the bathroom right before the bell rang so no one would see me going into the class. Family support got me through those difficult school years.

My mother had a knack for knowing when something wasn't right. She was my "knight in armor." She fought against a local public school that wasn't giving me a proper education. It caused the school to send me (they paid tuition) to Landmark School, a private school for learning-disabled students in 5th and 6th grades. The Landmark experience sent me in the right direction. I really don't know where I'd be today if it weren't for my mother and Landmark.

Seven years later, though, I still was very nervous about applying to college and then getting through college. I got acceptances from Boston College and Curry College, both in Massachusetts. I didn't make it to the University of Vermont. I haven't really had low times in college, but I've often thought I'd be much better off if I wasn't LD.

I've had to develop many strategies. I use the Academic Development Center a lot. I get accommodations. I get papers corrected by others. Knowing everything the school offers is very important. Talking to professors about my dyslexia helps, too. They understand what I need to make me successful in their class. Mostly, though, I have a lot of determination.

Writing papers and reading all the assigned material were my biggest challenges in college. I've always needed to spend more time on academics than others. I just need to be very disciplined.

I'm a nursing major now and I need to take my nursing boards soon. I'm really nervous. I need to just study, study, study. The nursing boards are multiple-choice and I'll have extended time and no reader. I'm not taking them orally. In 2004, the boards are changing to all essay questions. If only I could delay it until then. I'm hoping to go on to grad school in a few years, to get an MD or a nurse-practitioner degree.

Scott suggests:

❑ Learn to advocate for yourself. If something isn't working for you, talk to your parents or go to others you trust. It's a very hard thing to do, but it's a vital skill to have.

❑ Brush off negative comments from others.

❑ Understand how you learn best. It's an important piece of information. It will make learning easier.

❑ Just because you have dyslexia, it doesn't mean college is impossible. I did it and many others just like me did it. It takes dedication and the willingness to sacrifice other things.

❑ You need to have fun at college because, if you don't, you'll burn out. Learn to relax.

NATALIE NIELSON, recent graduate,
Brigham Young University

Natalie, 22, has a degree in Early Childhood Education. She is the only one of five children – she has two brothers and two sisters – diagnosed with dyslexia. In her sophomore year at BYU, the foreign-language department decided to accept American Sign Language into the curriculum. Natalie jumped at the opportunity. She now works for the California School for the Deaf, using signing skills on a daily basis.

My mother and prayer helped me get through the turbulent school years. My elementary years were just one struggle after another. I was in the slow reading group, remedial math, the last to be picked on the team, and went to my "special class" every afternoon. I took a lot of tests, talked to psychologists and wondered what was wrong with me. I knelt at my bed every night asking God for help. The prayers got me through the long days of not understanding my assignments, guessing at answers, staring at words which mean nothing to me, kids teasing and laughing at me and teachers pushing me aside.

It was at a special school for dyslexia where I found the answer to my nightly prayers. Here, I learned to read, spell, and write, using the Slingerland Multisensory Teaching Method—I transferred to this school after I was diagnosed in 3rd grade. But, mostly, I learned I wasn't alone. For the first time in my life, I was popular. I had friends with whom I could eat lunch. And, if I didn't do well in school, I knew there were areas in which I could shine—gymnastics, dance class, the school play and singing in a performing group. This made all the difference.

But when I mainstreamed back into public middle school, my self-esteem plummeted. I had a difficult time adjusting to the large, somewhat impersonal campus. I thank my mother for getting me through it. She was my friend. She focused on the things I did well. I got involved in community theater and started voice lessons. Never once did I doubt her love for me, or my worth in the eyes of God. She read to me every night. She drove me to all my tutors and rehearsals and corrected every homework assignment that came through the door. Yet, I still wasn't happy. Finally, we found a small, private school and I completed 8th grade there. Mom worked by my side and, together, we got my first "A" in English!

By the time I entered public high school, I was quite confident. The district didn't offer me any special tutoring or counseling because I wasn't in their

"Special Ed" program, but I learned to hold my own. My parents continued to hire outside math and English tutors. Again, my mother was my greatest source of support.

I knew I wanted to go to BYU because my parents and sisters had gone there. It was the only place I applied. I studied with a private tutor for the ACT, but it was a struggle getting permission to take the test with extended time. By the time I received the test results, the BYU admissions deadline had passed. I was devastated.

Once again, though, a prayer was answered. I got accepted to BYU on ONE condition, that I begin in the summer term. So, two weeks after high-school graduation—I was only 17—I packed up and went to college. For the first time, I was on my own. I didn't have anyone to correct my papers. No one to read to me. And no idea how hard college was going to be. I was frightened.

The Resource Center and good friends helped me overcome my fear. BYU has a great support group of counselors. One was assigned to me. She gave me several new techniques for note taking, studying and test taking. I learned how to skim a text, read the paragraph headings, go back and review the text and go back and ask myself questions. By the end of my college career, I was a pro at textbook skimming.

With hours of practice, I ended up getting "A's" and "B's" on my papers. One of my greatest lifesavers came during my sophomore year at BYU. The Foreign Language Department accepted American Sign Language into their curriculum. Until then, the math or foreign-language option had been a huge fear of mine. But, sign language, certainly I could do that. And I did. I got an "A" in every class. Today, I work for the California School for the Deaf in Fremont CA. I teach deaf kids who are dyslexic. I really care about them. I go to bed at night thinking about how I can help them.

I went to every study group I could and found a friend to call in every class in case I missed some notes or didn't understand an assignment. I visited the writing lab and used "SpellCheck" . . . a lot! My freshman year was challenging. My grades really plummeted because I was partying. I was in choir and I was in a sorority, too. When you're going through rush, it takes up all your time. I made that choice because I wanted to be involved. But once I figured out the system and learned a way of studying that worked for me, college became very manageable. I graduated with a 3.0. It was amazing. I had accomplished a life-long goal.

Natalie suggests:

❑ Look for the good things in yourself and make the most of them.

❑ Reach out to others. It's easy to feel self-pity and wallow in bitterness. But there's always someone out there who is less fortunate than you and whose problems are far greater.

❑ Give of yourself and you will find joy and happiness. That is the real success.

BRENDA BROWN, recent graduate, University of Arizona

Brenda, 22, got her degree in psychology with a minor in Spanish .

My roommates thought I studied too much. But if I didn't go that extra mile, my grades would have been very different than the "B's" and "C's" I was getting. Any leisure time I had, I spent with my friends and my boyfriend.

I didn't, however, sacrifice my love for keeping fit. I went to the gym daily. I studied there, too. I worked out on the bike and memorized note cards. For some reason, the gym helped me focus on what I was studying. On the bike, I felt less pressure about preparing for a test. On the days when I was frustrated with not being able to perfectly memorize what I'd been studying, I didn't get too upset because at least I was getting a workout. In the end, this keep fit/study program led to better health and better self-esteem.

S.A.L.T. counselors helped me plan each semester and select courses that were appropriate for my major and my minor. They also made sure I had the right number of units in each area so I could graduate in four-and-a-half years. I started in the S.A.L.T. program my freshman year and it really helped with my transition from high school to college. Each semester, when the class schedule came out, there was an asterisk next to several classes indicating that S.A.L.T. students did well in them. The counselors also knew which classes were extremely difficult or which faculty weren't as understanding.

Special accommodations helped tremendously at U of A. Once in awhile, my mind goes blank when I'm taking a test. I know what I want to say, but the words don't come out properly. With special accommodations, I could take my time and really concentrate. I took extended time tests (double time) in the Testing Accommodations Center. Actually, a few mainstream students took their tests there, too. Faculty were very trusting when I told them I was a S.A.L.T. student. They never asked for the official letter from the program. They gave me the accommodations I requested.

The best years of my life were in college. I got a good education, made wonderful friends and met a serious boyfriend I'm still dating. I became my own person in college. I learned a lot about myself, my values and what I enjoy.

An especially important lesson about my values came during my freshman year. I chose friends who smoked pot and partied. I ended up doing much worse those semesters than when I chose friends who studied seriously. I learned the hard way. Fortunately, my boyfriend and my best friend are 4.0 students. If I ever had questions, they were smart enough to answer them.

SUE PRINCETON, recent college graduate, Norwich University

Sue, 27, has a degree in Early Childhood Education. She graduated cum laude and has accumulated 12 units toward her master's in Special Education. She also teaches 1st grade at a school for learning disabilities. Sue tapped into the Resource Center on a daily basis. She used a reader, scribe, one-on-one tutoring and books/text on tape, recorded by an advisor. She has developed her own survival kit.

I just became a sponge for information. For a three-credit course, I'd go to the Learning Center for two hours a week. It wasn't uncommon after track practice to stay there until 10 p.m. If I didn't understand something, I asked the professor, the tutor or friends. Reading and writing aren't my strengths. I remember a psychology course, my sophomore year, where there was so much reading material, I got overwhelmed. My tutor offered to record the textbook on tape. Brilliant. Her familiar voice made learning so much easier. Another strategy I had was to sit in the front row in class so I could see and hear everything the professor said.

Thank goodness for my girlfriends. As a freshman at Bethany College (WV), they noticed I studied many hours in my dorm and in the Learning Center, but I wouldn't get good grades. Western Civilization was particularly difficult. I used taped lectures to help me understand the material and my roommates acted it out. The acting helped me visualize that time in history. My friends also knew track was my social arena. Most nights, I had to be in bed by 10-10:30 because of daily track practices. I asked my roommates to watch TV in another room. I owe a lot to my friends.

Then there were the off-campus obstacles. A few days into my freshman year, I opened up a checking account. But I was scared to write a check for fear I would misspell words. I came up with a neat solution. On a very small sheet of paper, I made a little list of numbers in word form. For example, 8 was eight, 11 was eleven, etc. I taped this to my checkbook. Plus, I learned to ask the sales assistant for a business card. Then I clearly could see the spelling of the company. It saves me any embarrassment.

After graduation from Norwich, I got certified to teach preschool through 3rd grade. That was a difficult time for me because I had to take the NTE (National Teachers Exam). The test was oral, but I failed the first time. The next time, I passed all the sections except General Knowledge. I took that section one more time before I passed the NTE in full. Now, I teach 1st-graders in a Catholic elementary school. The school specializes in learning disabilities and my firsthand experience with dyslexia is well received by parents and educators.

I also take summer classes at Cleveland State University in groups of 6-8 students. I already have 12 credits toward my master's in Special Education. It's a good fit for me.

Sue suggests:
- ❑ Find a college that meets your needs.

- ❑ Be honest about your learning difference. Know your strengths and work on your weaknesses.

- ❑ Don't give up

PRAGMATISTS
graduate students

ELIZABETH BALL, law student, Boston University

Elizabeth, 27, is a final-year law student. She completed her undergraduate degree at Carleton College, a small liberal arts school in Minnesota. She lives in Boston with her twin sister, who is not dyslexic.

I was lucky. I have a wonderful family. I have a supportive, academically involved mother. And I was popular as a child. I was able to build self-esteem early. I won scholarships in ballet and danced in the Nutcracker and Copeilla ballets. I acted in school plays. Plus, I have always loved athletics. I played varsity soccer in high school and college, and ran varsity track in college.

Achieving academic success was the number one thing in my family. My parents expected that I do my best. So I did. In high school, I just worked as hard as I possibly could. I never gave up. At that time, I didn't know I was dyslexic. In my senior class, I was ranked No. 3. And, despite my hatred of Spanish, I was the secretary of the Spanish club.

My most difficult years probably were the middle-school years. But it was more for social reasons. I didn't like my body. Because of my excessive ballet training, I went through puberty late. Then, at Carleton College, I had light-deprivation depression. I'm not sure if it was directly linked to my difficulties with Spanish, calculus and astronomy, or whether I'm simply prone to depression under strain. I know I have severe anxiety and a fear of failing academically. And, most recently, I had self-esteem problems because of Boston University's attitude toward students with disabilities. I was part of a class-action lawsuit against the university when they attempted to change policies in violation of the Americans with Disabilities Act. The outcome of the suit helped boost my self-esteem.

Practical and formal logic are, by far, the hardest college courses I've ever taken. But, I mastered them after hundreds of hours of practice problems. Then, I went on to become the teaching assistant for both classes. Calculus is very difficult for me and multiple-choice tests still are the bane of my existence. I love English and I've always excelled in it. But, I work very hard at writing my papers. In law school, I was picked to be a TA for the first-year writing program. I find that, once I master certain material, I'm a very good teacher. These are my strategies that have helped me along the way . . .

I function best in a completely silent room. My desk literally is in my closet at home. I live in a very quiet neighborhood and our apartment is on the third floor of a house. I don't even try to read anywhere else but in my bedroom. And, there can't be anybody or anything, not even my cat, in my closet when I'm working. I usually have on a small, loud fan to block out any potential sound or voice I may hear outside my closet door. I often drape a white table-cloth over my desk to help me concentrate. Even stray pencil marks on the desk can distract me.

When I'm in class, I sit in the very front row and watch the professor's lips as (s)he speaks. I follow every word. I try to write down everything because I can't hold more than a few words in my mind at once. If I can't keep up with the professor, I have no problem. I use a note taker for the "gaps." I also take advantage of all the accommodations available to me by law but I don't work through the LDSS (Learning Disabilities Support Services). I take my exams with double time. I take them in a separate, quiet room. I take a reduced course load and spread out my exams over the exam period. I don't use books on tape because I have auditory, as well as visual, dyslexia. I don't feel embarrassed or get discriminated against by faculty because grading is "blind". I'm my own advocate and it works for me.

I don't waste time socializing at school. But I make an effort to get involved in organizations I find intriguing. I was president of the Women's Law Association my second year of law school. And, I started an organization for law students with disabilities and served as its president. I'm proud when I do things that benefit myself and other people with dyslexia.

Above all, I listen to my body. As a law student, the first criteria for being able to do my work is my physical and mental health. I suffer from depression, migraines and back pain. If I have a migraine, I go to bed immedi-ately. Attempting to get things done when I'm in pain simply is a waste of my time.

Elizabeth suggests:
❑ Get accommodations for grad school entrance exams—GRE, GMAT, LSAT etc. I did for the LSAT and it helps.

BETH HENDERSON, Ph.D. student,
University of Southern California

Beth, 23, is a first-year doctoral student in developmental psychology. She completed her Associate degree at the College of San Mateo in California and her under-grad degree at USC.

Teasing, crying and self-loathing were daily events in grade school. I considered myself the proverbial "dumb kid." Being intelligent, bright and dyslexic was extremely frustrating. I knew I was as smart or smarter than the other kids, but I couldn't show that. They were reading chapter books by themselves, writing stories, climbing trees, catching balls and riding bikes around the neighborhood, things that were almost impossible for me. I couldn't understand why I was so different. I hated myself for being a failure. Temper tantrums weren't uncommon. I couldn't escape from the despair and disgust.

This cycle continued into middle school. Then, I finally found the key to set me free. It was long, delicate and silver. It was the flute. As soon as the silver mouthpiece touched my lips, I was home. I had found a way to express myself. Finally, my intellect and creativity were out in the open. Finally, I could be proud of myself.

It was a combination of influences that made my high-school experiences positive. Music definitely was a tremendous release and support for me. It provided an opportunity for me to participate creatively in school, as well as gain recognition for excellence. But, mostly, music allowed me to get in touch with my emotions. Music opened my heart in a very safe and wonderful way. The acute attention to detail required to achieve musical excellence was good for me, too, in terms of developing organizational skills and a critical, intuitive mind. Is it any wonder I'm now a research scientist?

My family support also was a key factor. My father recorded textbook assignments for me on tape. My mother really encouraged me to be my own person and to explore all of my creative options. I was treated as a responsible adult and behaved as such. Knowing someone believed in me was very energizing. It reminded me there wasn't anything I couldn't handle.

Having good social skills also played a part in my survival. I can't tell you how many free tutors I got from making friends with the "nerds." A large network of friends helped me cope with stress, and kept me active and alert.

And, laughter really was the best medicine.

Actually, I never thought of high school as something I needed to survive. I knew I was smart and that I had the skills to cope with my different processing mechanism. School, despite its challenges, has always energized me. I kept extremely busy with outside activities. But the most rewarding of all my activities was tutoring language arts to students in the Resource Specialist program during my junior and senior years. I gave them strategies on how to take notes, prepare for tests and survive when those around them didn't understand that they learned differently.

College has been purely about the joy of learning for me. I've made friends with a group of people who are academically successful and involved in campus activities. I've adopted their study habits and they provide me with support, release and a role-modeling system. As a senior last year, I was a resident advisor for 500 under-grad students, vice president of the Blue Key National Honors Society, a member of the Residential Student Leader Honorary Society and on the Deans' list, to boot. Now that I'm adjusting to the frenzied world of first-year, grad-school academia, I'm feeling very comfortable. I'm eager to learn.

My main coping strategy always has been knowing myself. I need to decide when I'm most productive in terms of being able to sit down and study. I need to create my ideal study environment and find good study groups to support my learning. I need to know what works for me—linguistics and statistics are logical. Astronomy, music theory, and math are challenging. I also have to learn to accept that I'm not perfect and that's OK.

I've been working as a graduate assistant in the Learning Resource Center, where I'm a paraprofessional education therapist. I do intakes, counseling, Slingerland remediation, testing and setting up accommodations. Through interacting with students like me, I realize how unique and gifted people with disabilities are. Most importantly, how "normal" they are. It makes me realize I'm really not "freaky" or "different." I still take all of my exams at the Center.

USC has been incredible in providing me with accommodations and support. We call ourselves the Trojan family. I've been lucky. Grad school is a huge time and energy commitment. Before I even applied to the doctoral program, I made sure I really knew in my heart exactly what I wanted to do. I did a lot of research on my program—developmental psychology—and I chose my advisor with the utmost care and discrimination. It makes all the difference in the world, especially during the dark times.

As for the term "disabled," it's totally arbitrary and relative. You can do anything you want to do. I remember my high-school English teacher telling me I would never pass the AP exam and would never make it to college. I got a 5 on the AP exam and now I'm a first-year, doctoral student.

Beth suggests:

❑ If you feel like an intelligent, creative and growing person, then you're a valuable member of society. You may process differently and you may see the world in different terms, but that's OK.

❑ Individual differences are what make life rich and special. Van Gough saw the world very differently. His interpretations on canvas are vivid and emotive treasures. Find your difference and make it a treasure.

C.L. BODIE, master's student, University of Oregon

C.L., 30, is in the Historic Preservation Program. She completed her Associate degree at West Valley Community College in California and her under-grad degree in art history at the University of California at Santa Cruz.

I was diagnosed with dyslexia at the age of 22. During middle and high school, I didn't think I was stupid, I just thought I was "missing a step." If anyone kept me going, it was my mom. She never lost faith in me. She would tell me constantly that I wasn't stupid and that I merely learned differently.

But I wanted to be like everyone else. Weeknights, I went to bed around 10 p.m. and got up at 5 a.m. to finish homework or to just keep up with reading material. I spent every moment of my time working on getting better grades. In the end, I got mostly "C's." My algebra teacher in my junior year knew I had a different learning style. He would go over and over a concept with the entire class until he saw that I wasn't confused. Besides that teacher, though, no other faculty member noticed. I took my tests with the constant distractions of rustling papers, people coughing and humming fluorescent lights. The tests always were timed and I never got through all the questions. It was brutal. I often wondered why life was so difficult and why I was so different. I wondered if it was going to be like this for the rest of the journey. I cried a lot. But I knew I wanted to go to college.

Now that I'm here at Oregon, I use sign language to figure out what I want to say or what is being said to me. I have 10 years of experience with signing.

Sign sometimes comes out through my hands when I can't figure out what I want to communicate . . . my hands know before my mouth. I was first introduced to this in high school. I went to a school that mainstreamed their deaf kids into hearing classrooms. And, in many cases, I had an interpreter in front of me. Most of the time, I understood the interpreter more than the instructor. In addition to this, I use extended time on tests, taped books, writing tutors and note takers. I also make a point of communicating early in the term with my professors, so there are no miscommunications.

Processing speed is a big issue in grad school. Since most of the reading material takes forever to get taped, I've learned to skim handouts, articles and chapters from books fairly quickly. I'll never read as fast as the requirements demand, but I do my best to cover most of the material. With writing, I start a paper far enough ahead of time because I always need a writing tutor or a friend to edit it before I turn it in. The best way I've found to write has been by trial and error, with help from an awesome writing tutor—they're hard to come by. Having a person read my paper and bleed all over it with a red pen has helped me see what I was doing wrong.

My only complaint about Academic Advising and Student Services is that I can't get a proofreader—the center needs more funding—even though this is my No. 1 priority in school. If I spend $75 and retake tests—as well as additional testing—to clarify my learning disability, I may get access to this. All I desire is one really good writing tutor. Instead, I've resorted to asking friends who, thankfully, don't see me as a burden.

Which brings me to computers. I can't function without a computer, period. I wish there were scholarships for students like me to obtain computers and software programs. Then I wouldn't be paying off an expensive credit card. Those of us who are learning disabled are pretty co-dependent on technology. I know there are computer labs on campus, but they're not always convenient to use, especially late at night. And I do appreciate Academic Advising & Student Services giving me a small note-taking computer (Alpha Smart) to use in class. It's great to carry around because I think so much better on a computer than on paper. But I still feel scholarships need to be made available.

I ended up buying a Macintosh and printer. The whole package cost me close to $2,000. It was a huge chunk of money. One computer program that has changed my life is "Power Talk/Plain Talk." The computer actually can read back to me what I've written. Before, I did this manually.

Just as an aside, the GRE is the most useless test to take for those who are learning disabled. The test only reassured me that I was disabled. I studied for months prior to taking it and I thought I was well prepared. I scored very low in the verbal section because I was unfamiliar with the words. I'm used to seeing them in sentences and, standing by themselves, they made no sense. The math/quantitative area was just another joke. Out of all three sections, I scored highest in logic because I could draw a picture to solve the problem . After six hours of torture, I remember sitting in my mom's car crying my heart out—she didn't want me driving after the test.The test has been so ego tearing and humiliating. It's no way of judging a person who has a processing disability.

I pleaded to have extra time on the test, but the authorities said that all learning disabled students were offered only double time, which was six hours. The authorities also refused to waive the GRE for me.

But now I'm in grad school and I don't even think about the GRE. I love grad school and recommend it to anyone who has the ambition and motivation to succeed, regardless of a disability. It took me two tries to get accepted. But I'm here now. My master's degree is a two-year program, but I'm doing it in three because I don't want to get overloaded. So far, I'm keeping up with the course work. Sometimes, though, it can be demanding. But I know I'll do fine. I take advantage of everything Academic Advising & Student Services offers. Before I applied to grad school, I asked myself if I really liked to learn. The answer was emphatically YES.

C.L.suggests:

❑ Learn to accept your LD as an "uncorrectable" (sic) characteristic. That's blunt and ugly, but it's truthful. It's like your skin color, it's unchangeable.

❑ After this acceptance, ask yourself these questions:
What are you going to do about it?
What skills do you have?
How do you learn best (visually, auditory, kinesthetically)?
What will help you learn better?
When these questions have been answered, go and accomplish them.

❑ Get yourself a computer. Technology will be your best friend. I know it's mine.

ALLISON BROWN, first-year medical student,
New York University

Allison, 23, completed her under-grad degree in biology at Stanford University. Allison created her own support system by using her circle of friends for study groups and editorial help. But she did run into roadblocks with teacher's assistants during introductory courses. She later realized a formal note from the DRC (Disability Resource Center) would have minimized her problems.

If I'd been born 20 years earlier, I wouldn't have made it as far as I have in the academic world. Word processing truly is a lifesaver for me. I also use the best resource I know—my friends—to proof my papers. Regarding the DRC, not until my senior year did I know it wasn't only for people with physical disabilities. That was a resource I wish I had taken the initiative to learn more about.

As an undergraduate in a big university like Stanford, I was pretty much on my own intellectually. And, at a place like that, how can you not have problems with self-esteem? I would look around me in lectures and realize that every head I saw once was crowned with its high school's valedictorian cap. In my first CIV (Western Civilization) section, words were casually thrown around by my "peers" that I had never even heard before. And everyone seemed to carry it off so effortlessly. The only thing that helped me feel worthy was holding on to previous exposure. I spent my high-school years in boarding school and, in that nurturing and stimulating environment, I learned who I was and how to express myself. I hung on to those memories at Stanford.

My undergraduate experience far exceeded any of my expectations. My classmates hardly ever overlapped with my circle of friends. In that way, I was able to create a supportive environment totally separate from my academic trails. The same was true of extracurricular activities. The Stanford I knew was such a cooperative environment—it almost has to be for anyone to survive its pressures and bureaucratic anonymity. I formed friends there who I will have for life.

This fall, I started medical school at NYU. The program is broken down into two segments: the first two years, I'm in actual classes and, the next two, I'm on the wards. Between graduation and starting medical school, I took a year off. I worked on a clinical research project studying hormone replacement, volunteered at a peer counseling center and traveled in the Middle East and Europe. (I was teaching English! in Jordan to people my own age. Needless to say, I didn't emphasize written work.)

I realize Stanford's biology program did a fantastic job preparing me for medical school. This first semester has been a wonderful experience, even though I'm working my tail off! I was very apprehensive about the "practicals" in anatomy. We had exactly one minute at each station to identify the tagged object on the cadaver and write down its name. That was very scary for me, but, because I was scared, I spent a huge amount of time studying for that part of the test. The first part was very hard and there were times when I knew the structure, but I just couldn't think of the word. But afterward, in talking to my classmates, I realized the same had been true for them. It was nice to know I wasn't alone, a feeling that was so different from the one I had growing up.

I was probably the first student in the history of my elementary school to be in the Special Education program and the Gifted and Talented Enrichment program simultaneously. I was lucky to have teachers who recognized I could benefit from both programs and to have a school system that would allow it.

Still, during grade school, my self-esteem was low. At first, as my classmates began to surpass me in 2nd and 3rd grade, I became extremely bossy. Eventually, as this felt worse and worse to me, I became the smart, quiet girl who would agree to anything they said. I kept trying to FEEL as smart as they were. Fortunately, years later, this turned around completely when I went to Italy for 8th grade. My parents, who were on sabbatical, put me in an Italian school. I was armed for the coming battle with a vocabulary of about 25 words. It was the hardest year of my life and the most fulfilling. I was forced to learn to cope, or break. I knew I was too strong for the latter, so I worked my tail off at the former, again with my parents' inexhaustible help.

The extensive role my parents played in my education—and the support from my teachers—kept me going through the tough years of school. Most of what I learned during school, I learned at home first. Once it was introduced in school, it was familiar, so not as stressful. My parents' patience and belief in me gave me confidence that couldn't help but carry over into school. They also helped me think of coping strategies. And, most importantly, I learned to practice those strategies in an environment where I felt comfortable before transferring them to the often-stressful school environment. Music and theater also were very important to me. They were ways for me to speak and express myself to people while still getting instantaneous interpersonal feedback. I felt in control of what I said while on stage. These activities kept me going through the difficult years.

One of the biggest difficulties always has been in-class essays, not only because of the spelling component, but also because of the time constraint. Just finding the right words to say what I want to say takes me a long time. (That sentence alone took me a few minutes.) Stanford professors were very understanding and gave me extended time. But the TA's for introductory courses were very strict about every little detail and any perceived advantage of mine was resented. I'm sure if I had gone to the trouble to get a note from the DRC, it would have been no problem. Thankfully, as I progress in my studies, spelling matters less and less as content has increased in importance. Scientific words and phrases are my downfall, but, thankfully, the professors usually are as bad as I am at spelling them. No one expects you to know how to spell "phosphofructokinase," but they're always surprised when you admit you don't know how many "L's" there are in "really."

I remember the days in grade school and junior high when one point was taken off for every spelling mistake. They said I just wasn't trying hard enough to learn the words. That definitely was not the case. Actually, when I lived in Italy, Italian words were easier to spell than English words because the language is 100 percent phonetic. In Italian, I always know the spelling because it's exactly the way it sounds. My problem with English is that more than one way of spelling will look totally correct to me.

Allison suggests:
   ❑ Challenge yourself. Show your talents in other ways while you perfect your coping strategies for dealing with what is hard for you.

   ❑ Create a support network, whatever that means for you, and USE IT (which often is the missing step).

PHILIP RAT, Ph.D. student, University of Iowa

Philip, 33, is a final-year student in rehabilitation counseling. He completed his under-grad degree in psychology at Appalachian State University and then went on to get his master's in rehabilitation psychology at the same university. Philip uses gutsy strategies to survive college.

Where possible, I convince professors to give me short-essay tests instead of multiple-choice. In under-grad school, I substituted a foreign language for statistics. Then, in grad school, I asked for special entry, which put me on probation for the first semester for my master's and doctoral programs. I have so many strategies.

I always meet in person with college admissions so they know where I'm coming from and what I expect from them. I keep up with the latest computer software programs. I use "Bookwise" for OCR, "IBM Voice" for screen reading and "Kurzweil" and "IBM" for voice recognition. I utilize the Learning Resource Center for books on tape, tutors and some extended time on tests.

Freshman and sophomore years were my most troublesome. I never do well in large classes. And reading is always a chore. Just fitting in those first years was hard. I mostly talked to faculty, Student Disability Services counselors and the school counselor. That seemed to work.

When it comes to faculty, I've had both good and bad experiences. Most would talk and work with me if I needed an accommodation. Of course, there were a couple of profs who didn't believe LD was real. Believe it or not, my worst experiences have been as a Ph.D. student. Some faculty believe only the best students should be in a doctoral program and if they have a disability that hampers them, they shouldn't be in the program.

But now I'm almost finished with my dissertation. Actually, I have to thank two Deans for a lucky break. They allowed my special entry under probation because my GRE scores were low. And I was granted probation on both master's and Ph.D. programs. But I had to achieve a 3.0 GPA the first semester of my master's program and a 3.5 the first semester of my Ph.D. program. I didn't prove them wrong.

Philip suggests:
  ❑   Develop coping strategies, use self-determination, and take

advantage of family support.

❑ Just keep at it. If you want to get into college, do everything you can. You may have to apply to several schools or go talk with admissions in person, but, in the end, it's worth it.

❑ If you don't want to go the college route—and the truly smart people like Bill Gates and Steve Jobs never did get a college degree—find another dream and follow it.

MARTY MONK, master's student,
University of Southern California

Marty, 30, is studying music education. He completed his under-grad degree in music percussion and performance at California State University at Northridge.

At USC, the Academic Support & Disability Services always advocates for me when a problem comes up. In a couple of classes, I have a reader. I also get help with proofreading and feedback on my papers. Most importantly, though, they offered me a learning assistant to help me with my master's project.

I know my limits, but, sometimes, I take on too much. I want to treat myself as if there's nothing wrong with me. At Cal State, I had a reader, note taker and tape recorder. I slowly tried to reduce my reliance on these helpers. I'm still not good in math. The way I overcome this is to do as much as I can every single day. Even if it's only a couple of minutes. Thankfully, there's no math requirement for my master's in music education.

I didn't have to take the GRE. I was put on "probation" for my first semester at grad school. I met with the Dean of the Music Department and was determined to stand my ground about being dyslexic. I was sure I was going to get knocked over because my grades weren't high. But, before our interview, I met with Academic Support & Disability Services and talked to them about my different learning style and special needs. At the interview with the Dean, I just explained what I wanted to do in grad school. I told him I was really interested in helping music appreciation students learn in a non-conventional way. Immediately, he pulled out a book he'd written on the same subject. BINGO, it was my lucky day. The chemistry was good. He liked my ideas.

I also managed to petition for a master's project instead of writing a thesis.

My project is "Teaching the Snare Drum to Children with Dyslexia," using the Orton Gillingham/Wilson methods. I state my case, write up lesson plans, implement my findings and summarize the results. I'm nearly 90 percent done. Actually, I'm taking three years to complete my degree, normally a two-year program, because I want to do a great job. It means a lot to me and to future music appreciation students.

Despite gloomy predictions—I was told early in my life that I was only going to make it so far in education—I will graduate with a masters in less than a year.

Marty suggests:

❑ Remember you are not the only one out there with dyslexia.

❑ You are a special person and will go as far as YOU want.

47 college students e-mailed me their survey responses. Some students I met in person and, a few, I talked to on the telephone. I wanted to find out how these college students with dyslexia were coping in schools across the country. Let's take a look at their responses.

Attitude

It turns out most students are asking for special accommodations and many are incorporating personalized coping strategies. The themes that best categorize their responses are as follows: conventionalists, pragmatists, independents and low profilers. Let me clarify further: conventionalists only use special accommodations to get through college, pragmatists use both special accommodations and personalized coping strategies, independents only use personalized coping strategies, and low profilers don't use either.

Character traits seem to alter the way these interviewees approach college. Those who embrace only special accommodations—conventionalists—look straight ahead. They keep motoring, looking neither right nor left, with one objective in mind—graduation. Pragmatic students also take a straight course, but with occasional stops and starts along the way incorporating additional special accommodations and/or new personal strategies. Independents are constantly looking left, right, above and below, trying to come up with improved strategies to make college more manageable, without tapping into conventional resources. Finally, Low Profilers also want to wear that cap 'n gown at graduation. They plod on, without setting off any alarm bells, and make it through college with little help or no help from the resource center.

This is what unfolded from the college-student survey:

Conventionalists (27%) rely heavily on special accommodations. Their stories are linked to an athletic or academic scholarship, or a necessity in pre-professional or grad-school programs, or simply a need to stay afloat. Some conventionalists seek out comprehensive LD support programs on campus, as a comfort zone.

Pragmatists (44%) have a lot in common with conventionalists, in that they both tap into what is offered at the Learning Resource Center on a formal basis. Pragmatists, though, try to balance the scales and, in doing so, incorporate their personalized coping strategies as part of "their" total plan.

Meanwhile, *Independents* (16%) are light on special accommodations, in the formal sense (sometimes it's done informally). In reality, they're rehearsing for the real world, the work place, where no special accommodations are given. Independents recognize what works for them and what doesn't, and, as they progress through school, come up with workable strategies.

The last group, *Low Profilers* (13%), are light in both personalized strategies and accommodations. In some ways they miss out on what's being offered at resource centers, from voice-recognition programs to help from counselors with course selection, to working closely with a learning assistant for a master's project. Low Profilers may be able to pull that extra "B+" if they get that little bit of help. But, then again, that's speculation.

Other factors undoubtedly contributed to their responses such as year in college, and previous school experiences.

Year in College

Whether one ranks as a freshman, sophomore or junior, this seems to affect those trying to strike a balance—primarily the pragmatists. For entering freshman, being different was not cool. It was more the norm to disassociate with the resource center, more the norm to handle work on your own, more the norm to play it as it comes. What isn't computed in all this is the extraordinary amount of reading material and paper writing, compared to high school. By the end of freshman year, some had learned the hard way and were flunking out of college. Sophomores also were testing the waters. But that's what college is all about.

Juniors, in the thick of it, were rocking and rolling. They had college under control, knew what they expected from the resource center, and determined how they wanted to supplement their own strategies. Seniors were ready to hit the real world (or move on to grad school). I have to say, grad students (and recent graduates) have some unusual stories and strategies. As seasoned students, some in their mid-20s and early-30s, they are not shy to come forth with unique plans and special accommodations. In some instances, they push the envelope with faculty and staff, and ask for never-before-requests. This trail blazing can only help future LD students.

Previous school experiences

Students who want to keep a low profile in college presumably have had ugly school experiences which have impacted their self esteem. Now in college, their attitude toward special accommodations range from: "I certainly don't want to be labeled like I was in school" to "I don't want to be placed in

Special-Ed classes again, or anything to do with the word special." For some conventionalists, too, past school experiences force them to look at colleges with all-embracing LD support services, and programs that offer special accommodations with NO hassle. For whatever reason, what was said in school—kindergarten through 12th grade—and what was inferred by teachers, alter the attitudes of a few respondents.

Gender, Family influences, Diagnosis,

I thought gender might have had an impact but it didn't. Nor did family views tarnish responses. But, I discovered that several students who felt they were at the bottom-of-the-pile in kindergarten through 12th grade, began to blossom when they were finally diagnosed with dyslexia in college.

My research also provides data on self esteem, resource centers, faculty, course work, and career choices. This is what I collected from the college-student responses:

91% of students say family support is essential when it comes to building and maintaining self-esteem
94% ask for special accommodations on a formal basis; some do it informally
75% use the Learning Resource Center on campus
61% say faculty is understanding
70% have a college 'social life'
61% are going on to grad school or are currently in grad school

For Schoolwork

40% say multiple-choice tests are the bane of their existence
31% say taking a foreign language is the most challenging school course
12% are taking American Sign Language as a "foreign-language"

Career choices

Social Sciences (40%) – teaching, nursing, medicine, counseling
Sciences (22%) – engineering, natural sciences, anthropology
Arts (20%) – advertising, marketing, drama, music, fiction writing
Law and Business (11%) – law, business, politics
Physical Sciences (7%) – sports or environment-related jobs

Self-esteem

Besides family support, students say that being in a club or varsity sport, the arts or drama, community service, religious or technology groups, help in maintaining their self-esteem. Only one respondent says her school helped with self-image. More often, teachers and school personnel comment: "You know, you're not college material, but there are other avenues to take."

Elementary school was horrible for some. For Ella Wass, there is a sense of panic in 2nd grade—everyone is trying to figure out why she is delayed in learning to read. For Alex Black, it stops being OK that she isn't reading in 4th grade. Her frustration shows up in problems with friends, social problems. T.J.Blanc's 3rd-grade teacher regularly asks her to stand up and read aloud, then says: "Oh I forgot you can't read. You can sit down." And, the stories go on.

But middle school, some say, is the worst time. Lea Brown hits a roadblock in 6th grade. His papers come back with red all over them. The teacher uses his work as an example of the wrong way to use grammar. Jerry Rambo goes from being in English honors to the skills class because teachers don't know where to place her.

Others say 11th & 12th grades are particularly threatening, with SAT preparation, re-testing for College Admissions, and college acceptances. Jack Peters feels like he's walking in the dark. He gets a "D" in English, then an "A" in trigonometry and an "A" in physics. Hope Stone fears she's in the lower part of her graduating class although there's no official ranking in her college prep school. Once the SAT scores are out, she knows.

More than half of the students I talked with say they have low times in college. Their coping skills vary. Almost always, they're on overload. When this happens, students reach for help at the resource center, network with faculty and tutors, take a deeper look at the workload, or put into place time-management skills. Alicia Vargas is failing in humanities because there isn't enough time to re-read the material. At Brown, she is no longer the "wonder women" she's been in high school. Maria Wolfe is set to graduate in four years, like any other mainstream student, but this puts her on "overload". She takes an extra year to complete her bachelor's at the University of Oregon. Alex Black's TA can't understand how she can misspell so many words in her weekly reading responses. This is after she's run it through the spell checker!

By direct contrast, Beth Henderson, Ella Wass and others flourish in college. For Beth, college is purely about the joy of learning. Now that she's adjusting to the frenzied world of first-year, grad-school academia, she's feeling very comfortable and eager to learn. Ella Wass doesn't know there's joy in learning until her junior year in college.

Academically challenging courses

More than 30 percent say a foreign language is the most difficult class in college. Now, more and more colleges are offering American Sign Language as a foreign-language option. Comments from students are positive. "It's a visual class; the signing is not confusing. There are no verbs to conjugate and no irregular spellings." This comes as a major breakthrough for students with dyslexia. Learning Resource Centers are telling students of this when they sketch out graduation requirements. C.L.Bodie has 10 years of experience with signing. As a master's student, she uses sign language to figure out what she wants to say or what is being said in class.

The volume of reading material in ALL classes is a major challenge for 95 percent of students in the survey, followed by writing papers and editing them. Spell checking comes out on top of the annoyance list! Meanwhile, 40 percent say multiple-choice testing is confusing. Sarah Rogers, at the University of Indianapolis, says some professors give questions that are too wordy, have answer choices that are too confusing, and overall present a threatening experience. A short-essay format is preferred. Buddy Turner a senior at Texas A & M doesn't like to be compared to other students in terms of how much he can cram in. He prefers tests that show his skill, offer more hands-on testing, ask him to read the specifications and solve problems, come up with solutions, and present findings. Just regurgitating information onto paper doesn't sit well with him, nor with most students.

A few say math is a problem—about 12 percent. They get help at the resource center or hire an off-campus tutor. Some look for colleges where there is no math requirement, but those colleges with no math requirement are rare. And, one respondent opts for a college where there is either a math or foreign-language requirement.

Learning Resource Center

Some 94 percent of students in the survey ask for accommodations, the most popular being extended time on tests/ exams. Students usually take tests in the Learning Resource Center unless faculty prefer their office or an adjacent office. Other accommodations include note takers, scribes, readers, tape recorders, textbooks on tape, tutors, and learning assistants to help with a senior or master's thesis.

In some centers, the learning assistant records a specific book, chapters from a book, newspaper and periodical articles for the LD student if they're not already in stock. Most students, though, order books on tape from RFB & D (Recording For the Blind & Dyslexia www.rfbd.org) through the learning center and complain bitterly that they don't arrive on time. In fact, sometimes they are a week or two late for the assignment or exam. I was told this is the norm and students tend to use this form of help as a last resource.

More than 90 percent ask for accommodations, but only 75 percent use the Learning Resource Center. Why the discrepancy? Some students prefer to advocate for themselves, by talking directly with faculty. They do this for two reasons: (1) they have the skills necessary to do the negotiating (2) they do not want to spend $75-100 on additional testing, or even be re-tested. (Psycho-education testing is not paid for by a health-insurance company.) To "join" the learning resource center, additional on-campus testing is required. Then a student can officially use all the services offered such as tutoring, advice on scheduling classes, advice on which profs look more favorably at LD students, support from the center when a conflict arises between faculty and student, and other accommodations (books on tape, a note taker etc.).

From what students told me, resource centers across the country are doing a good job of providing both emotional and academic support (of course, there are always some individual gripes). Most notable are the centers at the University of Arizona, the American University, Brown University, Landmark College, Denver University, University of Colorado at Bolder, University of Indianapolis, Southern Methodist University, University of Oregon, University of the Ozarks, and University of Southern California.

A surprisingly larger number of students are diagnosed with dyslexia in college these days. Often the Learning Resource Center does the testing. Lee Anthony doesn't know he has any kind of learning difficulty until his junior year in college, then he gets diagnosed. Just knowing there's an explanation for his problem makes all the difference. Carolyn Farmer gets a neuro-psych test done in her sophomore year and discovers she has dyslexia. It validates a lifetime of struggles. For Ana Sinto, the first three years at Brown are extremely difficult because she doesn't understand her problem, why she can't do well, why she is struggling. Then the Dean of Students suggests she get tested and her life seems to turn around. There are others stories, too, just like these.

Faculty

Attitudes come in all flavors. Faculty either go out of their way to help or behave as if dyslexia is not part of their vocabulary. Help comes because they may have taught previous LD students, or perhaps dyslexia is in their family. Either way, 61 percent of the college students I interviewed say faculty are understanding and listen to their special needs. For the other 39 percent, they have to work it out without any help or special support.

Being flexible with faculty seems to work well when discussing special accommodations with them. Sarah Rogers feels threatened by what her professor suggests, but goes along with "her" plan. Sarah normally takes extended time on tests in B.U.I.L.D. (Baccalaureate for the University of Indianapolis Learning Disabled) but her history professor says she can explain the material better than a reader in B.U.I.L.D. The professor insists Sarah take the test with her regular class. It's a tough call for Sarah. But, as a result of this, the professor is much more understanding of Sarah's needs, and Sarah learns to trust a faculty member.

This is not the norm with faculty, though. Since the Americans with Disabilities Act of 1990 most professors are aware of students' rights and act accordingly, but few go out of their way to help. This is how the system works at most colleges. At the beginning of each semester, an LD student gives his(her) professor a letter from the resource center outlining his(her) different learning style. This makes the request official and few altercations ensue. But where there's a gray area, where a student fails to hand in the official letter by a mid-term or the end of term, and then asks for extended time on tests/exams, some differences occur. Professors sometimes are not willing to make allowances, and understandably so. In essence, this letter is a student's "lifeline."

Social life

"What social life?" That's how most responses came in. About 30 percent aren't in extra curricular activities. Are they anti-social? No, but many are freshman or grad students who are testing the waters and are concerned with "overload" on fun activities. The overarching question is how to balance work with play. Some students say work is all-embracing and outside activities often tip the scales heavily in one direction. This needs constant fine-tuning.

Grad School

Approximately 61 percent of the students in the survey are applying to grad school or are already in grad school. The remaining are undecided. The GRE, GMAT, LSAT—standardized tests—are huge obstacles to grad school. They trigger SAT flashbacks. The good news is that improvements are in place. The GRE is taken electronically. A student can ask for extended time, ask for a reader and respond verbally. Even with these accommodations, though, students with dyslexia feel threatened. One student who avoids all the standardized test hoopla is Marty Monk. The Dean of the Music Department allows Marty to go on academic probation for the first semester of his master's program, but he has to maintain a 3.5 GPA for the first year. He does. Others say the amount of reading material is scary. Most say that personal determination and ambition rule. Plus, by grad school, they know the system.

Career choices

After many hours of interviewing and research I wanted to find the missing piece to the puzzle—"where do these young adults end up in the workplace?" This is what I discovered.

Some 40 percent say they'll graduate with a degree in nursing, teaching, counseling or medicine. Those statistics don't surprise me. I sense from their interviews a desire to help others, to counsel, to guide, to be understanding of people's needs, to have a sense of awareness. Students with dyslexia have compassion for others. These professions are sound choices.

Another 22 percent say they're majoring in engineering or anthropology. Again, those don't come as a surprise because several respondents enjoy investigative and scientific work, problem solving, analytical thinking and essential research. Given that dyslexic students are bright and curious, careers that are intellectually challenging are a natural choice. Parents in Silicon Valley CA, revealed that a large percentage of the top software designers in the valley have dyslexia. They may not send out error-free e-mails, but they sure come up with one-of-a-kind designs.

I was expecting more students to enter the field of the arts. With media coverage linking Tom Cruise, Cher, Whoopie Goldberg and Lindsay Wagner to dyslexia, I thought a larger number would be pursuing a career in film, drama or the arts. It turns out that 20 percent are going into advertising, marketing, drama, music and fiction writing. And, 7 percent plan to work in sports or environment-related jobs. Again, with notable athletes in the headlines—Magic Johnson, Carl Lewis, Greg Louganis and Bruce Jenner—I envisioned a higher number.

Only 11 percent of the students are studying law, politics or business. The amount of reading required in law school is probably a turn-off. A couple of students are getting an under-graduate degree in business, with a minor in science or sports, and a few are in poly-sci programs. I didn't find any student looking to be a court reporter, auditor, or reservation agent, the more structured, more methodical types of jobs. Students with dyslexia often don't have a knack for working with data and details, maintaining records, or performing data management and processing. Their talent lies in the social sciences, in investigative fields, in the arts. This conventional stuff is boring.

There's a pattern to these career choices, some sense of order. That last puzzle piece did the trick for me. I hope it answered your doubts, too.

POINTERS FROM COLLEGE STUDENTS FOR K-12 STUDENTS

❑ Don't listen to pessimism—either your own or someone else's.

❑ Find somewhere else to put your passion (not totally in academics). Then excel.

❑ Find out what makes you happy, then surround yourself with people who believe in you.

❑ Create a support network (whatever that means for you) and use it (which is often the missing step).

❑ Plan a different course if you're not fitting in with the norm. Find other ways to get to where you want to go.

About Your Different Learning Style

❑ Be honest about your learning difference. Learn to accept it as an "uncorrectable" (sic) characteristic. It's like your skin color, it's unchangeable.

❑ Find out the technical reasons why you are not succeeding, then find a school that will accommodate you.

❑ Remember, you can learn everything in your classes, you just have to approach it in a different way.

❑ Technology will be your best friend. Maximize it.

❑ Roll with the punches. Life is difficult for everyone is some way, shape or form.

About College

❑ You need to know there are LD programs where you get support without having to fight for it

❑ Find a college that meets your needs, then learning gets easier.

❑ Don't be afraid or embarrassed to ask for accommodations.

❑ Try to understand that others don't understand dyslexia. Then help them with that.

❑ Choose your battles wisely. You may not get through school in the "traditional" manner, but you'll make it.

❑ Anyone can do it. It's just a matter of will.

COPING STRATEGIES THAT WORK

❑ Network with faculty, TA's, the Learning Resource Center, advisors, tutors, friends. Gather as much information as possible. The more you gather, the easier your job becomes. In the real world, you have to network. Why not start in college?

❑ Get a letter at the beginning of the semester/quarter from the Learning Resource Center if you want special accommodations. DO NOT THINK faculty will drop dead for you when mid-terms pop up and you haven't made contact with them.

For Under-grad Students

❑ Take one course each semester where you either shine or feel relaxed (sports, drama, arts, music, computer, debating, etc.).

❑ Go part-time to avoid overload.

❑ Spend your junior year abroad in an English-speaking country— UK, Australia, New Zealand.

❑ Plan to graduate in five years.

❑ Consider taking three years for your master's, instead of the normal two.

For Tests

❏ If MC (multiple-choice testing) is a problem, ask to take short-answer tests instead.

❏ Ask for MC tests to be read to you and answered orally, whenever possible.

❏ Seek out courses that exclude MC testing.

❏ For the GRE—or other standardized tests—ask to be on academic probation for one semester instead of taking the exam.

For Computer Work

❏ Use the latest software programs in the resource center but note that software is constantly being updated. Check the Internet for links from LD sites, and search for similar software like those mentioned in my book—Dragon NaturallySpeaking, Kurzweil and IBM for voice recognition, IBM for screen reading, MicNote Pad for recording (Mac), Bookwise for OCR and Text Help / Windows 98 for spell checking—that you may prefer to use.

❏ Use a computer to take a written exam. This will help with spell checking.

For Language Arts

❏ When editing papers, get help at the resource center. Friends and parents are often too busy. Be conscious of time management because the center is not open at 2 a.m.

❏ For reading assignments (250+ pages per week in one class), ask for a reduced reading load, extended time, or to read a different type of textbook with similar content.

❏ If you need extra help on college-level reading, work with an Orton-trained tutor to understand your reading patterns (or a tutor in Special Education).

❏ Ask to do a research project instead of a research paper. There is less writing and less editing!

❏ For your thesis—senior or master's—ask to do a project instead. This will illustrate your practical adeptness and de-emphasize your writing skills. (William Hewlett of Hewlett Packard who was dyslexia, submitted the shortest masters thesis at MIT, 14 pages in total. It comprised of only equations!)

For FL (foreign language)

❏ Before applying to college, look for a school where there is no foreign-language requirement or where there is either a math or foreign-language option.

❏ If you are failing in your FL course, ask to be tested orally or do translations only.

❏ If FL is your weakness, select ASL (American Sign Language) as your FL requirement, even as early as in high school, but, most definitely, in college.

❏ Take classes on the cultural aspect of the FL, known as Reading Sequence. For example, take a course on the Japanese Education system or the role of women in China or Spanish folklore.

For Maths

❏ If math is a problem, ask for an alternate way to take the course or to be tested. Oral testing or a reduced number of questions often hit the spot.

❏ For statistics, ask to take it at a local junior college in the summer. Make it a single class so you can better concentrate on the information.

POINTERS FOR COLLEGE STUDENTS

❏ Check off those coping strategies on the POINTERS: Coping Strategies That Work list that you didn't know before. Then take action.

❏ Freshman, don't try to do it alone your first semester. Ask for help at the Learning Resource Center. Everyone at college is different. Diversity is what makes college unique.

❑ Grad students, use any coping strategies that improve your academic work. Remember, your negotiating powers are at their best. You're now a seasoned student!

For Course Work

❑ Take ASL (American Sign Language) as your FL (foreign language) requirement. Don't be a martyr and struggle with Spanish, Latin, German.

❑ If multiple-choice tests are the curse of your college life, ask for short-answer tests or oral testing.

❑ For reading assignments, use a time-management plan and a large calendar to schedule deadlines.

❑ For papers, break the project down into small components. Get help from the Learning Resource Center—friends are often on overload!

On Faculty, On Learning Resource Centers

❑ Realize that faculty are real people. Like the real world, some are nice, some are not that understanding, others lack empathy. Work around those who are giving you a hard time. Then try to educate them on dyslexia.

❑ Learning resource staff are the specialists on campus. If you need golf-course management, you'd go to a golf pro. If you need help with editing, time-management, etc., you need to stop by the Learning Resource Center.

And Finally

❑ Get a social life. Find time to have fun. There's something wrong if you can't break away from your work.

❑ Dreams are not a reality. But, they can be with some action on your part!

5 A FINAL NOTE

A FINAL NOTE

I hope these real-life stories will "lighten" your load, encourage you to move forward, and make you feel closer to friends and family with dyslexia. Here are some brief notes just to remind you again of some key points.

Dear parents:

I firmly believe that early testing is a good way to go. As early as 1st grade is the optimum time, if possible, especially if you have an inkling that something is not "right." Then if dyslexia is uncovered, you can move forward with a plan-of-action.

Please consider a short-term stay of 1 or 2 years for your child at a special school for dyslexia but put closure on the project. From my experience, it can turn a child around immeasurably. It rebuilds self confidence and makes schoolwork more manageable. More importantly, it will prepare your child to cope better when he or she returns to mainstream schooling.

Don't feel guilty about helping your dyslexic child with projects and homework. We all need a little help from time to time, some a little more than others. But, set aside quality time each week with your other children and with your spouse.

As your child matures, focus on developing good communication and time-management skills. Let your child know it's OK to have a different learning style. The more confident your child becomes with his or her dyslexia, the easier it will be for him or her in school, especially in college.

Dear siblings:

You appear to have your game-plan together. You're able to recognize your dyslexic sibling's strengths and talents. Oftentimes, you've learned from them and admire their qualities. You have no hang-ups about them learning differently, and you have a greater understanding of people with a disability. Because of your experience with your brother or sister, you're a better person.

I know it's hard to see your parents spend that extra time with your brother or sister, but speak up and let your parents know, you too, need some quality time. Be patient, though, and realize parents can't always be in two places at once.

Dear college students and those college bound:

What a great time to be applying to, and attending college. Research those colleges that are most suitable for your personality and those that have a clear understanding of your LD requirements.

Virtually all learning resource centers have the most recent software programs, and these centers will offer special accommodations with "no hassle." Use all the latest computer technology available. But, remember, you must hand in that letter from the Disability Office to your professors at the beginning of each term. It's your "life-line."

Continue to improve your communication and time-management skills. Take confidence-building courses such as public speaking. In essence, develop strengths that augment your academics.

Most importantly, know that college is a time to grow and a time to learn, to have fun, to socialize with friends, to play sports, to get involved in drama, fine arts or whatever your passion. Don't let your school work overload you. Reach out to the experts at the learning resource center. They're on campus for you, to help students like you get through college. Friends are great, but they, too, are often on overload.

Don't be embarrassed to say you learn differently. It's OK. Then go do it and enjoy your college-experience!

To all my readers:

People with dyslexia are truly creative individuals. They just happen to learn differently. Albert Einstein had dyslexia. Try to imagine what his parents said to each other every day!

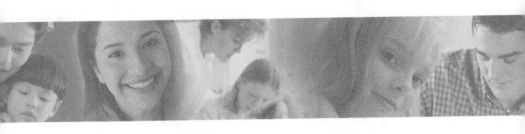

INDEXES

INTERVIEWS

school: He won't have the prestigious college degree to help him start off. It's going to be harder.

83 Nichole Courser, freshman, high school: Why isn't my brother like other kids I baby-sit?

85 Andrew Browne, freshman, Stanford University: I wish he would find more direction in schoolbooks.

86 Penelope Banks, recent graduate, Georgia Tech: Sometimes "it" prevents her from moving forward.

88 Colin Adams, junior, high school: I don't know if I could have moved our of our neighborhood school.

89 Athena Stamos, 7th grader: Why isn't my brother more like me?

90 Rachel Mason, freshman, high school: I just want to protect her.

91 Anne Finestien, sophomore, Stanford University: He'll probably end up making more money than me.

92 Scott Jacobson, graduate, Duke University: I'm very proud of her achievements.

93 Bobby Berg, freshman, Yale University: One thing I'm taking to college is the perseverance I've learned from him.

94 Laura Brighton, 4th-grader: I feel bad for him in spelling, because he has no clue what he's writing.

95 Marcus Oaks, sophomore, college prep school: I see him as CEO of a company.

97 Curt Wesley, recent graduate, University of Colorado: He's an "altogether" guy.

98 Camden Adams, sophomore, high school: So, he has dyslexia. It's no big deal!

99 Courtney Hennen, sophomore, high school: If there was no dyslexia in the family, there'd be a lot less yelling.

"My older sibling has dyslexia"

101 Debora Rosen, 8th-grader: I feel bad that my sister got stuck with the disability.

102 Ross Accordino, 8th-grader: I thought it didn't bother me that Mom was going to lots of meetings to find out about dyslexia. But, then it did.

103 Jessie Riving, 3rd-grader: Homework takes me about 20 minutes. For my brother, it takes two or three hours.

104 Maria Accordino, 7th-grader: I understand LD kids. I'm especially sensitive to those with a learning disability.

105 Lynn Curtis, 7th-grader: I'm my brother's "house" editor.

107 Julia Stone, recent MBA graduate: My sister will always be my best friend, dyslexic or not.

108 Theresa Jacobson, graduate, Duke University: Will our children have dyslexia? We're just newly weds.

109 Talia Laurance, 4th-grade: Sometimes I'm tired of hearing that she's an amazing artist.

110 Patrick Morgan, 4th-grader: Sometimes, I feel guilty that he's not a regular kid in a regular school like me.

111 Brendan Manning, 5th-grader: I did feel left out. Mom brought in a student to help with" magic-shows"

112 Annica Brown, sophomore, University of Pennsylvania: She's carefree and has a great sense of humor. I wish I was less inhibited.

CHAPTER 2
HOW-TO-COPE
PARENT-INTERVIEWS

239 Sam Lee, freshman, Southern Methodist University: I want to prove to people that I'm smart!

241 Nichole Childers, senior, University of California at Santa Cruz: I'm not ashamed of my dyslexia. It's just another part of me.

242 Carolyn Farmer, master's student, University of Michigan: I was a college drop-out. Now I'm a Psychiatric Mental-Health Nursing student!

244 T.J.Blanc, master's student, Auburn University: I quit school by my 16th birthday.

246 Helen Farr, junior, Syracuse University: "They" told me I wouldn't make it to a four-year college.

Low profilers

250 Madison Kendell, senior, Prairie View A & M: At 28, I finally had the courage to pursue a college degree.

252 Jerry O'Brien, former sophomore, Landmark College: Without a college degree, I'm regarded as "McDonald's material".

253 Maria Wolfe, senior, University of Oregon: By taking five years to graduate, college was manageable.

Independents

259 EllaWass, 4th-year Ph.D student, University of Washington: Coming from a highly academic family, my LD was a curse.

261 Patrick Karstens, recent graduate, University of Oregon: I work around my LD, instead of confronting it head-on.

264 Alice Wonderwater, master's student, Brown University: Brown was the first place I ever questioned my ability to write.

266 Hope Stone, recent graduate, Boston University: My family gave me constant support and believed in my abilities.

268 Cleo Amanda, master's student, Monterey Institute of International Studies: I wanted to see "life" in Germany. I was tired of being black and I had some issues with being female.

271 Lee Anthony, junior, University of Maryland at College Park: After graduation, I plan to work for the Peace Corps.

273 Michael John, medical student, University of California system: I'm living proof that an "almost" high school drop-out, can make it to medical school.

Pragmatists–under grad students

277 Jack Peters, junior, Brown University: I was walking in the "dark" in high school.

279 Alex Black, freshman, Stanford University: In 4th grade it stopped being OK that I wasn't reading.

282 Noah Andrews, sophomore, Southern Methodist University: I waited to be the last to read and then prayed time would run out.

283 Jerrie Rambo, junior, University of Maryland at College Park: Drugs and alcohol got me through middle school. By 9th grade, I dropped-out!

285 Lea Brown, freshman, Stanford University: I never leave messages on the white boards around the dorm.

287 Maureen Bardey, freshman, Oxford College at Emory University: Sometimes I wonder if I was adopted. All my siblings are gifted.

290 Ana Sinto, senior, Brown University: I'm determined to go on to medical school. But, no one else thinks I can do it.

291 Michael Levine, senior, University of Southern California: Sometimes I think I'm like a blind student. I need so much help.

293 Alicia Vargas, senior, Brown University: I got labeled before I even reached adolescence. I'm Latino and I have dyslexia.

295 Scott Jesser, senior, private Liberal Arts College, New Hampshire: My mother was my "knight in armor."

297 Natalie Nielson, recent graduate, Brigham Young University: I knelt at my bed every night asking G-d for help.

299 Brenda Brown, recent graduate, University of Arizona: My counselors help me plan each semester.

300 Sue Princeton, recent graduate, Norwich University: I was scared to write a check for fear I would misspell words. I came up with a neat solution.

Pragmatists–grad students

302 Elizabeth Ball, law student, Boston University: Practical and Formal Logic are, by far, the hardest college courses I've ever taken.

304 Beth Henderson, Ph.D. student, University of Southern California: Being intelligent, bright and dyslexic was extremely frustrating as a child.

306 C.L.Bodie, master's student, University of Oregon: I thought I was "missing a step" in high school. I didn't know I had dyslexia.

309 Alison Brown, 1st-year medical student, New York University: I'm pleased I wasn't born 20 years ago. Word processing is my lifesaver.

312 Philip Rat, Ph.D. student, University of Iowa: I always meet in person with college admissions so they know where I'm coming from and what I expect from them.

313 Marty Monk, master's student, University of Southern California: I didn't take the GRE. I was put on "probation" my first semester.

INDEX

British Dyslexia Association, 24
brothers, competitiveness between,
   85–86, 93, 97, 102
burnout
  in college, 294
  in high school, 154, 155–156, 182,
   306

C

campus visit, college, 199, 201,
   212–213, 225–226, 312
career choice, 322
career curriculum course, 212–213
Carnegie Mellon Fellowship, 294
Cat in the Hat (Dr.Seuss), 9, 44
Center for Special Services, 244–245
Center for Students With Disabilities,
   243
childhood, hurtful, 244, 250, 285–286
choir scholarship, 25
Choosing the Right College (duChossios
   & Stein), 224
church, as support system, 160–161,
   246
class scheduling, high school, 187
CLC. *See* Creative Learning Center
clinical psychologist, 21, 23, 25, 33, 36,
   43, 46, 48–49, 50, 59, 61, 65, 128,
   133, 139–140, 143, 155
Closed-Caption TV, 124, 133–134, 181
college
  burn-out in, 294
  conditional acceptance to, 211
  dropping out of, 243, 252, 289
  dyslexia friendly, 227–228
  extra year to graduate from,
   253–254, 255, 261, 271, 306
  pointers before applying to, 223
  studying abroad, 241, 263–264,
   268–269, 270, 277
college admission
  application form pointers, 226
  extracurricular activity as aid in, 187,
   223

recent testing need for, 187
  self-identifying during, 204, 205, 286
college experience
  academically challenging courses,
   319
  career choice, 317, 322
  college student summary on,
   315–322
  conventional student on, 231
  coping strategy, 324–326
  dyslexia diagnosis during, 317
  family support, effect on, 317
  foreign language in, 317
  gender, effect on, 317
  K-12 student pointers on, 323–324
  multiple-choice test, 243, 246, 254,
   262, 263, 283, 294, 312, 317
  pointers for, 326–327
  previous school experience, effect on,
   316–317
  self-esteem concerns during,
   317–318
  social life, 270, 285, 321
  year in college, effect on, 316
college faculty, run-in with, 260,
   263–264, 267, 280, 312
college "nirvana," 197–198
college search
  campus visit, 199, 201, 212–213,
   225–226, 312
  and degree of disability, 221
  and family attitude, 220–221
  and family financial situation, 221
  and home atmosphere, 222
  Learning Resource Center, 206, 218,
   225–226
  and maturity of student, 221
  parent networking during, 216
  pointers for, 224–226
  strategic planning parent in,
   193–194, 197–211
  sure-footed parent in, 195–195,
   212–219

146

local school district pays for, 142–144, 146–149

pointers for, 184

re-entry into public school from, 138–139, 141–142, 151

struggle for parent to pay for, 144–145

school psychologist, 29, 33, 35–36, 37, 38, 46, 48, 52, 53, 126, 136

scribe, 221, 225, 231, 292

self-advocacy

in college, 205, 245, 256, 289, 296

in elementary school, 18, 52

in high school, 169, 170, 179, 180

self-destructive behavior, 17, 46

self-esteem

building, 58, 65–67, 145, 149, 266, 290, 299

importance of, 133

low, 37, 39–40, 41, 46, 50–51, 55, 56, 58, 63–64, 103, 150, 259, 271, 297, 310

maintaining, 58, 67

positive, 57, 160–161

slipping, 73

self-identifying, on college application, 204, 205, 286

sense of humor, 262

shame, about having dyslexia, 242, 251, 295

sibling, mainstream

admiration for dyslexic sibling, 88

age of, effect on perceptions, 13, 114

birth order, effect on perceptions, 13, 77–78, 114

compassion for dyslexic sibling, 81

concern for dyslexic sibling, 104

on determination/perseverance of dyslexic sibling, 91, 93, 97, 99, 100, 112, 113

difficulty accepting dyslexic sibling, 36

dyslexia as non-issue for, 97–99

on dyslexic sibling's future, 77, 82, 83, 88, 97, 98, 99, 107, 115

exasperation of, 88

fear they may be dyslexic, 32–33, 104, 109

fortunate not to have dyslexia, 116

friends of, 116

frustration with dyslexic sibling, 81, 86, 87, 89, 96, 101

gender effect on perceptions of, 114

homework help by, 96

jealously toward dyslexic sibling, 32, 117, 138

learning about dyslexia, 82, 84, 90, 95, 116

mothering by, 80, 84, 86–87, 90

need for parent attention by, 36, 38, 79, 80, 81, 82, 83–84, 95, 102, 106, 111, 116, 133

nurturing/protective feelings of, 78, 80, 85, 90, 91

pointers for, 118

resentment of dyslexic sibling, 63, 80, 87, 96, 102, 103, 111, 133

respect for dyslexic sibling, 89, 91, 92, 93, 95, 97–102, 105–110, 113

summary of feelings of, 114–117

understanding of dyslexia by, 86, 90, 104–105, 112, 117

. *See also* family member; sibling, mainstream, and family

sibling, mainstream, and family

on family views/influences, 115–116

on input in decisions, 82, 84, 94, 109

on parents' handling of situation, 79, 84, 87, 88, 94

on special school decision, 80, 88–89, 100

. *See also* sibling, mainstream

single parent, 22–23, 41–42, 44–45, 60

sister, motherliness of older, 80, 84,
86–87, 90
Slingerland Multisensory Teaching
Methods, 38, 56, 89, 126, 155, 178,
297, 305
social studies assignment, 105
software
Bookwise, 312
Collier Encyclopedia, 172
DragonDictate, 213, 257
Dragon NaturallySpeaking, 231,
245, 287
IBM Voice, 312
Interactive Movie Book, 134, 181
Mavis Beacon Teaches Typing, 182
MicNote Pad, 231
Microsoft Encarta, 172
Oregon Trail, 135
Storybook Weaver, 134–135, 181
Talk and Word, 24
Text Help for Windows 98, 257
Treasure Mountain, 135
voice-recognition, 47, 213, 221, 231,
236, 245, 257, 287, 312
Special Education, 44, 47, 124, 250, 310
Special-Education tutor, 35, 39, 133,
186
Specialist Unit, off-campus, 53–54
Specific Learning Difficulty (SPELD),
159–160
speech therapy, 49, 239
SPELD. *See* Specific Learning
Difficulty
spell checker
as aid, 17, 127, 160, 172–173, 177,
182, 273, 274, 298
uselessness of, for severe dyslexic,
172–173
Spelling Dictionary (Lyons &
Carnahan), 247
spelling test
drilling student for, 160
modified, 127

sports
college, 198–200, 207, 261–262,
302
doing before homework, 171
elementary school, 146
high school, 35, 91, 92, 156, 169,
171, 174, 273, 282, 302
middle school, 89, 93–94,
106–107, 156
playing with sibling, 97–99
preschool, 20
and school work, 170, 299
spousal support, between spouses, 145
lack of, 34–35, 70
pointers for, 74
state law, 124
Statement, 53, 140, 159
Story Book Weaver (software),
134–135, 181
Strategic Alternative Learning
Techniques (S.A.L.T.), 195, 198, 204,
215, 216–217, 278, 299
Student Disability Services, 312
Student Life, 240
Studies Skill course, 202
study group, for reading assignment,
166, 260

T

Talk and Word (software), 24
TAP. *See* The Advanced Program
tape recorder, for aid in college, 233,
235, 241, 243, 244, 292, 304, 313
technical ability, of dyslexic child, 54,
103, 105, 149
technology, 182
headphone, 165
pointers for, 186
. *See also* computer; software
term paper writing, 294
test
multiple-choice, 243, 246, 254, 262,
263, 283, 294, 312, 317

ABOUT THE AUTHOR

A mother of a dyslexic daughter, Shirley Kurnoff found most LD books to be dry and clinical. After earning her master's degree in education from Stanford University, she put together the resource book she wished she'd had years ago. *The Human Side of Dyslexia: 142 interviews with REAL people telling REAL stories,* is the first of many interview-style family books that Shirley plans to write. Shirley lives in California with her husband and three children.

Print copies and/or an e-book version of *The Human Side of Dyslexia*
can be ordered on line at http://www.edyslexia.com. Purchase is also
available from the publisher by mail, fax or telephone.

London Universal Publishing
P.O. Box 2479 Monterey CA 93942
Tel: (831) 658 0288 Fax: (831) 658 0266

http://www.edyslexia.com